Certification Exam Review

FOR PHARMACY TECHNICIANS

Cheryl Aiken

Fourth Edition

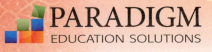
PARADIGM
EDUCATION SOLUTIONS

St. Paul

Senior Vice President: Linda Hein
Managing Editor: Carley Fruzzetti
Developmental Editor: Marybeth Lorbiecki
Director of Production: Timothy W. Larson
Production Editor: Carrie Rogers
Copyeditor: Suzanne Clinton
Cover and Text Designer: Dasha Wagner
Senior Design and Production Specialist: Jaana Bykonich
Indexer: Terry Casey
Vice President Sales and Marketing: Scott Burns
Director of Marketing: Lara Weber McLellan
Vice President Information Technology: Chuck Bratton
Digital Projects Manager: Tom Modl
Digital Production Manager: Aaron Esnough
Web Developer: Blue Earth Interactive

Care has been taken to verify the accuracy of information presented in this book. However, the authors, editors, and publisher cannot accept responsibility for Web, e-mail, newsgroup, or chat room subject matter or content, or for consequences from application of the information in this book, and make no warranty, expressed or implied, with respect to its content.

Trademarks: Some of the product names and company names included in this book have been used for identification purposes only and may be trademarks or registered trade names of their respective manufacturers and sellers. The authors, editors, and publisher disclaim any affiliation, association, or connection with, or sponsorship or endorsement by, such owners.

Photo Credits: Following the index.

We have made every effort to trace the ownership of all copyrighted material and to secure permission from copyright holders. In the event of any question arising as to the use of any material, we will be pleased to make the necessary corrections in future printings. Thanks are due to the authors, publishers, and agents listed in the Photo Credits for permission to use the materials therein indicated.

978-0-76386-785-0 (print)
978-0-76386-786-7 (digital)

BRIEF CONTENTS

Preface   ix

Introduction   Preparing for a High-Stakes Exam   3

Unit 1   Drugs and Drug Therapies   19

Chapter 1   Pharmacology for Technicians   21
Chapter 2   Pharmacy Conversions and Dosage Calculations   61

Unit 2   Pharmacy Duties and Regulations   81

Chapter 3   Pharmacy Law and Regulations   83

Unit 3   Dispensing Processes   105

Chapter 4   Prescription and Medication Order Dispensing   107
Chapter 5   Nonsterile Compounding   133
Chapter 6   Sterile and Hazardous Compounding   151
Chapter 7   Medication Safety and Quality Assurance   181
Chapter 8   Pharmacy Information Systems and Automation   203
Chapter 9   Pharmacy Inventory Management   215
Chapter 10   Pharmacy Reimbursement and Claims Processing   233

Appendixes   249

Appendix A   Common Pharmacy Abbreviations and Acronyms   249
Appendix B   Common Controlled Drug Substances   255

Index   259

* Study Supplements that can be accessed through the eBook/Navigator+ include: Top 200 Drugs, Top Hospital Drugs, Vulnerable Populations Resources and Drugs to Avoid, Common Palliative Care and Hospice Drugs, HIPAA Regulations Pertaining to Pharmacy Medical Terminology, and Tips for Multicultural Healthcare Service.

TABLE OF CONTENTS

Preface ix

**Introduction: Preparing
    for a High-Stakes Exam 3**
Why Become Certified? 2
State Practice Requirements 3
    Registration 3
    Licensure 3
    Certification 4
Choose the Right Exam 4
    Test and Certification Eligibility 7
    Test Preparation Strategies 10
    How and When to Study 10
    Prepare in Advance for Test Day 11
    The Day of the Exam 12
Tips for Taking Multiple-Choice Tests 13
After the Exam 14
    Grading of the PTCE 14
    Grading of the ExCPT 15
Recertification 15
Study Summary 16

**Unit 1
Drugs and Drug Therapies 19**

**Chapter 1
Pharmacology for Technicians 21**
Essential Knowledge for Technicians 22
Anatomical Classification of Drugs 23
Central Nervous System Agents 24
    Analgesic and Anti-Inflammatory Agents . . 25
    Antianxiety and Hypnotic Central
        Nervous System Agents 27
    Antidepressant and Antipsychotic
        Central Nervous System Agents 28
    Miscellaneous Central Nervous System
        Agents 31
Cardiovascular Agents 33
    Antihypertensive Agents 33
    Antihyperlipidemic (Cholesterol-Lowering)
        Agents 35
    Miscellaneous Cardiovascular Agents 36

Systemic Anti-Infective Agents 36
    Antibiotics and Sulfa Drugs 38
    Antifungals and Antivirals 40
Endocrine and Metabolic Agents 40
    Estrogens and Birth Control Agents 40
    Antidiabetic Agents 41
    Miscellaneous Endocrine Agents 43
Respiratory Agents 45
Gastrointestinal Agents 46
Renal and Genitourinary Agents 47
Hematological Agents 48
Biotechnology Drugs 50
Miscellaneous Drugs 51
Over-the-Counter Drugs 52
Holistic Health Medications and Dietary
    Supplements 54
    Homeopathic Medications 54
    Dietary Supplements 55
Reviewing Pharmacology 58
Study Summary 60

**Chapter 2
Pharmacy Conversions and Dosage
    Calculations 61**
Reviewing Conversion Formulas and
    Measurements 62
    Temperature Conversions 62
    Time Conversions 63
    Earlier Measurement Systems and
        Conversions 64
    Knowing the Metric System 65
    Reviewing Ratio-Proportion Equations 67
    Using Ratio-Proportion Equations to
        Convert Measurements to Metrics 68
Calculating Dosages 70
    Drug Ratio Strengths 70
    Calculating Tablet Dosages 72
    Calculating Dosages Using Body-Weight
        Ratios 73
    Calculating Dosages for Children 74

Applying Body Surface Area for Dosages . . 74
Calculating Liquid Dosage Amounts 75
Calculating Dilution Amounts 77
Study Summary 80

Unit 2
Pharmacy Duties and Regulations 81

Chapter 3
Pharmacy Law and Regulations 83
Pharmacy Oversight 84
Oversight Agencies and Organizations 87
FDA Drug Labels and Recalls. 88
Drug Recall Classifications
and Procedures. 89
Controlled Substances Regulations 90
Drug Classifications 90
Preventing Forgeries and Diversion 98
Disposal of Controlled Substances. 99
State Laws 100
The Courts and Professional Standards 101
Criminal and Civil Court Cases 101
Standard of Care 102
Ethics 102
Study Summary 103

Unit 3
Dispensing Processes 105

Chapter 4
Prescription and Medication
Order Dispensing 107
Reviewing Common Dosage Forms and
Routes of Administration 108
The Filling and Dispensing Roles of
the Pharmacy Technician 111
Generic Substitutions for Prescribed
Brand Drugs 111
Biologically Comparable Drug Products. . 113
Common Pharmacy Abbreviations 114
Patient Profile. 116
Patient Privacy and HIPAA Regulations . . 117
Components of a Prescription 117
Checking a Prescription. 118
Components of a Medication Order 122
Differences from a Prescription. 122
Checking the Medication Order 123
Filling a Prescription or a Medication Order . . 125
Prescription Filling 126
Medication Order Filling. 127
Final Check by the Pharmacist. 130
Study Summary 131

Chapter 5
Nonsterile Compounding 133
Types of Nonsterile Compounding 134
Basic Nonsterile Compounding Steps 135
Commonly Compounded Dosage Forms 139
Nonsterile Compounding Equipment. . . . 141
Common Techniques for Ingredient
Preparation and Blending 143
Compounding Calculations 145
Calculating with Concentration Percentage
Ratios 145
Using Alligation to Combine More than
One Concentration for a New
Concentration 146
Determining Beyond-Use Dating 148
Completing Nonsterile Compounding 149
Study Summary 150

Chapter 6
Sterile and Hazardous Compounding. 151
Sterile Compounding for Parenteral
Administration. 152
USP Chapter <797> 152
Types of Sterile Parenteral Drug
Products. 152
Medication Orders for Compounded
Sterile Products 153
Master Formulation and
Compounding Records 154
Cleanroom and Air Quality
Engineering Equipment 156
Aseptic Technique and Protective Garb. . . 157
Sterile Compounding Calculations 158
Overfill of Base Solutions 159
Calculating Sterile Compounding
Dilutions 161
Calculating IV Administration Flow
Rates and Volumes 164
The Sterile Compounding Process 167
Manipulating Needles and Syringes 168
Determining CSP Stability and
Beyond Use Date 171
Hazardous Compounding 172
Medical Surveillance. 174
Hazardous Compounding Engineering
Controls. 174
Nuclear Compounding 176
Waste Handling and Disposal 177
Study Summary 179

Chapter 7
Medication Safety
and Quality Assurance **181**
Medication Safety Systems 182
   FDA New Drug Oversight 182
   FDA Protective Actions for Released
      Drugs and Products 184
   Consumer Product Safety Commission . .189
Preventing Medication Errors 189
   Failure Modes and Effects Analysis 190
   Resources to Fight Medication Errors 192
   Technology, Automation, and
      Manufacturing Innovations 194
Technician Techniques to Reduce Errors 194
   Using NDC Numbers and Barcodes
      for Safety 195
   Times for Pharmacist Intervention 196
   Safety Processes at Every Step 197
Quality Control and Assurance 199
   Continuous Quality and Performance
      Improvement 199
   Staff Quality and Safety 199
   Patient Satisfaction 201
Study Summary **202**

Chapter 8
Pharmacy Information Systems
and Automation **203**
Pharmacy Computer Basics 204
Pharmacy Software Interoperability 204
Community Practice Information
   Technology and Automation 206
   E-Prescribing 206
   Prescription Processing 207
   Pharmacy Robotics and Automated
      Filling in the Community Pharmacy . . .209
   Point-of-Sale Cash Register, Sales,
      and Inventory Reports 210
Institutional Pharmacy Information
   Technology and Automation 211
   Electronic Records, Orders, and
      Administration Tracking 211
   Hospital Dispensing Robots and
      Automated Dispensing 212
   Sterile Compounding Automation
      and Administration 212
Study Summary **214**

Chapter 9
Pharmacy Inventory Management . . . **215**
Inventory Accounting 216
   Acquisition Costs versus Pharmacy
      Reimbursements .216
   Managing Inventory Value
      and Turnovers 219
Inventory Levels and Ordering Strategies 221
   Investigational Drugs 221
   Periodic Automatic Replenishment
      Levels and Reorder Ranges 221
   ABC Classification System for Stock
      Management 223
   Purchasing Relationships and
      Contracts 224
   Handling Purchasing Orders 226
   Processing Order Deliveries 227
   Handling Controlled Substances 229
   Drug Returns and Credits 230
Study Summary **232**

Chapter 10
Pharmacy Reimbursement
and Claims Processing **233**
Cash and Billing 234
Insurance Options 235
   Insurance Claims and Payment
      Structures 236
   Inputting Insurance Information 238
   Online Claims Submission 239
   Calculating Days Supply 242
   Otic and Ophthalmic Calculation
      Challenges 244
   Resolving Claim Issues 245
   Medication Assistance 246
Study Summary **248**

Appendix A
Common Pharmacy Abbreviations
and Acronyms **249**

Appendix B
Common Controlled Drug
Substances **255**

Index **259**

PREFACE

Certification Exam Review for Pharmacy Technicians
What Makes This New Edition Exciting?

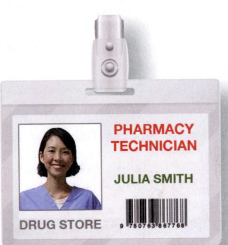

As a pharmacy technician, you want to build knowledge and establish a skills base for exceptional, safe service to patients. With certification, you will be able to continually advance in your career. *Certification Exam Review for Pharmacy Technicians,* Fourth Edition, has been updated to help you accomplish these goals. The fourth edition features include:

- Alignment with PTCE domains and ExCPT topical areas, covering the subjects in a logical order in clear language
- Instructor reviewed or written "Sample the Exam" questions at the end of chapters, with 120 new ones!
- Convenient eBook with study and assessment materials that are easily accessed through eBook links for the self-study course and through the Navigator+ learning platform for the instructor-guided course
- Numerous information tables and appendixes for organized studying and memorization
- Leading pharmacy topics covered in the rigorous new certification exams
- Updates on new standards for nonsterile, sterile, and hazardous compounding—encompassing revisions for USP Chapters <795> and new <800> guidelines
- Expanded sections on inventory and third-party billing

3-D
- New Biodigital™ 3D interactive diagrams of the human body systems in the pharmacology chapter for visualizing sites of pharmacological action
- Extensive instructor input in every aspect of the new edition

Web
- Web links for additional online pharmacy resources.
- Attractive margin features:

 Study Idea   Put Down Roots   Practice Tip   Safety Alert   Name Exchange

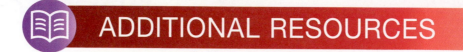

ADDITIONAL RESOURCES

The following student resources can be accessed through eBook links. The only exception is that students enrolled in an instructor-guided course may only access their chapter tests through the Navigator+ learning management system.

- **Supplemental Resources** include lists of Top 200 Drugs, Most Common Hospital Drugs, Common Palliative Care and Hospice Drugs, Vulnerable Populations Resources and Drugs to Avoid, HIPAA Regulations, and other useful study resources based on the most recommended pharmaceutical and medical websites.

- **New Digital Flash Card Sets** on pharmacy laws, generic/brand drug names, drug suffixes, controlled substances, and other information make studying these topics easy.

- A **Glossary** compiles key terms and definitions in one easy-to-access document.

- **"Sample the Exam" Chapter Tests** provide answers and answer rationale.

- An **Exam Generator** draws from a test bank of +1,000 questions and offers an infinite number of timed practice exams that simulate the PTCE with similar amounts of questions per each domain. Students can take a new exam as often as they like to judge their readiness for the real exam.

Instructor Resources

In addition to course planning materials, instructors receive the following resources in the Navigator+ learning management system:

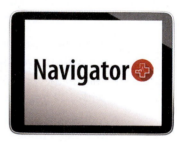

- **PowerPoint Slides** highlight key points of chapter content and can be downloaded and customized to meet your course needs.

- **Prebuilt Chapter Tests and Final Answer Keys** may be edited and instructors may add to these prebuilt tests directly in Navigator+ or by importing the provided RTF files into your own learning management system.

About the Author

Cheryl Aiken

Cheryl Aiken, BS, PharmD, RPh, is an assistant manager and pharmacy informatics specialist at the Brattleboro Retreat, a private psychiatric hospital in Brattleboro, Vermont. In addition to her work in the psychiatric field, she has served as a community pharmacist for independent and chain pharmacies, and as a staff pharmacist at the Brattleboro Memorial Hospital. She serves as the preceptor for IPPE and APPE Pharmacy Interns from Albany College of Pharmacy, Western New England College of Pharmacy and Husson University. In 2002, she helped establish an associate's degree and the Pharmacy Technician Training Program certificate at Vermont Technical College.

Acknowledgements

The quality of this body of work is a testament to the many contributors and reviewers who participated in the creation of *Certification Exam Review for Pharmacy Technicians*, Fourth Edition. We offer a heartfelt thank-you for your commitment to producing high-quality instructional materials for pharmacy technician students.

Textbook Consultants and Reviewer

Anne LaVance, CPhT—Past President of the Pharmacy Technician Educators Council (PTEC), Associate Professor Delgado Community College (New Orleans, LA); Board Member and Technician Committee Chair – Louisiana Society of Health-System Pharmacists (LSHP)

Robert J. Anderson, PharmD—co-author of the second and third editions of *Certification Exam Review for Technicians*. He has more than 40 years of experience in academia and pharmacy practice, having worked in both independent and chain community pharmacies. Dr. Anderson is a past member of the United States Pharmacopeia (USP) Expert Committee and Professor Emeritus at the Southern School of Pharmacy at Mercer University in Atlanta, Georgia. He is coauthor on the third, fourth, fifth, and sixth editions of *Pharmacy Practice for Technicians*.

Testbank Reviewers

Elina Pierce, MSP, CPhT—Director of Member Services of PTEC: Pharmacy Program Director and Instructor at Southeast Community College (Lincoln, NE); Senior Certified Pharmacy Technician; Pharmacy technician representative for Nebraska Pharmacists Association; 2010 Pharmacy Technician of the Year. She added 100 new "Sample the Exam" questions to Navigator+ (and self-study Quizzing Center).

Irene Banuelos-Villatoro, BS, CPhT, RPhT—Secretary of PTEC, Instructor at San Jacinto College North Campus (Houston, TX)

Andrea R. Redman, PharmD, BCPS—Pharmacist at Emory Healthcare (Atlanta, GA); Professor at Walden University (Minneapolis, MN), author of many clinical pharmacology research articles

Ashanti C. LaRoché, BA, CPht, SCAT-Certified—Assistant Professor of Delgado Community College Pharmacy Technician Program (New Orleans, LA); CTS Pharmacy Technician; nominated for NISOD Excellence in Teaching Award in 2015

Veronica Velasquez, BA, PhTR, CPhT—Treasurer of PTEC; Certified Instructor in Sterile Compounding and Aseptic Technique (SCAT) and Associate Professor in Pharmacy Technology Program, Austin Community College (Austin, TX)

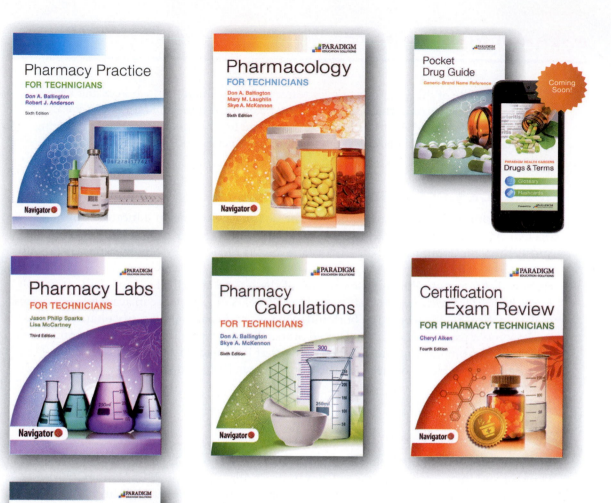

Paradigm's Comprehensive Pharmacy Technician Series

In addition to *Certification Exam Review for Pharmacy Technicians,* Fourth Edition, Paradigm Publishing, Inc. offers other titles designed specifically for the pharmacy technician curriculum:

- *Pharmacology for Technicians,* Sixth Edition
- *Pocket Drug Guide: Generic Brand Name Reference* available in print, eBook, or an app!
- *Pharmacy Labs for Technicians,* Third Edition
- *Pharmacy Calculations for Technicians,* Sixth Edition
- *Pharmacy Practice for Technicians,* Sixth Edition
- *Sterile Compounding and Aseptic Technique,* Second Edition

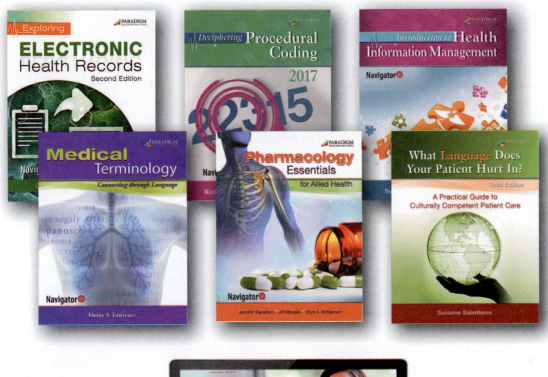

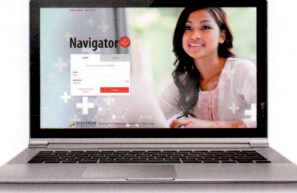

The *Navigator+* learning management system accompanies all new editions.

Related Health Career Titles

Additional titles in Paradigm's Health Career line of courses are particularly useful for pharmacy technicians:

- *Exploring Electronic Health Records*
- *Deciphering Procedural Coding*
- *Introduction to Health Information Management*
- *Medical Terminology: Connecting through Language*
- *Pharmacology Essentials for Allied Health*
- *What Language Does Your Patient Hurt In?: A Practical Guide to Culturally Competent Care, Third Edition*

Paradigm's all-new *Pocket Drug Guide* is available in both digital and print.

In print or as an eBook, the *Pocket Drug Guide* is a concise, convenient guide, which allows you to easily find and study the most common drugs from their brand or generic names.

In addition to the print book and eBook, the content will be available in a new digital format—the *Paradigm Health Careers Drugs & Terms app*!

A full glossary allows student to search by generic or brand name or by common use. This app encompasses more than 3,000 drugs and terms! Students are able to:

- Search the terms database by drug class or body system.
- Use flash cards included in the app to review Schedule II drug classes and common medical terminology.
- Create their own flash cards to practice identifying drugs and terms.

Plus, the embedded audio helps students master pronunciation!

Canadian Pharmacy Technician Supplement

This supplement assists Canadian students in understanding the differences between US and Canadian pharmacy practice. The supplement has four parts that can be read alongside specific chapters in this textbook:

- Part 1: Scope of Pharmacy Technicians in Canada (Chapter 1: The Profession of Pharmacy)
- Part 2: Drug Regulation in Canada (Chapter 2: Pharmacy Law, Regulations, and Standards)
- Part 3: Controlled Substances (Chapter 2: Pharmacy Law, Chapter 7: Community Pharmacy Dispensing, and Chapter 14: Medication Safety)
- Part 4: Top 100 Drugs Dispensed in Canadian Pharmacies (Chapter 4: Introducing Pharmacology)

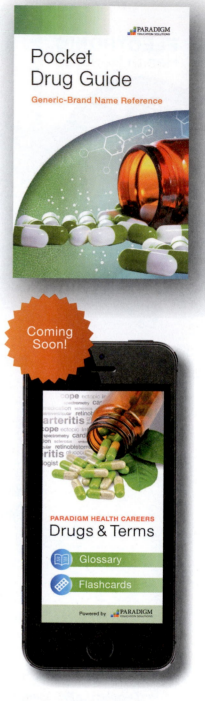

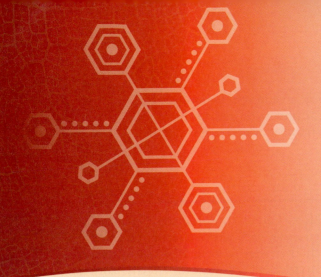

INTRODUCTION

Preparing for a High-Stakes Exam

Learning Objectives

1. Discuss the importance of certification for a pharmacy technician.

2. Understand the elements of certification, registration, and licensure.

3. Describe the major testing components of the PTCB and ExCPT examinations.

4. Make a study plan for the examination.

5. Use techniques for successfully taking a multichoice examination.

Access eBook links for resources and an exam generator, with 1,000+ questions.

A certification exam is a nationally recognized test used to measure competency in a professional area of practice. The exam's purpose is to protect the public interest by evaluating candidates' knowledge in a specific area. In this case, it is the knowledge necessary to perform the duties of a pharmacy technician. A nongovernmental agency develops the exam and implements the rules and policies related to certification based on criteria for the profession.

Certification Exam Review for Pharmacy Technicians, Fourth Edition, is intended to help you study for and pass a pharmacy technician certification exam. Two national exams are offered: the **Pharmacy Technician Certification Exam (PTCE)** and the **Exam for the Certification of Pharmacy Technicians (ExCPT)**. Individual states may recognize just the PTCE or both exams. Check your state's requirements before deciding which exam to take.

Certification recognizes that an individual has met predetermined qualifications in a specific area of study. A technician who successfully passes the exam may use the designation Certified Pharmacy Technician (CPhT) after his or her name. The Pharmacy Technician Certification Board's (PTCB's) associate director, William Schimmel, explained to an interviewer for *Pharmacy Times* that "national certification becomes a portable credential that can travel from state to state and job to job." Employers place a considerable value on certification because it demonstrates your knowledge as a technician and your commitment to your role in pharmacy. As we see things change in the profession and advanced roles for technicians open up, certification will open a number of new opportunities.

Why Become Certified?

Pharm Facts

According to the National Pharmacy Technician Association, there are more than 39,000 jobs for technicians available every year!

In a 2016 survey by the Pharmacy Workforce Center, three-fourths of pharmacy customers said that they would choose a pharmacy with certified technicians over one that does not have them. Parents with children were particularly likely to state this. These customers, and their employers, understand fully how the effective and safe delivery of pharmaceuticals depends on competent and knowledgeable technicians. Through certification, pharmacy technicians have demonstrated the ability, knowledge, and skills necessary to function effectively in a pharmacy team.

With certification, you become a marketable sales asset to any pharmacy, assisting in the care of patients and the success of the business or healthcare institution. You are open to increased responsibilities, job opportunities, and promotions, along with increased respect from your peers. In addition, certification offers a sense of accomplishment and the potential for greater job satisfaction.

As the profession of pharmacy advances, providing ever more medication therapy management and healthcare services, the possible career advancement opportunities multiply. There is an increasing need for qualified pharmacy technicians of many different experiences and skill sets ready to take on duties in pharmacy management, tech-check-tech roles, medication history profiles, medication reconciliation, insurance and billing, inventory, pharmacy informatics, patient assistance, hazardous drug handling, and nonsterile, sterile, and hazardous compounding.

Several organizations are currently working to improve training and education for pharmacy technicians. By the end of 2020, the PTCB will require all candidates seeking initial certification to complete a training program accredited by the American Society of Health-System Pharmacists and the Accreditation Council of Pharmacy Education (ASHP/ACPE) that includes both didactic coursework and practical experience. More information on the PTCB's new requirements is available at http://CertExam4e.ParadigmEducation.com/certification_changes.

Web

Pharm Facts

The ACPE is the Accreditation Council for Pharmacy Education that is working with the ASHP for program accreditation standards and certification.

ASHP, in partnership with individual state affiliates, is advocating in support of legislation at the state level that would require all pharmacy technicians to complete an ASHP/ACPE-accredited training program and earn PTCB certification as a prerequisite to licensure or registration by each state board of pharmacy and for practice in every hospital. The intent of the initiative is to improve patient safety and reduce medication errors through enhanced education and training. More information on the Pharmacy Technician Initiative is available at http://CertExam4e.ParadigmEducation.com/ASHPinitiative.

Web

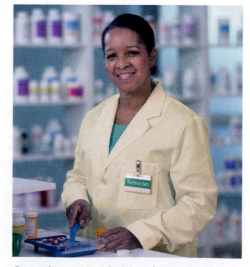

Once pharmacy technicians have passed their certification exam, they can proudly where the designation of CPhT.

State Practice Requirements

State pharmacy boards determine whether pharmacy technicians need to be registered, licensed, and/or certified. State requirements for pharmacy technicians may include one or all of these components. Many states stipulate a maximum ratio of technicians (including pharmacy interns) to pharmacists, which varies from 2:1 to 4:1. The ratio may be dependent on the number of certified pharmacy technicians employed at a site. Some states may use a higher technician-to-pharmacist ratio if at least one technician is certified. Only five states did not have laws regulating pharmacy technicians as of mid-2016: Colorado, Wisconsin, Pennsylvania, New York, and Hawaii, but likely it is only a matter of time until they do.

Study Idea

Since each state is different, call the office or visit the website of the your state board of pharmacy to find out the requirements for practice: registration, licensure, and/or certification.

Registration

In the majority of states, pharmacy technicians are required to be "registered," or listed on the state board of pharmacy's official list of pharmacy technicians before starting to practice in any licensed pharmacy. This is a way to control access to the restricted area of the pharmacy and track who is permitted to assist the pharmacist. Pharmacy technicians who are not registered, or have allowed their registration to lapse, cannot legally work in the restricted pharmacy area in these states.

Another of the main reasons for registration is to report and monitor any serious disciplinary action (such as stealing drugs or money) before the disciplined technician applies for another pharmacy technician job or is hired at another pharmacy within or outside the state. If a technician changes employment within the state, he or she must notify the board of pharmacy. Registration cannot be reciprocated or transferred to another state. States have varying continuing education requirements for annual re-registration.

There is no test required for registration, but the process generally includes an application to the state board of pharmacy and payment of appropriate fees. The application process may include a background check. Registration may be denied if the applicant has a history of criminal activity or charges related to drugs or alcohol use. Registration will be denied or revoked for actions that compromise the lawful activities of a pharmacy, and the state may levy fines against pharmacies that allow unregistered individuals in restricted areas. A majority of states also have training requirements, but these are not yet standardized across the states.

Licensure

Some states require pharmacy technicians to be licensed. Licensure is a more rigorous application process than registration. The process varies by state. Passing a licensure exam if often a key component. The license exam may be on state pharmacy laws or on the state laws plus practice in general. In addition, the license applicants may need to be certified and/or a graduate (associate degree or higher) of an accredited college program specializing in pharmacy technology. Individual states also have continuing education requirements for license renewal.

Web

Visit your state board of pharmacy website for information on individual state requirements. To learn more about state licensure requirements, visit the National Association of Boards of Pharmacy website at http://CertExam4e.ParadigmEducation.com/napb/pharmacyboards and click on Boards of Pharmacy.

Certification

You are ahead of the game to be seeking to pass a certification exam. More than half the states have made national certification either mandatory or preferred for licensure or practice, and the number of states making this a requirement is continuing to grow. In states with fewer requirements, employers are often making this requirement on their own to increase their business or facility rates of medication safety and efficiency.

There are strong financial reasons for becoming certified. Community pharmacies are increasingly expecting their technicians to be certified; it may be a requirement for initial employment (especially in large hospitals) or strongly encouraged within the first year of employment. Sometimes the cost of the exam and even training are covered for a valued employee.

Most hospital pharmacies require certification and will often expect prior experience or advanced training, especially if the technician will be working with sterile IV products and chemotherapy. Hospital accreditation depends on trained staffing. Some hospitals offer their own training or a monetary incentive.

Successful completion of a national certification exam qualifies you to work in a variety of pharmacy settings including retail, institutional, mail order, administration, and educational. Employer-specific examinations, such as those offered by some chain pharmacies may test an individual's ability to work in one specific pharmacy environment, but those exams are generally not comprehensive enough to demonstrate the skills needed to work in many different pharmacy environments. If certification is required, the state board of pharmacy determines which certification exam(s) will be accepted.

Choose the Right Exam

A certification exam for pharmacy technicians is a high-stakes, professional exam. The exam is similar to other high-level prerequisite tests, such as those for college or graduate school. To successfully complete the PTCE or ExCPT, it is important to become proficient in the knowledge and skills necessary to be a pharmacy technician and to practice good test-taking strategies.

Certification Exam Review for Pharmacy Technicians, Fourth Edition, is designed to prepare you for either test you choose. It includes 10 chapters that review the content of the nine exam subject areas developed by the PTCE. The book's three units categorize the 10 chapters into the three domains of the ExCPT. Overviews of the PTCE and ExCPT test plans and their domains are shown in Tables 0.1 and 0.2 on the next pages. The full plans can be found on the websites for the two tests noted on page 8 (PTCE) and page 9 (ExCPT).

TABLE 0.1   PTCE Testing Content—90 Questions (80 Scored)

Book Chapter	Subject Domain	Description	Category Weight
Chapter 1	1. Pharmacology for Technicians	• Generic and brand names of medications • Common indications, doses, side effects, and contraindications • Drug interactions • Knowledge of over-the-counter (OTC) drugs, herbals, and dietary supplements	13.75%
Chapter 3 Appendix B, Supplement	2. Pharmacy Law and Regulations	• Drug Enforcement Administration (DEA) regulations • US Food and Drug Administration (FDA) recalls • Infection control standards • Omnibus Budget Reconciliation Act (OBRA) requirements • Hazardous drugs • Health Insurance Portability and Accountability Act (HIPAA) • Risk Evaluation and Mitigation Strategy (REMS)	12.5%
Chapters 5, 6	3. Sterile and Nonsterile Compounding	• Infection control (hand washing; personal protective equipment, etc.) • Handling and disposal requirements • Beyond-use dating • Procedures • Equipment • Documentation of sterile and nonsterile compounds	8.75%
Chapter 7, Appendix A	4. Medication Safety	• Error-prevention strategies • Patient Package Inserts (PPIs) and MedGuides • Pharmacist referrals • High-risk medications • Approved labeling • Abbreviations	12.5%
Chapter 7	5. Pharmacy Quality Assurance	• Use of National Drug Code (NDC) and barcoding for medication dispensing and inventory control • Infection control procedures (personal protective equipment, needle recapping, etc.) • Risk management guidelines • Customer satisfaction measures	7.5%
Chapters 2, 4	6. Medication Order Entry and Fill Process	• Intake, interpretation, and data entry • Calculations • Filling and dispensing processes • Labeling • Packaging requirements	17.5%
Chapter 9	7. Pharmacy Inventory Management	• Use of NDCs, lot numbers, and expiration dates • Formulary and approved drug lists • Ordering, receiving, storage, and removal	8.75%
Chapter 10	8. Pharmacy Billing and Reimbursement	• Third-party reimbursement policies and plans • Resolution • Coordination of benefits	8.75%
Chapter 8	9. Pharmacy Information System Usage and Application	• Computer applications in the dispensing of prescriptions and medication orders • E-prescriptions	10.0%

TABLE 0.2 ExCPT Testing Plan—100 questions (and 20 Pretest Questions)

Book Chapter	Subject Category	Description	Category Questions
Chapters 3, 4, 7, 8, 9, 10	1. Regulations and Pharmacy Duties		35%
		• Overview of technician duties and general information including federal and state laws, regulations, and standards	(14%)
		• Controlled substances, including knowing the schedules and product, rules of dispensing and documentation	(10%)
		• Other pharmacy laws, such as HIPAA, generic substitutions, child-resistant containers, labeling, among others	(11%)
Chapters 1, 2	2. Drugs and Drug Therapy		11%
		• Drug classifications, dosage forms, routes of administration, OTC drugs, NDC numbers	(4%)
		• Commonly prescribed medications	(7%)
Chapters 2–10	3. Dispensing Processes		54%
		• Prescription information, including the parts of the prescription, gathering information from patient and missing information from prescriber, interpreting abbreviations, refill authorization	(8%)
		• Preparing and dispensing prescriptions, including measuring, calibrating instruments, communicating with patients, record keeping, safety procedures, properly inputting and responding to computer alerts, patient education materials, auxiliary labels, third-party claims processing	(29%)
		• Calculations, including conversions, dosage quantities, days supply, compounding calculations (ratio strengths, w/w%, s/v%, v/v%, dilution/concentrations, mEq), and business calculations	(7%)
		• Nonsterile and sterile compounding, unit dose, and repackaging, including proper aseptic technique, compounding procedures, labeling, vials and ampules, expiration and beyond use dates, different parenteral routes of administration	(10%)

Pharm Facts

The PTCE is the more long-standing and recognized of the two tests. ASHP accredited programs encourage or require students to take this exam.

Pharmacy Technician Certification Exam

The most popular and recognized national certification is the Pharmacy Technician Certification Exam (PTCE), sponsored by the PTCB. The examination grew out of efforts by two states (Michigan and Illinois), the ASHP, and the American Pharmacy Association to develop technician standards. The board developed the PTCE based on task analyses of the actual work of pharmacy technicians in both the retail and hospital pharmacy settings. In 2001, the National Association of Boards of Pharmacy joined this coalition to offer a certification program for pharmacy technicians.

The PTCE for pharmacy technician certification is accepted by all 50 states and the District of Columbia as a legitimate certification for the profession, and in almost half of the states it is the only test mentioned as a practice standard. Five states require or will only accept the PTCE. Since 1995, the PTCB has granted over 585,000 certifications.

Some states specifically require PTCB certification to be eligible to practice—Arizona, Louisiana, North Dakota, Texas, and Wyoming (as of November 2016), with more moving in this direction. Hospitals and institutions favor the PTCE.

Exam for the Certification of Pharmacy Technicians

An alternative test evolved out of the efforts of the National Community Pharmacists Association, National Association of Chain Drug Stores, and the National Healthcareer Association (NHA). The Exam for the Certification of Pharmacy Technicians (ExCPT) is offered through the NHA, which offers other healthcareer certification exams as well. Although the ExCPT is similar in content to the PTCE, it has a little more focus on retail pharmacies and is not recognized in all states.

Clearly, there is a need for all states to have more consistency in technician training and examination requirements. The National Association of Boards of Pharmacy is working toward this goal in its Model State Pharmacy Act and Model Rules initiative for all states.

Test and Certification Eligibility

Both certification exams require the applicant to be a graduate of high school or to have passed the General Education Development (GED) test or some other equivalency test. You may also have achieved a foreign or alternative diploma recognized by your state and the American Association of Collegiate Registrars and Admissions Officers that indicates sufficient secondary education proficiency. (If you have not yet attained this diploma but will be in the next 30 days, the NHA will allow you to sit for the exam. If you pass, you can be granted a provisional certification for up to 12 months to complete the educational requirements if other eligibility criteria have been met.) Eligibility requirements for the two national certification tests differ slightly.

PTCE Eligibility and Scheduling

Certification by the PTCB requires a disclosure of all criminal and state board of pharmacy violations. Many academic pharmacy technician programs do a screening of students and also have them pass a drug test. Instructors do not want to train students at risk of drug abuse and then place them in situations where they may be tempted to misuse or steal drugs. Though PTCB certification does not presently require pharmacy-related educational training and work experience, by 2020 all applicants will receive it expected to have completed an ASHP-accredited pharmacy technician education and training program. See Table 0.3 for an example of PTCE requirements.

TABLE 0.3 PTCE Requirements

- High school diploma or GED
- No felony convictions
- No drug- or pharmacy-related convictions, including misdemeanors (Misdemeanors must be disclosed.)
- No denied, suspended, revoked, or restricted registration or licensure, consent order, or other restrictions by any state board of pharmacy
- No admission of misconduct or violation of regulations of any state board of pharmacy

The PTCB also requires all exam certification applicants and certified personnel to be in compliance with all their policies, including their Code of Conduct, summarized in Table 0.4. The PTCB standards and expectations are outlined on its website and include following all PTCB, federal, state, local, and employer rules and laws; upholding professional standards; delivering safe medications and recognizing practice limitations in deference to the pharmacist; maintaining and respecting patient and professional confidentiality; providing truthful representation of one's actions and credentials; following appropriate safety procedures and standards; and avoiding conflicts between patients and employers, among other standards.

For more information, visit http://CertExam4e.ParadigmEducation.com/PTCB and its code of conduct page: http://CertExam4e.ParadigmEducation.com/Conduct.

There are a few steps involved in scheduling to take the PTCE. First, you must apply online at http://CertExam4e.ParadigmEducation.com/Application1. Be prepared to pay the testing fee (which in 2016 was $129).

Web

If the application is accepted, authorization to schedule an exam will arrive via email and be valid for 90 days. Because the test must be taken at a computer-based testing site at one of the Pearson Professional Centers and military testing centers, you must schedule with Pearson VUE via telephone at (866) 902-0593 or online at http:// CertExam4e.ParadigmEducation.com/Application2.

A confirmation of the test date and place will be sent via email within 24 hours. Candidates who need special testing accommodations must call (800) 466-0450.

TABLE 0.4 Code of Conduct and Ethical Expectations for Pharmacy Technicians

The PTCB Code of Conduct expects its certified technicians to:

- maintain high standards of integrity and conduct,
- accept responsibility for their actions,
- continually seek to improve their performance in the workplace,
- practice with fairness and honesty,
- encourage others to act in an ethical manner consistent with PTCB standards and responsibilities.

Web

Source: Pharmacy Technician Certification Board website at
http://CertExam4e.ParadigmEducation.com/PTCB

The NHA Code of Ethics expects its certified professionals to:

- use their efforts for the betterment of society, the profession, and the members of the profession,
- uphold the standards of professionalism and be honest in all professional interactions,
- continue to learn, apply, and advance scientific and practical knowledge and skills, staying up-to-date on the latest research and its practical application,
- participate in activities contributing to the improvement of personal health, our society, and the betterment of the allied health industry,
- continuously act in the best interests of the general public,
- protect and respect the dignity, privacy, and safety of all patients.

Web

Source: *National Healthcareer Association Certification Candidate Handbook* at
http://CertExam4e.ParadigmEducation.com/NHAHandbook

Each certification exam testing site has a secure, comfortable, properly lit, temperature-controlled environment. You will be given one hour and fifty minutes to complete the 90-question examination.

The PTCE is organized into nine domains or sections, each of which is weighted differently. Skills and knowledge from both the community and institutional settings are required to pass this examination, including basic compounding knowledge and skills. Out of the 90 multiple choice questions, only 80 are scored. Each question comes with four possible choices. Only one answer is correct. *You should answer every question whether you are sure of the answer or not*, because the final score is based on the total number of questions answered correctly rather than the percentage of correct answers. Educated guesses are encouraged. After the exam, in the final 10 minutes, you will take a post-exam survey and receive your unofficial results onsite.

ExCPT Eligibility and Scheduling

In addition to the secondary education requirement, all ExCPT candidates must have completed a pharmacy technician training program from a state-recognized institution within the past five years. In lieu of this, you can have passed an employer-based academic training program that has been approved by the state board of pharmacy or have 1,200 hours of employer-supervised, pharmacy-related experience within any one year of the past three years. Those with pharmacy-related training in the military are also eligible. The student must prepare a "candidate profile" and agree to an attestation statement before sitting for the exam.

The NHA also sets out a high standard of expectations for all its allied health certifications in its NHA Code of Ethics, and it further outlines specifics of behaviors expected for pharmacy technicians to attain and maintain certification. These include, among many other standards, that pharmacy technicians "assist and support pharmacists in the safe and efficacious and cost effective distribution of health services and healthcare resources;" "continually enhance professional knowledge and expertise;" and "respect and support the patient's individuality, dignity and confidentiality." The list has been adapted from the American Association of Pharmacy Technicians Code of Ethics. For more information, go to the NHA website at http://CertExam4e.ParadigmEducation.com/NHA.

To take the ExCPT, you also need to apply and show that you meet the test criteria, which you can do online at http://CertExam4e.ParadigmEducation.com/Application3.

Once you receive approval to schedule, you can select an available date and time at your school if it is an NHA-affiliated school offering the test or at the nearest PSI testing center (PSI is an international company specializing in testing). Call (800) 733-9267, or schedule online at http://CertExam4e.ParadigmEducation.com/Application4.

There is an NHA test fee (which in 2016 was $115) that may be accompanied by additional PSI fees. NHA-affiliated schools often include the fee for the exam in the costs of the school program. If special testing accommodations are needed, you must fill out a form at the NHA website: http://CertExam4e.ParadigmEducation.com/Application5.

Though the ExCPT can also be taken as a paper test at some sites (bring two number 2 pencils and an eraser!), it is generally offered as a computer-based examination. Test takers are given two hours and ten minutes to complete the 100 multiple-choice questions (and 20 pretest questions) from a large test bank.

Pharm Facts

The cost to take the ExCPT has generally been less than the PTCE.

Web

Test Preparation Strategies

Preparation is an important part of taking a high-stakes exam. There are three areas of preparation: study, preparation for thorough knowledge of the subjects, and test-taking skills. This section discusses important exam preparation skills and strategies. The main chapters review the pharmacy knowledge and skills needed by technicians interwoven with study ideas.

Practice exams can help to determine where to focus your study efforts. That is why *Certification Exam Review for Pharmacy Technicians*, Fourth Edition, offers end-of-chapter and final test with exam-like questions and an end-of-course test generator that provides a nearly infinite number of timed mock exams with the same proportion of questions per domain as the PTCE.

How and When to Study

Study Idea

Do not cram at the last minute—set up a study schedule over the course of a few weeks to prepare for the exam.

Do not wait to study until just before the exam. Talk to graduates from your program and other certified pharmacy technicians about their experiences studying for and taking the exam and get their tips. Cramming raises test anxiety and harms the memory. Start studying now to become familiar with the skills and concepts on the exam.

Budget Time to Study

Make a timeline and plan, schedule in a few hours each day to study uninterrupted by family or friends. Spread your review over a period of weeks. Focused reviews conducted over time are more effective than cramming at the last minute. As a certified pharmacy technician, you will use this information for years to come, not just on the exam. By developing your skills and knowledge slowly over time, you will retain more information and improve your recall in the future.

After taking the pretest at the end of this introduction, you will know which areas require less attention and practice and which need more.

Study Idea

Carry your flash cards with you wherever you go, and any time you have a few minutes, review the drug brand and generic names.

Study Resources

Study well all the tables in each chapter and the appendices, memorizing some. This course also includes other key supplements, such as "Top 200 Drugs, "HIPAA Regulations," Cmmmon Drugs to Avoid for Vulnerable Populations," and others. These can be accessed through eBook links. Additional resources include digital flashcards, a full book glossary, and the computer-graded "Sample the Exam" questions at the end of each chapter. Then at the end of the course, take the final and generate timed exams to simulate the actual exam experience. The Paradigm Health Careers *Drugs & Terms* smartphone app can help you study generic and brand drug names and medical terms.

Study Groups

Study groups can also be an effective way to review and discuss information. If you work in a pharmacy, ask your colleagues for help. If you do not work in a pharmacy, ask a local pharmacy if you may shadow one of their

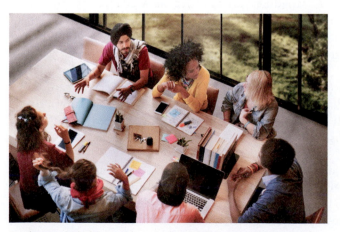

Study groups help provide associates for encouragement and to hold each other accountable for set times to study.

technicians. (You may do this through your program or have to register with the state board of pharmacy to be behind the pharmacy counter.) Getting hands-on experience to observe and assist in the work of practicing pharmacists and pharmacy technicians is an excellent way to study for the exam.

Ask your instructors to identify areas where you need to focus your attention. If you know a pharmacist well or work with one, ask for help in areas like pharmacology and pharmacy calculations.

Develop Relaxation Techniques

Taking a high-stakes professional exam can be stressful. Cheer yourself on like an athlete, and practice relaxation techniques if you start feeling anxious to keep your mind clear. Deep breathing, positive thinking, and visualization exercises can help prepare the body and mind for the challenge and allow you to focus on studying and the exam questions. It may be helpful to drive by the test site before the exam to become familiar with the area so you know where it is.

Prepare in Advance for Test Day

Study Idea

Form a study group with others studying to work out problems together, share tips, and quiz each other with flash cards.

Think of preparing for the exam as you would for a trip. Get the proper directions and know where you will park if you are driving there. The night before the exam, pack all the items needed for the test. Depending on which exam you take, you will need a government-issued photo identification, such as a valid passport, driver's license, US Armed Forces identification card, or nondriver identification issued by your state Department of Motor Vehicles. (The Take Note on page 12 lists approved IDs.)

You are allowed to bring certain items, such as religious apparel and comfort aids, to the PTCE test site, including the following:

- cough drops
- eyeglasses, eye patches, magnifying glasses
- hearing aids
- canes, crutches, casts, braces, slings, walkers
- medical devices attached to the body
- wheelchairs and other mobility devices
- required medications (unwrapped and not in a container)

Practice Tip

Remember, the name on your identification must be identical to the name provided to the testing center when you registered.

Pack only the necessary items. You will not need pencils, paper, calculator, phone, or anything else. Anything needed to take the exam will be provided at the test site. You will be supplied with a secure locker to store items not permitted in the exam area. No electronic devices such as cell phones, tablets, or calculators are allowed in the testing room. Calculators will be provided online or will be available upon request from the testing monitor.

Follow Good Sleeping and Eating Habits

Pharm Facts

Tissues, earplugs, and noise-canceling headphones must be provided by the testing center for the PTCE, if needed.

The night before the exam, do not pull an all-nighter cramming for the exam. Get a good night's sleep. Set the alarm and wake up on time, refreshed and ready. Eat a nutritious meal or snack before the test to help maintain energy. Avoid eating high-fat foods or excessive sugar before the exam, as these foods can make you groggy or sleepy in the middle of the test.

Be sure to bring valid identification, which is defined as an unexpired, government-issued ID that has a photograph and signature. If the identification does not include a signature, a secondary ID will be required. This could be a social security card, credit/debit/ATM card, or employee/school ID. The testing center may also require biometric identification, such as a fingerprint scan or a palm vein scan.

The Day of the Exam

Study Idea

Allow plenty of time to get there, even if you have to wait. It is better to not have the stress of cutting it close, and you can study while you wait, stretching your mind like an athlete stretches the body before going into a race.

Don't be afraid of the exam or that feeling of pretest jitters. They show instead that your body and mind are recognizing a challenge and are preparing to meet it, like an athlete before a race. So don't fear it; lean into it and use the energy. Use the sense of stress to motivate yourself to study ahead of time, and understand that stress is a natural part of the process and should be used as an asset to to help you focus.

Breathe, breathe, breathe, and stretch before you sit down, just like an athlete. Be on the top of your game, and go for it! Your mind, which has been trained and prepared, will run for you and do that exam.

Arrive Early

On the day of the scheduled exam, you should arrive 30 minutes early (having made sure ahead of time that you have the directions and know where to park). Getting lost and/or missing the starting time will result in the cancellation of your appointment and loss of your exam fee.

Table 0.5 provides a list of key things to do on the day of the exam.

TABLE 0.5 The Day of the Exam

Get enough sleep the night before the test. Also, make sure to get adequate sleep the week before the test.
Dress casually and comfortably. Take extra time to plan what to wear.
Check the directions to the site and bring the proper ID(s) and anything else necessary.
Arrive at the testing center early, and choose a comfortable work area.
Before the test, go the bathroom.
Pump yourself up and tell yourself you can do it! Breathe deep to fill your brain with oxygen, and do this any time you feel stressed while taking the test.

Study Idea

Test stress can be good! It can help you rise to the challenge. Become your own cheerleader for this event. You can do it!

The Testing Environment

At the exam site, you will be provided with an erasable board to serve as a scratch pad. A calculator will be available on the exam computer. Practice with and become proficient using your computer's calculator so this does not slow you down during the exam. You are not allowed to ask the exam site staff questions concerning the test content. There are no scheduled breaks. If you must leave the testing area to use the restroom, you will not be given additional time to complete the test. You must present identification to re-enter the test area. Remember, cell phones, calculators, recording devices, and photography equipment are not allowed in the test area.

Web

You will be given time to view a tutorial before the exam. You must agree to all PTCB or NHA testing policies prior to starting the appropriate exam. You may download the tutorial in advance from the Pearson VUE website: http://CertExam4e. ParadigmEducation.com/Pearson-tutorial. This may help to reduce test anxiety.

Tips for Taking Multiple-Choice Tests

Study Idea

Slow down and read the entire question to make sure you know what the question is asking before answering. You can guess on an answer and flag it; then after you have finished them all, go back for second thoughts.

One of the advantages of taking a multiple-choice test is that the correct answer is provided in the list of possible answers. There is no penalty for guessing. Pace yourself so you can answer every question. If you are unsure of the correct answer, follow some standard test-taking tips to choose a best-guess response.

- Plan your time. You will have two hours to answer 90 multiple-choice questions for the PTCE, or 2 hours and 10 minutes for 100 multiple choice questions and 20 pretest questions for the ExCPT. Do not get stuck on a troublesome question. If you are not sure of an answer that doesn't require calculations, answer the question in 30 to 60 seconds, select an answer, flag the question, and move on. Return to the question later.

- Read the whole question before answering. Make sure you understand what the question is, and take the question at face value. Do not waste time looking for trick questions.

- *Answer the question in your head before reviewing the choices.* This will prevent you from being influenced by the answers provided.

- Remember there is *only one best answer listed*, although more than one answer may appear to be correct. So look for the most complete answer. When writing multiple-choice questions, one correct answer and three distractors are provided. The distractors are usually terms you know but not fully right.

- *If you do not know the answer, use a process of elimination.* Eliminate the most obviously wrong answer first, then the second, and make your best decision from the remaining two choices. This tactic gives you a 50% chance of selecting the correct answer.

Study Idea

Do not get stuck on one question because you feel it is ambiguous, misleading, or deficient. Guess the answer; move on; then note your concern at the end of the exam in the comment section.

- In calculation questions, the distractors may use the correct numbers in incorrect ways and often include answers you might get if you are unsure how to do the calculation or make a mistake with the decimal point. Solving the problem before you look at the choices provided helps eliminate distractors.

- Do not look for patterns in the answers. Computerized tests are written without concern for answer placement.

- If you are still unsure of the correct answer, select the longer or more descriptive answer of the remaining choices, although a good test writer will make all of the answers approximately the same length.

- If the answer set presents a range of numbers and you are not sure of the correct answer, it often works to eliminate the highest and lowest choices and select from the middle range of numbers.

- Watch out for negative words in a question. Be alert for words such as *not* or *except* or *only*. These questions ask you to identify the false statement instead of the true statement. Read the question carefully and make sure you understand what is asked.

- Beware of questions and answers that contain absolutes, such as *always, never, must, all,* and *none*, which severely limit the meaning of the item. Answers that contain absolutes are often incorrect except in terms of safety, aseptic procedures, and identifying the strictest laws.

- Become familiar with the computerized timed testing process and take simulated practice tests with the eBook's exam generator. It is there to help you get comfortable with the exam process.

- If you feel a question is ambiguous, misleading, or deficient in accuracy or content, fill out the comment section at the end of exam. This may help your grade if the question is found to be faulty.

Table 0.6 summarizes some key tips to consider while taking the certification exam.

TABLE 0.6 During the Exam

Listen, read, and follow directions carefully.
Read each question carefully. Do not skim or you can miss key words, especially negatives! Make sure to follow the computer screen prompts.
Answer easy questions first, and come back to the more difficult questions.
Never leave a question unanswered. Use the process of elimination! There is no penalty for guessing.
Manage your time.
Change your answer only if you are certain you made a mistake. Your first answer is usually correct.
Do not leave the testing area unless you must.

After the Exam

After completing the exam, you will receive your results immediately as pass or fail. Your numerical score will be sent to you or made available online at a later date. Each exam has its own scoring system.

Grading of the PTCE

The results you receive at the test site are unofficial results. The official results will be emailed to you and/or posted on the PTCE website in two to three weeks. Questions for the PTCE are weighted based on level of difficulty. According to the PTCE scoring blueprint, the possible scores range from 1,000 to 1,600, and 1,400 or higher is passing. The PTCB reports that since its inception, the test has been rigorous with numerous math and drug questions. An average of 57% of the scored exams qualify the test takers for certification.

With the new ASHP standards, the test has become even more rigorous. Unsuccessful candidates may appeal their scores or a specific testing item by completing an appeal form and submitting a review fee. The review fee may be refunded if the appeal is successful.

You can take the PTCE four times, though you must wait 60 days between attempts for the second and third try and six months for the fourth attempt (you must reapply and pay the fee each time). The official certificate that recognizes you as a Certified Pharmacy Technician (CPhT) will arrive in the mail in four to six weeks, and you can use it immediately.

Grading of the ExCPT

The ExCPT is immediately graded, and students at the PSI testing centers find out whether they passed or not. The scores are also confidentially posted on the NHA website within two days. The scores range from 200 to 500, converted from the raw test scores and weighted question system. A passing score is 390 or above.

Candidates who do not pass the ExCPT are allowed to retake the exam after four weeks. You can log into your account at the NHA website for a diagnostic of your test and recommendations for improvement. Those who successfully pass the ExCPT will receive a formal CPhT certificate and wallet card within 7–10 business days of the exam date.

Recertification

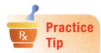

Practice Tip

For PTCB recertification, 10 credits may be related college courses, but 10 must be pharmacy specific. Free credits can be found at Power-Pak C.E. For registration, go to http://CertExam 4e.Paradigm Education.com /PowerPak.

Web

Recertification is required by both the PTCB and NHA every two years to maintain certification status. To be recertified for either, you must earn 20 hours of technician specific credit in pharmacy-related, approved continuing education (CE), and both require one hour of continuing education to come from pharmacy law. PTCB recertification also requires one hour of continuing education in medication or patient safety.

Acceptable CE topics include drug distribution, inventory control, managed healthcare, drug products, therapeutic issues, patient interaction, communication, interpersonal skills, pharmacy operations, prescription compounding, calculations, pharmacy law, preparation of sterile products, and drug repackaging. Certificates of participation must be obtained for each CE program. Pharmacy-related continuing education may be provided by a professional pharmacy or related healthcare organization on appropriate topics.

Certification may be revoked if a technician is convicted of a felony or a crime involving "moral turpitude" (involving problems with honesty, morals, or justice), including illegal sale, distribution, or use of controlled substances or prescription drugs; or for making false statements in connection with certification or recertification. Refer to the exam website or the board of pharmacy in your state for more information.

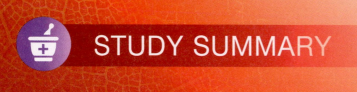

STUDY SUMMARY

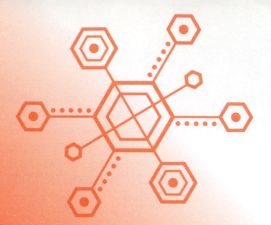

- Check the requirements for practice in your state and what possible changes to these requirements are coming down the pipeline.

- Remember that the PTCB is integrating new professional pharmacy technician standards that will be fully implemented by 2020 that require the passing of an ASHP/ACPE-accredited training program and national certification.

- Hospitals favor hiring those who have passed the PTCE. They are also seeking additional training in sterile and hazardous compounding from those who want jobs in these areas. The PTCB is working on a certification for this advanced position.

- As you study, imagine the vast number of career opportunities that certification opens up, which would be unattainable without the CPhT certification.

- Strategize on which national certification exam suits your current and future career plans—the PTCE or the ExCPT—and schedule your appointment.

- Make a realistic study plan that spaces out the chapters, with sufficient time for studying each and testing by chapter section.

- With each chapter, study the tables, appendices, and supplements, and take the end-of-chaper tests.

- Leave a few weeks to take a number of mock timed exams for yourself with the exam generating program, which provides tests with questions in similar proportions to the PTCE. These will help build your confidence.

- Remember the tips for succeeding at multiple-choice questions and the power of the process of elimination. If you don't know the answer for sure, knock out all the options that you know are wrong and choose from what is left.

- Don't be afraid of test-taking stress. Like an athlete, use that adrenaline to do better than you would have done without it.

- Be confident. If you have practiced, you will do well.

- Pack for the test the night before, prepare early, eat a good breakfast, and arrive a half hour ahead of time with the proper ID(s) and registration materials.

- Take the test and succeed!

ADDITIONAL RESOURCES

To see how much you remember, take the Study Skills test that can be accessed the the Ebook link for the self-study course and through Navigator+ for individuals enrolled in the instructor-guided course.

THINKING BEYOND THE EXAM

1. Many state boards of pharmacy are considering adopting new rules and regulations concerning the certification, registration, or licensure of pharmacy technicians. Find out what your state board of pharmacy is considering. Write a brief paragraph or essay explaining your choice to seek certification or your thoughts your state's qualifications for practice.

2. Why is a chain store's technician exam not adequate to earn the national designation of CPhT? Write a brief paragraph.

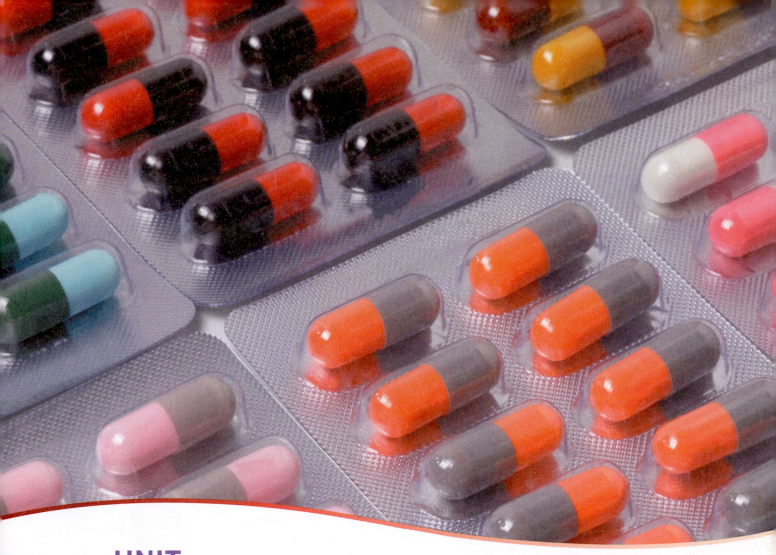

UNIT

1 Drugs and Drug Therapies

Chapter 1   Pharmacology for Technicians   21

Chapter 2   Pharmacy Conversions and Dosage Calculations   61

19

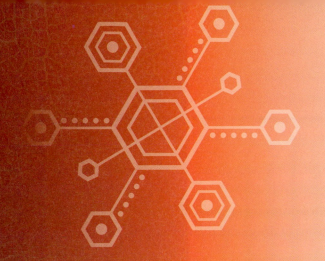

1

Pharmacology for Technicians

Learning Objectives

1   Define pharmacology and the scientific disciplines encompassed by pharmacology.

2   Explain how drugs are organized by anatomical systems.

3   Identify the generic names, brand names, and indications for the most frequently prescribed drugs in community and hospital pharmacy practice for various bodily systems.

4   Know the side effects and adverse reactions for central nervous system, cardiovascular, anti-infective, endocrine, respiratory, gastrointestinal, and renal drugs.

5   Name drugs that can interact with cholesterol-lowering drugs to cause muscle fatigue.

6   Discuss unique patient counseling recommendations for bisphosphonates.

7   Identify a serious, life-threatening drug interaction caused by erectile dysfunction drugs.

8   Identify common medications that require auxiliary labels and administration instructions.

9   Identify drug families by suffix similarities.

10 Understand the labeling requirements and the technician's role with over-the-counter drugs, homeopathic remedies, and dietary supplements.

Access eBook links for resources and an exam generator, with 1,000+ questions.

There are many drugs on the market for many indications. This chapter reviews and discusses the basic pharmacology of the most commonly dispensed drugs in the community and hospital pharmacy. The pharmacy technician should have a clear understanding of the generic and trade names of the most common medications, their primary indications, and common side effects. Technicians also need to know the common auxiliary warning labels that accompany these drugs and which commonly prescribed drugs are controlled substances or are on lists of high-risk drugs. This knowledge is important to function effectively in the pharmacy and is also covered on the certification exam. Essential pharmacological information is necessary to better understand the drug utilization alerts and enhance patient education and compliance with the prescribed medications.

Essential Knowledge for Technicians

Pharm Facts

The PTCE domain 1 on pharmacology will be 13.75% of that certification exam. The ExCPT topical area 2 on drugs and drug therapy will be 11% of that certification exam.

Put Down Roots

Pharmacology comes from the Greek word *pharmakon,* or "drug," and the Latin suffix *-logia,* or "study of."

Pharmacology is defined as the scientific study of drugs and how they work (the mechanism of action) along with side effects, adverse reactions, and drug interactions. In its broadest sense, pharmacology encompasses specialized scientific disciplines about drugs, including:

- **therapeutics**—appropriate uses of drugs for targeted medicinal purposes
- **pharmacodynamics**—mechanisms of drugs and their biochemical and physiological effects
- **toxicology**—symptoms, mechanisms, detection, and treatment of poisonous effects and side effects
- **pharmaceutics**—various dosage forms and routes of administration and their drug-releasing capabilities
- **pharmacokinetics**—movement of drugs within the body: absorption, distribution, metabolism, and elimination (ADME) of drugs from the body, and harmful drug interactions
- **pharmacognosy**—natural sources of drugs and herbs

It takes pharmacists numerous years of studying these basic and applied elements of pharmacology for thousands of drugs before they begin to practice, which is why patient questions about drugs must always be directed to the pharmacist.

In most cases (88%), prescribers will write a prescription for a brand name drug—which is easier to remember and spell—though a generic drug that is bioequivalent will be dispensed. Therefore, the pharmacy technician must be aware of the correct substitutions and situations when generic drugs can be legally substituted for brand name drugs and when they cannot. Unless otherwise noted, you will find the brand name drug listed as a proper name with the first letter capitalized, and the generic drug/ingredient will not be capitalized. Sometimes, however, a generic drug will be mentioned with the brand name in parentheses. There are also generic drug brands.

Technicians also need to know each drug's **primary indications**, or the common intended uses to treat specific diseases, and each drug's **contraindications**—the specific situations *in which the drug should not be used* because it will be harmful to a patient.

For every intended drug action, there are related unintended reactions, or **side effects**, that must *always* be considered. They can be mild or severe, such as varying intensities of nausea, constipation, diarrhea, itchiness and other skin reactions, drowsiness, pain, muscle aches, headaches, shakiness, and numbness.

Drug interactions occur when a drug affects the intended indication of another medication or reacts poorly with it. Interactions can happen between a prescribed drug and another prescribed or nonprescribed drug, food, or multiple drugs. Drugs in combination can cause many difficulties as they react together, and their side effects build up.

Even vitamins, nutrients, or herbal supplements can interfere with or enhance a drug's potency or cause intense reactions; so *the vitamins and supplements a patient is taking must be added to the patient profile and also considered.* Finally, a drug to address one disease might make another disease or condition the patient is experiencing worse.

Adverse drug reactions (ADRs) are injuries or severe harmful responses due to a single dose or an extended use of a drug. ADRs can arise from side effects, contraindications, allergic reactions, and wrong use, or they may result from combining a drug with one or more other medications, vitamins, or herbal supplements. These events can range in severity from an extremely unpleasant experience of shaking, vomiting, hives, and other occurrences to paralysis, blindness, and death. That is why technicians must look so carefully at the patient profiles of medications, allergies, history of use, and software alerts. The technician serves as the first line of inquiry and defense against prescription errors, while the pharmacist counsels and makes the final decisions.

Web

The Institute for Safe Medication Practices (ISMP) has created lists of high-alert medications for community and ambulatory healthcare settings, long-term care settings, and acute care settings. These can be found at the ISMP website at http://CertExam4e.ParadgimEducation.com/ISMP. There are also lists designed to address medication concerns for vulnerable populations, such as the elderly (Beers Criteria) and pregnant women. A study supplement on these lists for vulnerable populations and other drug lists can be accessed through eBook links.

Anatomical Classification of Drugs

To study and remember common generic and brand name drugs, it is often easiest to consider them according to their classification by anatomical system or organ and by their pharmaceutical action. For example, metoprolol succinate (Toprol XL) and lisinopril (Prinivil, Zestril) are found in the cardiovascular (heart-blood system) category, and both are used to treat high blood pressure, but each lowers the blood pressure in a different way. The generic names of certain classes of drugs for specific indications often share the same suffix at the end of their generic names. (Notice the *-pril* at the end of lisino*pril* and related drugs enala*pril* and rami*pril*.)

Each generic drug name is also known as its **US Adopted Name (USNA)**. The identifier is chosen by the USNA Council to be simple, informative, and unique. The USNA generic names cannot be owned or branded by any company.

As you memorize the generic drug names, it will be easier if you can learn them in their families, as can be seen in Table 1.1. A great resource list of generic drug name prefixes and suffixes can be found at the end of the chapter.

TABLE 1.1   Sample of Common Generic Name Suffixes with Drug Class/Category

Suffix	Generic Examples	Class/Category
-sone	dexamethasone, methylprednisolone, prednisone	Corticosteroid, anti-inflammatory
-cillin	amoxicillin, ampicillin, nafcillin	Penicillin-derivative antibiotics
-dipine	amlodipine, nicardipine, nifedipine	Calcium channel blockers, cardiovascular

Drug Facts and Comparisons® (F&C) is a primary reference for substituting generic for brand name drugs organized by bodily systems and indications. It provides factual, up-to-date information on drug product availability, indications, administration and doses, pharmacological actions, contraindications, warnings, precautions, adverse reactions, overdoses, and patient instructions. *F&C* is available as a hard-bound copy and as an online subscription for eAnswers.

Following the lead of the *F&C*, here are some of the categories this chapter will explore that make studying and memorizing easier:

Central Nervous System (CNS) Agents
- Analgesic and Anti-Inflammatory Agents
    - Antianxiety and Hypnotic Agents
    - Antidepressant and Antipsychotic Agents
    - Miscellaneous CNS Agents

Cardiovascular Agents
- Antihypertensive Agents
- Antihyperlipidemic Agents
- Miscellaneous Cardiovascular Agents

Systematic Anti-infective Agents
Endocrine and Metabolic Agents
- Estrogens and Birth Control Agents
- Antidiabetic Agents
- Miscellaneous Endocrine Agents

Respiratory Agents
Gastrointestinal Agents
Renal and Genitourinary Agents
Hematological Agents
Biotechnology and Miscellaneous Drugs
Over-the-Counter and Homeopathic Drugs
Dietary Supplements

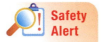

Safety Alert

Make sure to read all black box warnings as you get to know the drugs you will be working with.

For the hospital setting, the American Hospital Formulary Service (AHFS) serves as a primary reference for drug information. Although there is some overlap with community pharmacies in terms of drugs dispensed, drugs used in hospital settings include injectable antibiotic and biotechnology drugs.

Black box warnings—which show up in pharmacy reference materials, patient education materials, directions from the manufacturer, FDA, and drug reference collections—highlight dangerous side effects, interactions, and use.

Central Nervous System Agents

3-D

The central nervous system (CNS) consists of specialized nerve cells called neurons, which are located in the brain and spinal cord. Neurons within the CNS communicate with other neurons primarily through chemicals known as neurotransmitters, such as serotonin, norepinephrine, dopamine, acetylcholine, and histamine to name a few. Prescribed drugs often alter the neurotransmitter activity at the neuron level to produce medicinal effects, which also produce side effects that must be considered. (See a 3-D diagram of the CNS at http://CertExam4e.ParadgimEducation.com/3D-01.)

Analgesic and Anti-Inflammatory Agents

Analgesic medications are used to relieve or reduce pain, whereas anti-inflammatory drugs work to reduce swelling (see Table 1.2). Many analgesic drugs are narcotics, which can substantially affect mood and behavior. Narcotics have significant contraindications and restrictions since they can cause insensibility or stupor.

All narcotics are listed by the DEA as controlled substances because of their addictive characteristics—they can cause greater tolerance (a need for higher doses for the same effects), physical and psychological dependence, and addiction. Because of this, controlled substances are differentiated by their addictive qualities into the DEA Schedules with different legal requirements for security and documentation, and technicians need to know commonly prescribed drugs on these schedules (see Appendix B).

Analgesic Medications

Common analgesics are the **opiates**, which are drugs from the opium poppy plant, including heroin (illegal), morphine, and codeine (note the suffix *-ine*).

TABLE 1.2   Common Analgesic and Anti-inflammatory CNS Agents

Generic Name	Brand Name	Classification
Pain Relief		
acetaminophen	Tylenol, Panadol, Anacin, and more	Non narcotic analgesic
buprenorphine/naloxone	Suboxone, Subutex (no naloxone)	Narcotic analgesic/antagonist
codeine	various trade names	Narcotic analgesic
fentanyl	Duragesic, Actiq	Narcotic analgesic
hydrocodone/APAP*	Lortab, Norco, Vicodin	Narcotic analgesic
hydromorphone	Dilaudid	Narcotic analgesic
lidocaine	Lidoderm	Anesthetic analgesic
methadone	Dolophine	Narcotic analgesic
morphine	MS Contin, MSIR	Narcotic analgesic
oxycodone	OxyContin, Roxicodone	Narcotic analgesic
oxycodone/APAP	Percocet, Endocet	Narcotic analgesic
tramadol/APAP	Ultracet, Ultram (no APAP)	Central analgesic
Anti-Inflammatory		
celecoxib	Celebrex	COX-2 inhibitor
ibuprofen	Motrin, Advil	NSAID*
meloxicam	Mobic	NSAID
naproxen	Naprosyn, Aleve	NSAID

*NSAID (nonsteroidal anti-inflammatory drug) and APAP (acetyl-para-aminophenol) are explained in the next section.

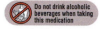

Opioids are synthetically made narcotics that offer opium-like effects of reduced perception and reaction to pain, and increased pain tolerance. Opioids often include opium substances but are chemically designed to have varied or extended opium-like effects. Medications that fall into this category are the ones that will be described: hydrocodone, oxycodone, and other related drugs (note the suffix *-one*). These are Schedule II drugs with no refills permitted. Opioids should not be taken with central nervous system depressants (which will be covered later) or alcohol.

Prescription drug abuse is the number one drug problem in the United States, and hydrocodone combination abused drugs (Lortab, Norco, and Vicodin) are far and away the most often prescribed drugs. Hydrocodone is the generic ingredient name for a powerful opioid narcotic pain reliever. Oxycodone (OxyContin, Roxicodone) also offers strong, narcotic pain relief. Many hydrocodone, oxycodone, and codeine preparations contain acetaminophen, which increases their analgesic effects.

No refills are permitted for Schedule II narcotics, such as oxycodone or morphine. Methadone (Dolophine) is another opioid used for pain, but it is also used to detoxify those with opioid dependence. Suboxone is a combination brand name drug (buprenorphine and naloxone) that is primarily used to treat narcotic addiction.

Safety Alert

Oxycodone is available as both an immediate-release generic drug and a long-acting brand name drug (OxyContin). Beware these differences to avoid medication errors.

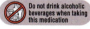

In the hospital setting, injections of morphine, meperidine (Demerol), and hydromorphone (Dilaudid) are commonly used for temporary relief of severe pain. The latter are also Schedule II drugs. For terminally ill hospice or cancer patients, around-the-clock narcotics, administered via infusion pumps, liquids, or controlled-release solid dosage forms or patches are commonly and appropriately used to provide comfort and pain relief.

Narcotic analgesics can cause stomach upset and constipation. So it is recommended that these medications be taken with food, and if constipation occurs, which it often does, a stool softener or short-term laxative is typically recommended.

Narcotic analgesics are generally considered CNS depressants, and they can cause drowsiness. It is best to avoid using them with other CNS depressants, such as psychiatric medications, over-the-counter (OTC) sleeping medications, or alcohol. **Adjuvant medications** are helper medications. They are not strictly used for pain, but they help in pain management and may be prescribed along with a pain reliever. Some common adjuvants are antidepressant and antiseizure medications, muscle relaxants, sedatives, and sleep-enhancing drugs.

TAKE NOTE

Prescription drug abuse in a national epidemic, and technicians are on the front lines of the struggle to save lives. Such drug abuse is considered to have contributed to the deaths of celebrities Prince, Michael Jackson, Corey Haim, Heath Ledger, Anna Nicole Smith, and Whitney Houston. But one must also remember the thousands who are not famous who die each year from similar addictions and abuses of prescription medications.

A 2015 Boston Medical Center study showed that over 90% of patients who nearly died of opioid overdose *received a refill or new opioid prescription immediately afterwards.* Part of the problem is that there has been no system to alert the physicians of the overdose.

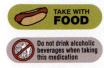

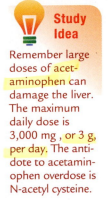

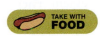

Nonnarcotic analgesics, often found in OTC medications, are used for milder pain conditions, such as in **acetyl-para-aminophenol (APAP)**, also known as acetaminophen (Tylenol). It is a nonnarcotic analgesic found in many prescription and OTC products. It is used for children and adults as a fever reducer and pain reliever (for headache and arthritis) that will not upset the stomach. Acetaminophen is considered generally safe to use during pregnancy. However, large total daily doses (such as more than three grams per day—five to six extra-strength tablets per 24 hours) for the average person *can damage the liver*, especially if combined with alcohol. When APAP is therapeutically combined with a narcotic, the therapy often offers better relief for pain than either drug alone and allows for lower dosing of the narcotic.

Additional nonnarcotic pain relief medications include lidocaine (Xylocaine) and tramadol (Ultram). Lidocaine is a localized pain reliever that can numb an area and can come as a patch (Lidoderm) that is worn for 12 hours and then removed for 12 hours. It is a prescription drug but not a controlled substance. Tramadol is a narcotic-like substance that is frequently prescribed as around-the-clock pain medication. It was reclassified as a Schedule IV drug in 2014 by the DEA. It should not be taken with alcohol, narcotics, or sedatives, or if these have been used in the last few hours. Use of non-narcotic pain relief medications may reduce the required dose or frequency of the more potent and addicting narcotic medications.

Anti-Inflammatory Medications

Some of the most common CNS agents are **nonsteroidal anti-inflammatory drugs (NSAIDs)** as shown in Table 1.2. They include ibuprofen and naproxen. *If a patient is allergic to aspirin, NSAIDs cannot be dispensed*. NSAIDs come in a variety of common prescription and OTC forms. NSAIDs are used to treat not only short-term pain and headaches but also chronic conditions, such as rheumatoid arthritis, migraines, and backaches. In conditions where swelling and pain are linked, many of the NSAID medications, such as ibuprofen (Motrin), handle both.

These anti-inflammatory agents are nonnarcotics but can cause serious gastrointestinal (GI) bleeding if taken in large doses for an extended period of time, especially in older individuals. It is recommended that NSAIDs always be taken with food, milk, or a snack. Be aware that NSAIDS may increase the blood-thinning effects of aspirin when taken at the same time. Celecoxib (Celebrex) is less likely to cause the GI side effects and bleeding, but it is much more costly. If a patient is allergic to sulfa drugs (drugs containing sulfur derivatives), Celebrex is contraindicated.

A number of anti-inflammatory drugs are **steroids**, or complex synthetic substances that can resemble human hormones. **Corticosteroids**, such as cortisone and prednisone, resemble the hormone cortisol. Short-term use of steroids can be effective, but they can be detrimental if used long-term. These anti-inflammatory agents are described in the section on the endocrine system.

Antianxiety and Hypnotic Central Nervous System Agents

Antianxiety and hypnotic drugs are **psychoactive drugs**, medications that modify brain functions to influence mood, perception, and consciousness. Individuals often experience greater anxiety and depression when they cannot sleep. **Hypnotic** drugs are those that induce sleep. The commonly dispensed antianxiety and sleep medications listed in Table 1.3 are also CNS depressants, so they have the same limitations

TABLE 1.3 Common Antianxiety and Hypnotic Central Nervous System Agents

Generic Name	Brand Name	Classification
Antianxiety		
alprazolam	Xanax	Benzodiazepine
clonazepam	Klonopin	Benzodiazepine
chlordiazepoxide	Librium	Benzodiazepine
diazepam	Valium	Benzodiazepine
lorazepam	Ativan	Benzodiazepine
Hypnotic (anti-insomnia)		
eszopiclone	Lunesta	Non-benzodiazepine
temazepam	Restoril	Benzodiazepine
zolpidem	Ambien	Non-benzodiazepine

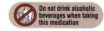
Do not drink alcoholic beverages when taking this medication

as the narcotic analgesics, such as not mixing them with psychiatric medications, OTC sleeping medications, or alcohol.

The psychoactive drugs in the **benzodiazepine (BZD)** family (the "**benzos**") are used to treat anxiety, panic attacks, seizures, and insomnia. (Notice the common suffix *-pam* or *-lam* in the generic drugs in Table 1.3.) They include diazepam, known as Valium, the old-fashioned solution for soothing nerves. (Diastat is a rectal dosage form of diazepam used for emergency treatment of seizures.) Like the opioids, the benzo drugs are also an enormous part of the prescription drug abuse problem. They generate some degree of physical or psychological dependence if used long-term. Benzos are all Schedule IV drugs. Drugs in the benzo family and other CNS depressants should not be taken with opioids. This combination can lead to unresponsiveness, extreme dizziness, and slowed and difficult breathing.

The non-benzodiazepine sedatives zolpidem (Ambien) and eszopiclone (Lunesta) are used for insomnia and have interactions similar to the benzos. Because of their dependence profile, the listed non-benzo hypnotics have been classified at the Schedule IV level. Refills of C-IV drugs must occur within six months of the original prescription date—limited to five refills. Prescriptions must be monitored for early refills and abuse. Most of these medications are recommended for short-term or "as needed" (or nightly) use. In practice, though, many are used on a long-term, routine basis for anxiety or insomnia. The FDA has recommended dosage reductions in women and older individuals for zolpidem (Ambien) and eszopiclone (Lunesta) because of next-day drug hangovers that adversely impact safe driving.

Study Idea

Notice that names of drugs in the benzo family generally end in *-lam* or *-pam*.

Antidepressant and Antipsychotic Central Nervous System Agents

Antidepressant and antipsychotic drugs (as listed in Tables 1.4 and 1.5) generally act directly on the neurotransmitters, such as serotonin, norepinephrine, and dopamine, to achieve a therapeutic effect.

These drugs can work for a period of time and then lose their effectiveness as the body develops a tolerance. Also, some of these drugs can **bioaccumulate**, or collect in the fat cells of the body, resulting in the development of side effects after taking a drug for some time. Patient education and compliance are important while taking antipyschotics and antidepressants; a patient may experience **withdrawal symptoms**—that include anxiety, sweating, nausea, and shaking—if the drug is stopped abruptly. These drugs should always be tapered off.

Antidepressants

Among the most common CNS agents currently used in the United States, 12 are used to treat depression. As shown in Table 1.4, these drugs work through different mechanisms (listed by classification), and the specific type and dose must be tailored to each patient to achieve the correct therapeutic response. *Antidepressants carry black box warnings because of the increased risk of suicidal thoughts and behavior in children, adolescents, and young adults.*

Several analgesic and muscle relaxing prescription (and some OTC) drugs, such as tramadol (Ultram) and cyclobenzaprine (Flexeril), can cause unsafe levels of serotonin when used with certain antidepressants, such as fluoxetine (Prozac), sertraline (Zoloft), and paroxetine (Paxil), causing confusion and agitation, among other symptoms. They should not be taken together. Alcohol should not be used with these drugs either.

Some antidepressants block the reabsorption of serotonin so that more of the secreted serotonin circulates for positive effects. Several antidepressants, including

TABLE 1.4 Antidepressant Agents

Generic Name	Brand Name	Classification
amitriptyline	Elavil	Tricyclic
citalopram	Celexa	SSRI*
doxepin	Sinequan	Tricyclic
duloxetine	Cymbalta	NE/5HT* reuptake inhibitors
escitalopram	Lexapro	SSRI
fluoxetine	Prozac	SSRI
imipramine	Tofranil	Tricyclic
mirtazapine	Remeron	Serotonin receptor antagonist
nortriptyline	Pamelor	Tricyclic
paroxetine	Paxil, Paxil CR	SSRI
phenelzine	Nardil	MAOI*
sertraline	Zoloft	SSRI
tranylcypromine	Parnate	MAOI
trazodone	Desyrel	Serotonin receptor antagonist
venlafaxine	Effexor, Effexor XR	NE/5HT reuptake inhibitors
vortioxetine	Trintellix	Multi-serotonin agonist/antagonist

*Note: SSRI = (selective serotonin receptor inhibitor), NE = (norepinephrine), 5HT = (serotonin), MAOI = (monoamine oxidase inhibitor)

Prozac, generically known as fluoxetine, work in this way. These drugs are known as **selective serotonin reuptake inhibitors (SSRIs)**. Drugs like fluoxetine, venlafaxine (Effexor), and duloxetine (Cymbalta) may cause insomnia if given at bedtime. Venlafaxine and duloxetine should be used cautiously in patients with high blood pressure as they can raise blood pressure levels.

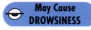

The generic amitriptyline (Elavil), a **tricyclic antidepressant (TCA)**, is an older antidepressant drug that offers a mild tranquilizing, soothing action. It is still used for depression, to enhance the effect of pain medications, and to prevent migraine headaches. This drug commonly causes drowsiness and is sometimes prescribed as a sleep medication for insomnia. Amitriptyline can cause a dry "cotton" mouth and blurry vision.

Trazodone has a different mechanism from some of the other drugs but is also used as an antidepressant. The side effects of trazadone are similar to other antidepressants, including dry mouth, vision changes, and drug "hangover." Because it can cause drowsiness, it is sometimes prescribed for insomnia. Patients taking trazodone should avoid sun exposure, and males should be warned about the risk of priapism, or a prolonged painful erection. Also, trazodone can cause cramps in ankles and feet and some loss of small motor function after prolonged use in some patients.

Antipsychotics

Antipsychotic drugs are the medications used to manage disordered thought and personality behaviors, and common ones are listed on Table 1.5.

The first antipsychotic drugs developed, including chlorpromazine (Thorazine) and thioridazine (Mellaril), were used to treat schizophrenia. The drugs are rarely prescribed today because of the higher incidence of side effects, such as blurred vision, dry mouth and related dental problems, and dementia-like symptoms. Other drugs and formulations have encountered success with fewer difficult side effects due to the blockage of certain brain functions.

TABLE 1.5 Antipsychotic Central Nervous System Agents

Generic Name	Brand Name	Classification
aripiprazole	Abilfy	Atypical
brexpiprazole	Rexulti	Atypical
chlorpromazine	Thorazine	1st generation
fluphenazine	Prolixin	1st generation
haloperidol	Haldol	1st generation
lurasidone	Latuda	Atypical
olanzapine	Zyprexa	Atypical
quetiapine	Seroquel, Seroquel XR	Atypical
risperidone	Risperdal	Atypical
thiothixene	Navane	1st generation
trifluoperazine	Stelazine	1st generation
ziprasidone	Geodon	Atypical

Aripiprazole (Abilify), olanzapine (Zyprexa), quetiapine (Seroquel), and risperidone (Risperdal) are considered atypical antipsychotic drugs because they target specific neurotransmitters. These drugs are often used to enhance the antidepressant effects of traditional antidepressants. In addition to modulating the mood swings of bipolar depression (excessively low mood, energy, and activity) and mania (excessively high mood, energy, and activity), these drugs are used in adults to treat schizophrenia (mental and emotional fragmentation and faulty reality perception) and severe agitation.

Atypical antipsychotic drugs may cause or aggravate metabolic syndrome, characterized by obesity, hypertension, Type II diabetes, and hyperlipidemia. These agents should be used cautiously in elderly patients due to potential cardiovascular adverse reactions. If the patient experiences any rigidity, tremor, or involuntary muscle twitching, the physician should be notified immediately. Alcohol should not be used while taking these drugs.

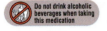

Miscellaneous Central Nervous System Agents

Additional drugs that help regulate or stimulate the CNS are listed in Table 1.6. They include many ways to soothe or heal overactive or misfiring neurons and other nervous system disorders.

TABLE 1.6   Miscellaneous Central Nervous System Agents

Generic Name	Brand Name	Classification	Indication
amphetamine salts	Adderall	CNS stimulant	ADHD
carisoprodol	Soma	Skeletal muscle relaxant	Muscle spasms
cyclobenzaprine	Flexeril	Skeletal muscle relaxant	Muscle spasms
lamotrigine	Lamictal, Lamictal XR	Anticonvulsant, mood stabilizer	Seizures, bipolar disorder
gabapentin	Neurontin	Anticonvulsant, analgesic	Pain, seizures
divalproex sodium	Depakote, Depakote ER	Anticonvulsant, mood stabilizer	Seizures, bipolar disorder
lisdexamfetamine	Vyvanse	CNS stimulant	ADHD
memantine	Namenda	Brain receptor antagonist NMDA receptor antagonist	Alzheimer's disease
methylphenidate	Concerta, Ritalin	CNS stimulant	ADHD
metoclopramide	Reglan	Prokinetic agent	Nausea, heartburn, gastroparesis
ondansetron	Zofran	Serotonin receptor antagonist	Nausea, vomiting
pregabalin	Lyrica	Anticonvulsant, analgesic	Pain, seizures
promethazine	Phenergan	Antidopaminergic	Nausea
ropinirole	Requip	Dopamine receptor agonist	Restless legs
sumatriptan	Imitrex	Serotonin receptor agonist	Migraine headache
tizanidine	Zanaflex	Skeletal muscle relaxant	Muscle spasms
topiramate	Topamax	Anticonvulsant	Migraine headache, weight loss, epilepsy

The diagnosis of attention deficit hyperactivity disorder (ADHD) is on the rise in pediatric patients. It manifests itself in difficulty focusing or concentration, overactivity, and difficulty in impulse control. The usually prescribed drugs, such as methylphenidate and amphetamines, stimulate rather than depress the CNS, and this actually helps support the brain in focusing attention and behavior. Common side effects are insomnia and loss of appetite. These drugs should be taken in the morning or early afternoon.

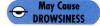

Methylphenidate is available as both an immediate-acting drug (Ritalin) and as a longer-acting drug (Concerta). Adderall and Adderall XR (short- and long-acting formulations) are combinations of amphetamine salts (amphetamine and dextroamphetamine). Lisdexamfetamine (Vyvanse) is also prescribed for ADHD. Amphetamines, or "uppers" as they have been called, are very dangerous for their addictive qualities. The DEA places them in the Schedule II category—no refills are authorized without a new prescription.

Abuse of these drugs is a real problem. New uses for older drugs include the use of guanfacine (Tenex and Intuniv) and clonidine (Kapvay and Catapres) for ADHD in children to augment or even replace traditional stimulants. These agents originally were used to treat hypertension.

To slow the progression of moderate to severe Alzheimer's disease, other CNS agents, such as memantine (Namenda) and donepezil (Aricept), are used. Memantine is sometimes used in combination with donepezil, but drowsiness is a common side effect. Donepezil is metabolized in the liver, so it is susceptible to drug interactions. The main side effects are gastrointestinal, such as diarrhea, nausea, and vomiting.

Epilepsy is a disease where a patient suffers from seizures, which are spasms with an overfiring of the neurons of the brain and nervous system. Patients are given anticonvulsant (antiseizure) medications that try to calm the nervous system by inhibiting the overly rapid and excessive firing of neurons. The most common drugs for treating epilepsy are phenytoin (Dilantin), divalproex sodium (Depakote), and lamotrigine (Lamictal). (See Table 1.6).

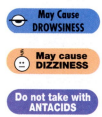

Gabapentin (Neurontin) and pregabalin (Lyrica) were initially used to control seizures. Today, though, these drugs are primarily used to reduce nerve pain associated with diabetes, chronic pain, shingles, and spinal cord injuries. Pregabalin is sometimes prescribed for fibromyalgia, or severe chronic muscle fatigue. (It is a C-V controlled substance.) The most common side effects of these anticonvulsant drugs are drowsiness, dizziness, and swelling of the ankles. OTC antacids, such as Mylanta or Maalox, interfere with the absorption of these drugs, particularly of gabapentin and pregabalin. It is recommended that pregabalin be administered at least one hour before or two hours after the patient takes antacids.

Muscle relaxants, which reduce muscle strain and pain, include carisoprodol (Soma), cyclobenzaprine (Flexeril), and tizanidine (Zanaflex). These drugs are commonly prescribed with narcotic analgesics and antianxiety drugs. They are indicated for short-term treatment of muscle spasms; however, they are often used long-term. The combination of muscle relaxants and narcotic analgesic increase the risk of sedation and respiratory depression in patients to long term use must be monitored.

Sumatriptan (Imitrex), which is a serotonin receptor agonist, is used to treat occasional migraine headaches. It is available in various dosage formulations and must be used with caution in patients with heart disease and women of childbearing potential. There are many serotonin receptor agonists in this class used to treat migraines, and all have the suffix *-triptan*.

Study Idea

There are many drugs in the serotonin agonist class to treat migraines, and all have the suffix *-triptan*.

Metoclopramide (Reglan) is used to treat heartburn and slow stomach emptying in diabetics as well as severe nausea and vomiting resulting from chemotherapy. It is commonly given 30 minutes prior to each meal and at bedtime; it can cause some severe abnormal muscle movement with long-term use. Ondansetron (Zofran), which is also used for chemo-induced nausea, is available as an oral disintegrating tablet (ODT), a syrup, and an injection for pediatric patients or those too sick to swallow tablets. Promethazine (Phenergan), a dopamine antagonist, is commonly used in tablet, liquid, injection, or suppository forms for the treatment of nausea and vomiting from a viral illness or migraine headache.

Ropinirole (Requip) is commonly prescribed at bedtime to treat "restless legs syndrome" (involuntary twitching of the legs). Common side effects with all these miscellaneous CNS drugs are drowsiness and dizziness; as with most CNS drugs, alcohol must be avoided.

Cardiovascular Agents

3-D

Heart disease is a major health threat in the United States and includes conditions like hypertension. The complications of untreated or undertreated high blood pressure include kidney failure, stroke, and heart attack. The risk of heart disease may be partly genetic, but hypertension is often the result of lifestyle choices as well, such as smoking, unhealthy food choices, being overweight, and lack of exercise. Elevated cholesterol is an important risk factor for hypertension and general heart disease. For a 3-D diagram of the cardiovascular system, go to http://CertExam4e. ParadgimEducation.com/3D-02.

Antihypertensive Agents

There are many **antihypertensive agents** (see Table 1.7) that work to lower blood pressure by dilating blood vessels, slowing heart rate, and increasing the elimination of salt and fluid from the body. Often, more than one drug is needed to reach the desired blood pressure range, usually below 140 mm Hg for the systolic reading.

Drugs known as **calcium channel blockers (CCBs)** stop calcium from entering the cells of the heart and blood vessels, making them more flexible and able to relax and widen, lessening blood pressure. The most commonly prescribed CCB is amlodipine (Norvasc), and it can cause headache, fast heart rate, and sometimes ankle swelling.

Beta-adrenergic blockers (beta blockers) are drugs for heart conditions that stop the blood pressure–raising effects of the hormone epinephrine (also known as adrenaline), which makes your heart beat faster. Beta blockers can make the heart beat slower with less force, and they include atenolol, metoprolol, and the newest agent, nebivolol (notice the suffix *-olol*). Some are also used for glaucoma and migraines.

Metoprolol succinate is available in an extended-release dosage form; metoprolol tartrate is in an immediate-release dosage form. These different salts cannot be interchanged. They are generally well tolerated, but a patient must not run out of these medications—if the drug is withdrawn for 48 to 72 hours, blood pressure can rebound to unsafe levels, leading to severe chest pain or even a heart attack. Diabetics who are prone to low blood sugar (hypoglycemia) must use these drugs with caution because the drugs can mask symptoms of low blood sugar.

Diuretics, which reduce water retention, are also prescribed for high blood pressure. They are addressed in the renal (kidney) section to follow.

Study Idea

The names of many ACE inhibitors end in *–pril*, wheras the names wheras the names of many ARBs end in *-sartan*.

Angiotensin-converting enzyme (ACE) inhibitors reduce blood pressure and prevent heart failure by blocking or reducing the liver's production of a hormone that constricts the blood vessels. Their first cousins, **angiotensin receptor blockers (ARBs)**, block the reception and action of the constrictive hormone. So these drugs help keep the vessels more open—for more blood flow and lower blood pressure. These drugs also protect the kidneys from the damage caused by diabetes and hypertension. However, ACE inhibitors and ARBs *can cause the body to retain potassium* and must be used with caution by patients also taking potassium supplements or potassium-sparing diuretics (covered in Table 1.7) and by patients with declining kidney function.

The most common side effect of the ACE inhibitors *is a drug-induced dry cough* caused by the buildup of bradykinin, an irritating chemical, in the lungs. If the cough continues, an ARB is usually prescribed. The most *serious adverse effect of ACE inhibitors is angioedema*, a swelling under the skin that can be a life-threatening allergic reaction manifested by a swelling of the tongue, lips, or eyes. If these symptoms occur, the drug must be discontinued immediately, and the patient should be referred to emergency care.

TABLE 1.7 Common Antihypertensive Cardiovascular Agents

Generic Name	Brand Name	Classification
amlodipine	Norvasc	CCB*
atenolol	Tenormin	Beta-adrenergic blocker
benazepril	Lotensin	ACE inhibitor
chlorthalidone	Hygroton	Diuretic
diltiazem	Cardizem, Dilacor	CCB
enalapril	Vasotec	ACE inhibitor
furosemide	Lasix	Diuretic
hydrochlorothiazide	Hydrodiuril	Diuretic
lisinopril	Prinivil, Zestril	ACE inhibitor
losartan	Cozaar	ARB*
metoprolol	Lopressor, Toprol XL	Beta-adrenergic blocker
nebivolol	Bystolic	Beta-adrenergic blocker
nifedipine	Procardia, Adalat	CCB
olmesartan	Benicar	ARB
propranolol	Inderal, Inderal LA	Beta-adrenergic blocker
ramipril	Altace	ACE inhibitor
torsemide	Demadex	Diuretic
verapamil	Calan, Isoptin	CCB

*Note: CCB=(Calcium channel blocker) and ARB=(Angiotensin receptor blocker). Diuretics are discussed in the renal section.

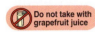
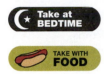
Antihyperlipidemic (Cholesterol-Lowering) Agents

Antihyperlipidemic drugs are cardiovascular drugs that fight the buildup of **lipids** by lowering the patient's level of dangerous **cholesterol** (fatty acids) and **triglycerides** (three fatty acids combined with glycerol). Cholesterol consists of two main types of fatty acids: **LDL (low-density lipoprotein)**—bad cholesterol—and **HDL (high-density lipoprotein)**—good cholesterol.

Antihyperlipidemic agents, commonly referred to as **statins** (see Table 1.8), prevent the production of "bad cholesterol." Statins are called **HMG-CoA reductase inhibitors**. They can lower LDL cholesterol up to 50% or more. Statins should not be taken with grapefruit juice as this may decrease metabolism of the drug and increase the risk of side effects. Muscle fatigue is a common side effect, especially when these drugs are combined with other agents, such as gemfibrozil, verapamil, diltiazem, macrolide antibiotics, and amiodarone.

Nicotinic acid (Niaspan) is a B_3 vitamin with a broad spectrum of activity. In large doses, it lowers the amounts of LDL and triglycerides in the body. It also improves HDL, the "good cholesterol." Nicotinic acid is available as a prescription and OTC drug, but patients should be made aware that liver function should be tested periodically in patients using this drug. The dose must be slowly increased over several weeks to avoid flushing (warmth, redness, itching, tingling of skin) and headaches. Flushing can be prevented by pre-dosing with aspirin 30 minutes prior to taking nicotinic acid. The dose is usually taken at bedtime with a snack.

Fenofibrate (TriCor) lowers triglycerides rather than cholesterol and is usually well tolerated. However, it must be used with caution with statins, warfarin, and other blood thinners.

Omega-3 fatty acids are effective in lowering the triglycerides. Salmon is high in omega-3 fatty acids and can help naturally lower triglycerides. Natural fish oil, or a fish oil supplement, is effective in lowering triglycerides. For patients who are allergic or intolerant to seafood, Lovaza is a "prescription only" omega-3 fatty acid.

TABLE 1.8 Common Antihyperlipidemic Cardiovascular Agents

Generic Name	Brand Name	Classification
Cholesterol- and Triglyceride-Reducing		
atorvastatin	Lipitor	Statin
ezetimibe	Zetia	Blocks cholesterol absorption
fenofibrate	TriCor	Decreases triglycerides
lovastatin	Mevacor	Statin
niacin	Niaspan	Decreases triglycerides
omega-3 fatty acid	Lovaza	Decreases triglycerides
pravastatin	Pravachol	Statin
rosuvastatin	Crestor	Statin
simvastatin	Zocor	Statin
simvastatin-ezetimibe	Vytorin	Statin/blocks cholesterol absorption

Miscellaneous Cardiovascular Agents

In addition to drugs to fight high blood pressure and cholesterol, other cardiovascular agents (see Table 1.9) are used to treat arrhythmia (abnormal heartbeat), heart failure, and angina pectoris (severe chest pain). The agents for heart failure all work differently and are sometimes used in combination with each other or with the ACE inhibitors or ARBs discussed previously. Carvedilol (Coreg) is commonly used as a primary drug in the treatment of heart failure. It is also available as a controlled release dosage formulation (Coreg CR). Nonspecific beta blockers *must be used with caution in patients with asthma and chronic obstructive pulmonary disease (COPD)*. All beta blockers should be used with caution *with other drugs that lower heart rate.*

TABLE 1.9 Common Miscellaneous Cardiovascular Agents

Generic Name	Brand Name	Classification	Indication
carvedilol	Coreg	Alpha/beta blocker	Heart failure
digoxin	Lanoxin	Inotropic agent	Heart failure
isosorbide	Imdur, Ismo, Isordil	Vasodilator	Angina pectoris, heart failure
nitroglycerin	Nitrostat, Nitrolingual	Vasodilator	Angina pectoris

Study Idea

Nitroglycerin is available as a sublingual tablet, sublingual/oral spray, oral time-released capsule, topical ointment, and intravenous infusion.

Digoxin (Lanoxin) is an older drug that helps a weak heart beat stronger. While in use, the patient's serum blood levels should be monitored to prevent toxic levels and side effects, including abnormal heart rhythms (arrhythmias). The drug can slow down the heart rate and cause nausea and vomiting when toxic levels are reached, especially if blood potassium levels are low.

Isosorbide (Imdur, Ismo, Isordil) belongs to the nitrate family. The **nitrates** all work similarly—they dilate the blood vessels, particularly those of the heart, to increase oxygen and blood flow, to relieve chest pain, and/or reduce the workload on the heart. Nitrates *can all cause headaches and a dangerous drop in blood pressure when combined with erectile dysfunction drugs*, including the well-known brands of Viagra, Levitra, and Cialis. Nitroglycerin is the most commonly known drug of this group.

Nitroglycerin is often taken at the first sign of chest pain, with repeated doses every five minutes for three doses. If chest pain continues, the patient is advised to take a crushed aspirin tablet and get to the emergency room as quickly as possible. Nitroglycerin sublingual (under the tongue) tablets are sensitive to air and light and should be replaced every three to six months. (*Because of the need for its use in emergencies, nitroglycerin should never be dispensed in a child-resistant container.*)

Systemic Anti-Infective Agents

3-D

Anti-infective agents include antibiotics, sulfa drugs, antifungals, and antivirals (see Table 1.10). For a 3-D view of the lymphatic-immune system, go to http://CertExam4e.ParadgimEducation.com/3D-03.

TABLE 1.10   Common Anti-Infective Agents

Generic Name	Brand Name	Classification
Infection		
amoxicillin	Amoxil	Aminopenicillin
amoxicillin-clavulanate	Augmentin	Aminopenicillin
ampicillin-sulbactam	Unasyn	Aminopenicillin
azithromycin	Zithromax (Z-Pak)	Macrolide
cefazolin	Ancef	Cephalosporin
ceftazidime	Fortaz, Tazicef	Cephalosporin
ceftriaxone	Rocephin	Cephalosporin
cephalexin	Keflex	Cephalosporin
ciprofloxacin	Cipro	Fluoroquinolone
clindamycin	Cleocin	Lincosamide
ertapenem	Invanz	Carbapenem
doxycycline	Doryx, Vibramycin	Tetracycline
gentamicin	generic only	Aminoglycoside
levofloxacin	Levaquin	Fluoroquinolone
meropenem	Merrem	Carbapenem
metronidazole	Flagyl	Antiprotozoan
nafcillin	generic only	Penicillinase-resistant penicillin
penicillin	Veetids	Natural penicillin
sulfamethoxazole/trimethoprim	Bactrim, Septra	Sulfonamide
vancomycin	Vancocin	Glycopeptide
Fungal Infection		
amphoteracin B	Ambisome	Polyene
fluconazole	Diflucan	Antifungal
Viral Infection		
abacavir	Ziagen	Anti-HIV—nucleoside reverse transcriptase inhibitor
acyclovir	Zovirax	General antiviral
atazanavir	Reyataz	Anti-HIV—protease inhibitor
darunavir	Prezista	Anti-HIV—rotease inhibitor
efavirenz	Sustiva	Anti-HIV—non-nucleoside reverse transcriptase inhibitor
emtricitabine/tenofovir	Truvada	HIV nucleoside analog reverse transcriptase inhibitor
oseltamivir	Tamiflu	Influenza
ritonavir	Norvir	Anti-HIV—rotease inhibitor
tenofovir	Viread	Anti-HIV—nucleoside reverse transcriptase inhibitor
valacyclovir	Valtrex	General antiviral

When a patient does not complete an anti-infective therapy to kill all of the microorganisms, those that survive will reproduce, creating more resistant bacteria by natural selection, decreasing the effectiveness of the antibiotic. Consequently, stronger doses of the antibiotic or additional drugs need to be prescribed, which, in turn, creates a higher risk of side effects. Due to drug resistance, the required dose of amoxicillin to treat ear infections in children has doubled in the past 30 years. A more serious example in the hospital environment is the development of methicillin-resistant *Staphylococcus aureus* (MRSA), which can be so unresponsive to antibiotics that it can cause death.

Pharmacy technicians should stress the importance of completing the entire course of antibiotic therapy to reduce the incidence of antibiotic resistance and recurring infections.

Antibiotics and Sulfa Drugs

Since antibiotics kill or weaken bacteria, they *also kill good bacteria and commonly cause side effects, such as diarrhea and yeast infections.* Yogurt or probiotics often offset the diarrhea, but yeast infections may require treatment with OTC or prescription drugs. Also, with many antibiotics and sulfa drugs, *the patient should take precautions in the sun because these agents cause sun sensitivity.* Some kinds of antibiotics *may lower the effectiveness of birth control*, so patients on birth control medications must be made aware of this.

Among the most common anti-infective drugs is penicillin (Veetids, Pen VK) and its derivatives: amoxicillin (Amoxil) and amoxicillin-clavulanate (Augmentin) and, in the hospital, ampicillin-sulbactam (Unasyn). These are commonly used to treat upper respiratory (breathing), sinus, and ear infections in children and adults. Ampicillin-sulbactum (Unasyn) and nafcillin are used in the hospital to treat infections resistant to traditional penicillins. It is important to check for penicillin allergies.

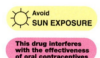

Safety Alert

It is important for the technician to double-check the allergy history in the patient profile prior to dispensing any antibiotic prescription—looking especially for penicillin allergies.

The cephalosporins are antibiotics synthesized to be like penicillin, and they are generally well tolerated. Fewer than 5% of those allergic to penicillin develop a rash with cephalosporins, but the patient (or parent) should be advised of the possibility. However, *if the patient has an anaphylactic reaction (severe allergy) to penicillins, cephalosporins should be avoided too.* Each of the different cephalosporins—such as cefazolin (Ancef), ceftazidime (Fortaz, Tazicef), ceftriaxone (Rocephin), and cephalexin (Keflex)—fights activities against different microorganisms. With the exception of cephalexin, most cephalosporins are administered by the intravenous route. They are frequently used in both the community and hospital settings.

For individuals with penicillin-related allergies, other antibiotics are also commonly used, such as azithromycin (Zithromax Z-Pak). Azithromycin works by stopping bacteria from making their own proteins. It is commonly prescribed in tablet (Z-Pak) or suspension form for the treatment of upper respiratory infections in children and adults. Azithromycin has the advantage of a five-day course of therapy (instead of a two-week or longer regimen), which may improve patient compliance. The drug should be taken with a meal or snack to lessen GI side effects. Unlike some antibiotic suspensions, which should be refrigerated, this one can be kept at room

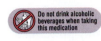

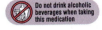

temperature. Azithromycin commonly interacts with other drugs, so the medication profile and use must be particularly assessed by the pharmacist.

Clindamycin is an alternative antibiotic for use in patients who are allergic to penicillin; it can cause severe diarrhea. Clindamycin is commonly prescribed for a dental infection as it has anaerobic coverage, which is common in the oral cavity. If patients develop serious bloody diarrhea, they should contact their physicians immediately, because they may have developed colitis from the antibiotic or a *Clostridium difficile* infection. In the hospital, clindamycin and metronidazole are used to treat or prevent severe anaerobic infections post-surgery. They are also used topically to treat acne in adolescents and adults. Metronidazole is also frequently prescribed for five to seven days to treat vaginal infections. *The use of alcohol with this drug could cause severe nausea.*

The fluoroquinolones are a class of potent antibiotics that include ciprofloxacin (Cipro) and levofloxacin (Levaquin). They *should not be taken with milk, dairy products, or antacids.* In rare but serious cases, these drugs can cause ruptured tendons or severe tendinitis with strenuous exercise, which the MedGuide describes. As with many drugs, they are available as an injection in hospitals for serious infections as well as eye and ear drops. Ciprofloxacin and levofloxacin may interact with diabetes medications for lowering blood sugar, which can cause decreases in blood sugar to dangerous levels.

Doxycycline (Doryx) is an all-purpose antibiotic commonly used to treat various bacterial infections, including acne. It is in the family of tetracycline antibiotics. These *must not* be taken by pregnant or nursing patients, those on birth control, or children younger than 8 years of age. In addition, they must not be taken at the same time as dairy, antacids, iron, or calcium supplements. Patients should particularly avoid sun exposure as they may burn more quickly.

Several antibiotics listed in Table 1.10 are commonly used in the hospital and administered intravenously. Technicians working in a hospital will become familiar with the intravenous antibiotics and how to prepare them as sterile products. Ampicillin-sulbactam (Unasyn) and nafcillin (only generic is available) are used to treat infections resistant to traditional penicillins. Clindamycin is particularly effective to fight post-surgery infections caused by anaerobic bacteria (those that do not require oxygen for growth). It is administered intravenously in hospitals and in other dosage forms in the community pharmacy after dental surgery. It is tolerated by patients allergic to penicillin but can cause ongoing diarrhea. If patients develop bloody diarrhea, they should contact their physician immediately.

Metronidazole is also used intravenously in the hospital after surgery as an agent against protozoa and anaerobic microorganisms. It is frequently prescribed as an oral tablet for five to seven days to treat vaginal infections as well. The use of alcohol with this drug could cause severe nausea, elevated heart rate, vomiting, and warmth/redness under skin, and even death. Again, it must be emphasized, *alcohol of any kind, must be avoided for up to 72 hours after last use.*

Vancomycin (Vancocin) is commonly the drug of choice to treat methicillin-resistant *Staphylococcus aureus* (MRSA)—this is the bacterium responsible for many hard-to-treat infections in the hospital. If the MRSA infection is vancomycin-resistant, meropenem (Merrem) and other antibiotics serve as alternatives. Gentamicin (only generic is available) is an intravenous antibiotic that is frequently used in combination with other antibiotics to treat serious infections. Kidney functions and drug blood levels must be carefully monitored with both vancomycin and gentamicin to adjust dosing. *At toxic levels, these drugs can cause some degree of hearing loss*; care must be taken to ensure accurate dosing levels.

Sulfa Drugs

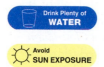

In addition to antibiotics, **sulfa drugs** (sulfur-based medications) also fight bacterial infections (as well as some fungal infections). The most commonly prescribed sulfa drug is a combination of sulfamethoxazole and trimethoprim (Bactrim, Septra), which when combined have mutually beneficial effects on fighting bacteria. This drug is commonly used to treat urinary tract infections (UTIs) and ear infections. Sulfa drugs should be taken with large quantities of water and must be used cautiously with blood thinners and other drugs. Sunscreen precautions should be recommended.

Antifungals and Antivirals

Antifungals fight microorganisms that reproduce with spores. Commonly prescribed drugs to fight them are listed on Table 1.10.

The antifungal drug fluconazole (Diflucan) is commonly prescribed as a one-time or short-term oral treatment for fungal yeast infections. Amphotericin B is an intravenous antifungal used in hospitals to treat systemic fungal infections. It must be infused slowly over six hours.

Practice Tip

HIV medications are usually dispensed in the manufacturer's packaging to protect them from moisture and sunlight.

For viral herpes infections, acyclovir (Zovirax) and valacyclovir (Valtrex) are used topically (Zovirax Ointment), orally, and intravenously. Oseltamivir (Tamiflu) is an antiviral drug used for flu outbreaks in both children and adults in a five-day therapy.

A few commonly prescribed agents for treating HIV, which the technician should be familiar with, are listed in Table 1.10. These are the nucleoside/nucleotide revers transcriptase inhibitors (NRTIs), the non-nucleoside reverse transcriptase inhibitors (NNRTIs), and the protease inhibitors. These drugs make it difficult for the virus to replicate itself. Many HIV treatments come as combinations products with three to four drugs in one tablet. Patients should follow labeled instructions and not miss a dose.

Endocrine and Metabolic Agents

3-D

The **endocrine** system is the network of glands that secrete hormones into the circulatory system to regulate bodily functions, including metabolism, or the processes of producing energy from nutrients. Various endocrine and metabolic agents are frequently prescribed in the community pharmacy. These drugs vary from hormones and birth control medications to drugs that treat bone loss, diabetes, thyroid conditions, inflammatory diseases, and gout (see Table 1.11). For a 3-D diagram of the endrocrine system, go to http://CertExam4e.ParadgimEducation.com/3D-04.

Practice Tip

Patients need to be reminded that antibiotics may interfere with birth control.

Estrogens and Birth Control Agents

In menopausal and postmenopausal patients or those who have had a hysterectomy, reproductive hormone production drops dramatically, producing hot flashes, insomnia, and emotional imbalance. Hormone-replacement therapy with estrogen is often used to reduce the symptoms. The major side effect of estrogens is nausea, and there is a concern about the increase in the risk of stroke and cancer with long-term (over five years) use.

There are many prescription birth control medications available on the market. Most contain reproductive hormone combinations of **estrogen** and a progestin (a synthesized **progesterone**) to simulate pregnancy and thereby prevent ovulation. Users may experience some of the weight gain and mood swings of pregnancy.

TABLE 1.11 Common Hormonal Agents

Generic Name	Brand Name	Classification
Hormone Replacement Therapy		
conjugated estrogen	Premarin	Sex hormone
estradiol	Estrace, Estring, Femring, Vagifem	Sex hormone
medroxyprogesterone	Provera, Depo-Provera	Sex hormone, contraceptive
Birth Control		
ethinyl estradiol-norethindrone	Loestrin 24 Fe	Contraceptive
ethinyl estradiol-norgestimate	TriNessa, Tri-Sprintec	Contraceptive
ethinyl estradiol-drospirenone	Gianvi	Contraceptive
ethinyl estradiol-etonogestrel	NuvaRing	Contraceptive
ethinyl estradiol-norelgestromin	Ortho Evra, Xulane	Contraceptive
levonorgestrel	Plan B	Emergency contraceptive
norethindrone	Ortho Micronor, Nor-QD, Aygestin	Contraceptive, sex hormone

Most birth control therapies include three weeks of active medication and one week of placebo or iron tablets. Newer birth control pills, such as Seasonale and Seasonique, are available in 91-day supply packs that offer the convenience of menses once every three months.

NuvaRing is a once-a-month birth control device (in place for three weeks, out for one week) where hormones are slowly released intravaginally through a self-inserted ring dispenser; this drug should be refrigerated when stored. Ortho Evra is a birth control arm patch that also slowly releases the hormones over seven days. It is about the size of a Band-Aid and is worn on the inside of the upper arm or hip and is changed once a week.

In patients over age 35 who smoke, birth control medications may increase the risk of a stroke. The FDA mandates that manufacturers provide and pharmacists dispense a MedGuide with each birth control prescription. Plan B One-Step, made of the hormone levonorgestrel (Take Action and Next Choice), which contains the progestin levonorgestrel, is an OTC drug marketed for use after sex and may be obtained by women of any age. The treatment is most effective if taken within 72 hours of intercourse.

Safety Alert

If patients mention severe side effects from birth control, such as intense depression or break through bleeding, recommend that they immediately consult the pharmacist and their provider.

Antidiabetic Agents

Diabetes is one of the fastest growing chronic diseases in the world, especially in the United States. Diabetes drugs (see Table 1.12) all lower blood sugar but by different mechanisms of action. With Type I diabetes (previously known as juvenile diabetes), the body has stopped producing insulin, and patients need daily doses of insulin for replacement. Type II diabetes, also called adult onset diabetes, is where the body does not use insulin properly so blood sugar levels go up and down. They must be modulated with oral medications or adjusted with injections of insulin. Most diabetics have this form. Patients need nutrition and lifestyle changes, oral medications, and/or insulin injections.

TABLE 1.12 Common Diabetes-Controlling Agents

Generic Name	Brand Name	Classification
acarbose	Precose	Alpha-glucosidase inhibitor
exenatide	Byetta	GLP-1 Agonist
glimepiride	Amaryl	Sulfonylurea
glipizide	Glucotrol	Sulfonylurea
glyburide	DiaBeta, Micronase	Sulfonylurea
insulin aspart	Novolog (fast acting)	Insulin
insulin detemir	Levemir	Insulin
insulin glargine	Lantus, Toujeo	Insulin
insulin glulisine	Apidra	Insulin
insulin lispro	Humalog (fast acting)	Insulin
insulin neutral PH	Humulin N, Novolin N	Insulin
insulin regular	Humulin R, Novolin R	Insulin
liraglutide	Victoza	GLP-1 Agonist
metformin	Glucophage	Biguanide
pioglitazone	Actos	Thiazolidinediones
sitagliptin	Januvia	DPP-4 inhibitor

Insulins

Many types of insulin are available on the market today. Insulins that controls blood sugar between meals and during sleep are called long-acting or **basal insulins**. Insulins that controls blood sugar during eating are called fast-acting or **bolus insulins**. Rapid-release insulins are recommended to be taken 15 minutes prior to meals. Some rapid-release insulins can be sold without a prescription. Insulin must be refrigerated prior to use, and an open vial/pen must be used within a certain period of time once out of the refrigerator. Helping the patient locate the manufacturer-recommended beyond-use instructions will prevent patients using subpotent insulin.

Many insulins now come in a pen form in strengths other than U-100, including U-200, U-300, and U-500. For patient convenience, the dose of insulin is dialed into the pen and administered, doing away with the need for needles and syringes. Make sure patients are dispensed pen-needles to administer insulin with their insulin pen. Some insurance companies, however, will not pay for insulin pens, so make sure to check before dispensing insulin pans.

Insulin glargine (Lantus) is one of the most commonly prescribed basal insulins; it is often taken at bedtime. It does not peak or trough but simply provides a level reduction of blood sugar over a 24-hour period.

Many insulins are prescribed separately or as mixtures of a rapid-release and slower release insulin to be administered with syringes or pens. Be aware that Novolin and Humulin insulins are different from Novolog and Humalog insulins, and they should not be substituted for each other. Humalog and Novolog are fast-acting, shorter lasting insulins that should be used with meals or for treating a high blood sugar.

Safety Alert

Insulin mix-ups and misspellings are the most common source of medication errors.

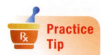
Prescriptions are required for diabetic supplies, and needle and syringe prescription requirements vary by state. Medicare Part D plans cover diabetic supplies, but allowed quantities vary and depend on whether the patient is insulin dependent. Medicare Part B may cover insulin supplies with a prescription and proper documentation and diagnostic codes from the prescriber.

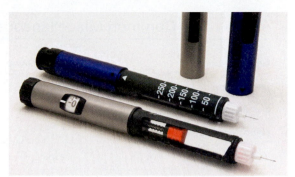

Many patients find using an insulin pen, such as the ones pictured above, more convenient than using an insulin vial and syringe.

Antidiabetic Drugs

All drugs for Type II diabetes work to modulate or lower blood sugars but by different mechanisms of action. Often more than one drug is needed to attain target levels.

The most common antidiabetic drugs are the sulfonylureas, a class of drugs that stimulate the cells of the pancreas to produce more insulin—think of "squeezing a sponge" to imagine the action. Sulfonylurea drugs include glipizide (Glucotrol) and glyburide (DiaBeta, Micronase). A patient's blood sugar level has to be monitored carefully (often self-monitored) to prevent hypoglycemia (low blood sugar) caused by having too much insulin. *The sulfonylurea drugs can cause sensitivity to the sun and may interact poorly with other drugs* (such as the antibiotic Cipro).

Other diabetes drugs have varying chemical bases for different types of actions. Metformin (Glucophage) is the most frequently prescribed Type II diabetes. It is available in both an immediate-release and extended-release form. The drug should be taken with food, and the patient may need to take a vitamin B_{12} supplement while taking long-term metformin. Sitagliptin (Januvia) is a relatively new treatment for Type II diabetes. It is most effective at controlling blood sugars after a meal. It is sometimes prescribed as Janumet, a combination of sitagliptin (Januvia) and metformin. Pioglitazone (Actos) must be used with caution in patients with heart failure.

Exenatide (Byetta) and liraglutide (Victoza) are newer long-lasting agents that are injectable in either daily or weekly formulas. Their main side effect is nausea and vomiting. Liraglutide is also available as a weight loss agent in a higher dosage.

Miscellaneous Endocrine Agents

The body has numerous other hormonal glands and metabolic mechanisms that can go awry and may require medication, as you can see in Table 1.13.

For the treatment of bone loss, or osteoporosis, **bisphosphonates**, such as alendronate (Fosamax), are used. Bone loss often occurs in postmenopausal women or men over age 75 who do not receive enough calcium. Bisphosphonates slow down the cells that break down bone, and they are most commonly taken once weekly or monthly. Only water (not a caffeinated drink) should be taken with them. To increase absorption and minimize esophageal (food tube) erosions in care-facility patients, these drugs must be taken first thing in the morning, on an empty stomach, and not while the patient is in a reclining position. This may present a problem in a bedridden patient.

Thyroid systems often go askew, especially as people age. The thyroid hormones released by the thyroid gland have important functions to influence energy levels and metabolism, growth, body temperature, muscle strength, appetite, and the health of many organs.

TABLE 1.13 Common Miscellaneous Endocrine and Metabolic Agents

Generic Name	Brand Name	Classification
Osteoporosis, Hypercalcemia		
alendronate	Fosamax	Bisphosphonate
Hypothyroidism		
levothyroxine	Levoxyl, Synthroid	Thyroid hormone
Hyperthyroidism		
methimazole	Tapazole	Thyroid reduction
Anti-inflammatory		
allopurinol	Zyloprim	Xanthine oxidase inhibitor
methylprednisolone	Medrol Dosepak	Corticosteroid
prednisone	Deltasone	Corticosteroid

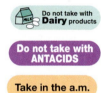

Hypothyroidism is when the thyroid is not active enough and completely stops producing the thyroid hormone. People have very low energy or a great deal of fatigue. Hypothyroidism is very common with age, especially in women. Many physicians and some patients may request a brand name drug, such as Synthroid (generic levothyroxine), due to better tolerance or a more reliable therapeutic effect. If Synthroid is prescribed as "brand necessary," it is considered a DAW prescription when billing an insurance provider. Thyroid replacement medications should be taken in the morning or on an empty stomach to increase absorption. They must not be taken at the same time as dairy, antacids, iron, or calcium, or within two hours of ingestion of these substances.

Hyperthyroidism is the opposite condition, where the thyroid is overstimulated and active, which is less common but even more dangerous. It can lead to racing heartbeats and anxiety, bulging eyes, and even blindness. A common medication is methimazole (Tapazole). Patients should not take alcohol, which can cause serious problems.

Cortisol is a hormone that the adrenal glands produce that helps the body deal with stress and inflammation. Corticosteroids—including dexamethasone (Decadron), prednisone (Deltasone), and methylprednisolone (Medrol Dosepack)—resemble cortisol and are used to treat a variety of inflammatory diseases, such as rheumatoid arthritis, asthma, allergic reactions, poison ivy/oak, ulcerative colitis, Crohn's disease, and gout.

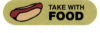

Corticosteroids should be taken with food and may interfere with blood sugar or blood-thinning medications. Cortisteroids are usually prescribed for short-term use because prolonged use can increase the risk of high blood pressure and blood sugar, appetite and weight gain, muscle weakness and bruising, glaucoma or cataracts, stomach ulcers, and hallucinations. It is important to note that corticosteroids are not the same types of steroids as the anabolic steroids used by athletes. Some patients with chronic inflammatory conditions may be on lifelong therapy or may use high doses of cortisteroids for a short time for acute flare-ups. Allopurinol is a xanthine oxidase inhibitor, used to treat gout, preventing the formation of painful urate crystals. For more accute attacks of gout, colchicine and NSAIDs are used to treat the inflammation and pain.

Respiratory Agents

3-D

Asthma, **chronic obstructive pulmonary disease (COPD)**, allergies, and coughing constrict the airways and cause inflammation, which results in shortness of breath and wheezing and decreases oxygen saturation in the blood. To aid breathing, a relaxing of the airways needs to occur. Table 1.14 contains a variety of common respiratory drugs used for relaxing and opening the airways. For a 3-D view of the Respiratory System, go to http://CertExam4e.ParadgimEducation.com/3D-05.

TABLE 1.14 Common Respiratory Agents

Generic Name	Brand Name	Classification
Asthma, COPD		
albuterol	ProAir, Ventolin, Proventil	Bronchodilator
budesonide-formoterol	Symbicort	Combination
fluticasone-salmeterol	Advair	Combination
levalbuterol	Xopenex	Bronchodilator
COPD		
ipratropium	Atrovent	Anticholinergic
ipratropium-albuterol	Combivent	Combination
tiotropium	Spiriva	Anticholinergic
Asthma, Allergy		
fluticasone	Flonase, Flovent	Inhaled steroid
montelukast	Singulair	Leukotriene receptor antagonist
mometasone	Asmanex	Inhaled corticosteroid

Practice Tip

Patients need to be reminded to keep inhalers and nebulizers clean and to rinse their mouths after using corticosteroids to prevent a fungal infection in the mouth called thrush.

Albuterol (ProAir, Ventolin, and Proventil), levalbuterol (Xopenex), ipratropium (Atrovent), and tiotropium (Spiriva) all work in different ways to open the breathing passageways (bronchodilators) and lungs of patients with asthma or COPD. Albuterol is the fastest acting bronchodilator and should be used for acute attacks. Albuterol may be prescribed as a tablet, syrup, metered-dose inhaler (MDI), propellant spray for inhaling, or sterile solution for a nebulizer, which mists it for inhaling.

The side effects of albuterol and its derivatives include increases in heart rate and blood pressure. Overuse may cause patients to develop a tolerance so that other medications need to be considered. Ipratropium and tiotropium both cause dryness in the mouth, throat, and eyes. These drugs are inhaled into the lungs and provide relief for shortness of breath. The brand Combivent combines ipratropium and albuterol. In essence, all of these drugs provide symptomatic relief only.

The mixed formulations of budesonide-formoterol (Symbicort) and fluticasone-salmeterol (Advair) combine a passage-opening substance with a corticosteroid that reduces the swelling that causes difficulty breathing in asthma and COPD. Decreasing inflammation should reduce the number of acute attacks and the need for the use of short-acting agents, such as albuterol.

Antihistamines fight the body's histamine responses to allergies, such as itchiness, redness, nasal mucus or runny nose, swelling of airways, and coughing. Montelukast (Singulair)—available in tablet, chewable tablet, and granular forms—works against asthma and allergies to neutralize and prevent the release of chemicals that cause symptoms like bronchoconstriction.

For less intense diseases and symptoms, physicians and pharmacists often recommend that the patient select OTC nonsedating antihistamines, such as loratadine (Claritin) or fexofenadine (Allegra). Nasal sprays that provide intranasal steroids like fluticasone (Flonase, Flovent) and mometasone (Nasonex) are used routinely to prevent seasonal allergy symptoms from developing. These drugs are now available without a prescription.

Gastrointestinal Agents

3-D

The digestive system—the gastrointestinal (GI) system, which includes the esophagus, stomach, the small intestine, and the large intestine—develops common ailments, so there are frequently prescribed medications (as shown in Table 1.15). For a 3-D view of the gastrointestinal system, go to http://CertExam4e.ParadgimEducation.com/3D-06. The most often prescribed gastrointestinal agents are the **proton pump inhibitors (PPIs)**, which work to prevent stomach acid production. These include esomeprazole (Nexium), lansoprazole (Prevacid), omeprazole (Prilosec), and pantoprazole (Protonix). Taken with NSAIDs, proton pump inhibitors treat and prevent NSAID-induced ulcers. Also, drugs that suppress acid secretion given with multiple antibiotics will effectively treat *Helicobacter pylori* infections that cause ulcers.

A family of drugs known as **histamine-2 antagonists (H_2 blockers)**, such as famotidine (Pepcid) and ranitidine (Zantac), work to slow down the release of more acid in the stomach.

PPIs and histamine-2 antagonists are well tolerated, with only occasional reports of side effects like headache and dizziness. However, PPIs, such as omeprazole, can interfere with beneficial effects of the blood-clotting prevention drug clopidogrel (Plavix). These drugs should not be taken together, even if they are spaced 12 hours apart.

Long-term use of PPIs has been reported to increase bone loss, especially in older women, so an OTC calcium supplement may be recommended to accompany these drugs. Some other gastrointestinal agents that are also used, such as promethazine, ondansetron, and metoclopramide, were previously listed in Table 1.6—Miscellaneous Cardiovascular Agents.

Treatment of inflammatory bowel disease involves GI drugs that work locally, such as sulfasalazine, olsalazine, and mesalamine. Related to sulfa drugs, these agents work in the colon to treat and prevent ulcerative colitis. Patients may also receive corticosteroids orally or via rectal enema or suppository. Most common side effects include headache, nausea, fatigue, and skin rash.

Severe ulcerative colitis may need to be treated with biological response modifiers like infliximab (see biotechnology drug section for more information). Irritable bowel syndrome (IBS) is another chronic gastrointestinal tract ailment with stomach pain, gas, diarrhea, and/or constipation. New agents, such as lubiprostone, linaclotide, and eluxadoline, taken with fiber supplements, antidiarrheals, and antispasmodics help relieve symptoms (see Table 1.15). Fiber supplements, antidiarrheals, laxatives, and probiotics will be discussed in the OTC drugs section.

TABLE 1.15 Gastrointestinal Agents

Generic Name	Brand Name	Classification
dicyclomine	Bentyl	Antispasmodic
eluxadoline	Viberzi	Antidiarrheal for IBS-D*
esomeprazole	Nexium	PPI*
famotidine	Pepcid	H$_2$ antagonist*
lansoprazole	Prevacid	PPI
linaclotide	Linzess	Anticonstipation for IBS-C*
lubiprostone	Amitiza	Anticonstipation for IBS-C
mesalamine	Asacol, Lialda, Pentasa, Rowasa	Intestinal anti-inflammatory
omeprazole	Prilosec	PPI
olsalazine	Dipentum	Intestinal anti-inflammatory
pantoprazole	Protonix	PPI
ranitidine	Zantac	H$_2$ antagonist
sulfasalazine	Azulfidine	Intestinal anti-inflammatory

*Note: IBS-D = (Irritable Bowel Disease-Diarrhea), PPI = (Proton Pump Inhibitor),
H2 antagonist = (Histamine-2 antagonist), IBS-C = (Irritable Bowel Disease-Constipation)

Renal and Genitourinary Agents

3-D

The renal system, or urinary system, includes the kidneys, bladder, ureters, and urethra. The genitourinary system includes both the genital reproductive system and the urinary tract. Male and female genitourinary systems have different difficulties. For a 3-D view of the male system, go to http://CertExam4e.ParadgimEducation.com/3D-07. For the female system, go to http://CertExam4e.ParadigmEducation.com/3D-08. The most frequently prescribed renal and genitourinary agents are the diuretic drugs for all populations and the drugs to address erectile dysfunction (ED) and prostate problems for men (see Table 1.16).

Take in the a.m.

Diuretics, sometimes called "water pills," work with the kidneys to eliminate excess salt and water from the body by dilating (widening) blood vessels. They are used to treat swelling from water retention, high blood pressure, and heart failure. Diuretics should be taken in the morning or early evening. Most can cause a loss of potassium, which can cause muscle cramps or, in severe cases, irregular heart rates. Potassium loss can be offset by consuming potassium-rich foods, such as fresh citrus fruits and bananas, or taking potassium supplements. Hydrochlorothiazide and furosemide (Lasix) act at different sites of the kidney, and their onset, duration of action, and potency differ. Diuretics that contain triamterene (Dyazide, Maxzide) or spironolactone (Aldactone) are considered potassium-sparing, meaning that they maintain healthier levels of potassium.

TABLE 1.16   Renal and Genitourinary Agents

Generic Name	Brand Name	Classification
Diuretics, Prostate Disorder		
finasteride	Proscar	5-Alpha reductase inhibitor
furosemide	Lasix	Loop diuretic
hydrochlorothiazide	Esidrix, HydroDIURIL, Oretic	Thiazide diuretic
spironolactone	Aldactone	Potassium-sparing diuretic
tamsulosin	Flomax	Alpha blocker
triamterene-hydrochlorothiazide	Dyazide, Maxzide	Combination, potassium-sparing
Erectile Dysfunction		
sildenafil	Viagra	Phosphodiesterase inhibitor
tadalafil	Cialis	Phosphodiesterase inhibitor
vardenafil	Levitra	Phosphodiesterase inhibitor

Practice Tip

A pregnant pharmacy technician, or one trying to get pregnant, should not handle finasteride. See Appendix B.

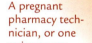

Do not take this drug if pregnant or planning to become pregnant

Many antihypertensive drugs listed in Table 1.7 are available in combination with a diuretic. However, diuretics must be used with caution with ACE inhibitors, digoxin, and lithium. The pharmacist needs to assess the potential for drug interactions.

Erectile dysfunction drugs include the well-known and marketed brand drugs Viagra (generic sildenafil) and Cialis (generic tadalafil). These drugs vary by onset and duration of action. Rare side effects include changes in blue/green color vision and prolonged painful erections (priapism). *A life-threatening drop in blood pressure (hypotension) can occur if these agents are used with any nitrate.*

Benign prostatic hypertropy (BPH), or an enlarged prostate not due to cancer, is treated with tamsulosin (Flomax) and finasteride (Proscar). Tamulosin is a common **alpha-adrenergic blocker**, and a common side effect is first-dose syncope (or drop in blood pressure causing fainting), so tamsulosin is usually prescribed as a bedtime dose. Finasteride is a 5-alpha-reductase inhibitor that blocks the conversion of testosterone. Finasteride can decrease hair loss producing baldness but also sexual function. Some patients complain the side effects last for a sustained period after ceasing use of the drug. In addition, *the drug can pass in the semen and may harm a resulting fetus. It should not be used if a couple is trying to conceive a child*, or if a man is sexually active without contraceptives with a woman of child-bearing age.

Hematological Agents

Hematological drugs include those dealing with blood cell production, quality, and clotting. Table 1.17 lists frequently prescribed hematological medications. The hematological agents discussed in this section will focus on drugs used to treat

TABLE 1.17 Common Hematological Agents

Generic Name	Brand Name	Classification	Indication
alteplase	Activase	Fibrinolytic	Acute ischemic stroke, myocardial infarction
apixaban	Eliquis	Factor Xa inhibitor	Prevent blood clots
clopidogrel	Plavix	Antiplatelet drug	Prevent blood clots
dabigatran	Pradaxa	Thrombin inhibitor	Prevent blood clots
enoxaparin	Lovenox	Thrombin inhibitor	Prevent blood clots
heparin	generic only	Thrombin inhibitor	Prevent blood clots
reteplase	Retavase	Fibrinolytic	Acute ischemic stroke, myocardial infarction
rivaroxaban	Xarelto	Factor Xa inhibitor	Prevent blood clots
tenecteplase	TNKase	Fibrinolytic	Acute ischemic stroke, myocardial infarction
warfarin	Coumadin	Blood thinner	Prevent blood clots

Safety Alert

The list of negative drug interactions for warfarin is long, so great care must be taken with the medication profile and any nonprescription drugs and supplements.

thromboembolic (blood clot) disorders. Biotechnology drugs used for hematologic diseases will be discussed in the next section and vitamins in the OTC drugs section.

Warfarin (Coumadin) is a drug that is used both short- and long-term to prevent blood clots in high-risk patients. Patients on this drug are less likely to clot but more likely to bleed profusely. With blood thinners, toxic levels are not far from the therapeutic levels, so patients must be closely monitored on a routine basis with a blood test to measure the international normalized ratio (INR) to see how well it clots. The therapeutic level for warfarin is between 2.0 and 3.5. *Warfarin creates serious adverse reactions when taken with many other drugs and supplements, so technicians and pharmacists must be very careful to watch for drug utilization review alerts* and have them resolved by the pharmacist. (Be careful with all warfarin or Coumadin questions on the certification exam because of this.) Warn patients against taking St. John's wort with warfarin or any anticlotting agent.

Because blood thinners are so difficult to modulate at just the right levels, some prescribers write Coumadin as "brand necessary" (DAW). This drug (and other blood thinners) is *very susceptible* to drug interactions, such as with aspirin (a mild blood thinner) and many herbal drugs (such as ginger, ginkgo, and ginseng). When other drugs are added to the regimen or when dosages are adjusted, the pharmacist must assess the potential for serious interactions.

Warfarin works by inhibiting vitamin K–dependent clotting factors. *Vitamins and diets that are high in vitamin K can impair the pharmacological effect of warfarin.* Newer agents have been introduced more recently to prevent clot formation, including dabigatran (Pradaxa) and rivaroxaban (Xarelto), which are faster acting and do not require regular blood testing. The disadvantage to these new agents is the cost. (Should there be an overdose of Pradaxa, there is a new antidote called Praxbind.) Clopidogrel (Plavix) often works to decrease the risk of blood clots by inhibiting blood platelets. Diet does not affect this drug, but the use of proton pump inhibitor drugs for the stomach can interfere with its therapeutic effect.

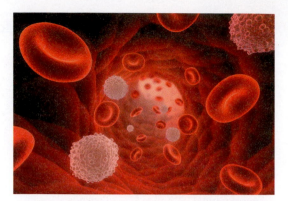

Heparin (generic only) is an anticlotting drug that is administered intravenously and subcutaneously to treat and prevent blood clots. It is used especially for lungs and legs in hospital settings. Frequent blood tests are required for IV heparin patients to monitor against the major side effect—excessive bleeding.

Warfarin and heparin work to prevent drug clotting, but consequently they can also cause excessive bleeding if there is an injury. They are also very prone to causing adverse drug reactions when interacting with many other drugs.

Enoxaparin (Lovenox) is used as an injection to prevent blood clots. It is particularly used in high-risk surgeries or for **bridging therapy** to prevent blood clots after surgery while waiting for the slow-acting warfarin to take effect (usually in one week). Enoxaparin has been shown to be as effective as heparin, and it requires no blood tests and causes less bleeding.

Patients who come to the emergency department of the hospital with an acute myocardial infarction (heart attack) or acute ischemic stroke may be given an intravenous dose of a fibrinolytic, such as alteplase, reteplase, or tenecteplase, to dissolve the clot. The major risk with *these drugs is bleeding or hemorrhagic stroke*. Combining these drugs with heparin can increase the risk of bleeding.

Biotechnology Drugs

Numerous drugs developed through biotechnology are used for a variety of medical conditions: (1) to treat anemia from chronic kidney disease or cancer chemotherapy, (2) to boost white and red blood cell counts for those at risk of an infection or experiencing severe fatigue, and (3) to treat inflammatory diseases. The most common drugs are shown in Table 1.18.

Infliximab (Remicade, Remsima, Inflectra), adalimumab (Humira), and etanercept (Enbrel) have a wide spectrum of uses, from severe rheumatoid arthritis to GI inflammatory diseases, such as Crohn's disease, to severe psoriasis that is unresponsive to conventional therapy.

With the exception of adalimumab (Humira) and etanercept (Enbrel), the technician working in a community pharmacy will not be exposed to these costly and potent agents, although hospital technicians most likely will.

Biotechnology drugs are also available to stimulate the production of a body's white blood cells (WBCs), which are needed to boost immunity, and red blood cells (RBCs) to carry oxygen. Cancer, chemotherapy, and radiation therapy can all cause damaging effects to white blood cells, red blood cells, or both. Low WBC counts increase the risk of infections, and low RBC counts increase the risk of fatigue.

Technicians working in a hospital or servicing a cancer or dialysis clinic need to be familiar with bone marrow colony-stimulating factors, such as darbepoetin alfa (Aranesp), epoetin alfa (Procrit), and filgrastim (Neupogen). These are life-saving drugs for patients undergoing chemotherapy, which can depress the bone marrow and subsequent immune system function.

Pharm Facts

Infliximab (Remicade, Remisima, Inflectra) is an intravenous biologic drug used for treating autoimmune and inflammatory diseases like Crohn's disease and rheumatoid arthritis.

TABLE 1.18 Biological and Immunological Agents

Biological Name	Brand Name	Classification	Indication
adalimumab	Humira	Inhibits inflammation	Inflammatory disorders
darbepoetin alfa	Aranesp	Bone marrow stimulating agent	Anemia from kidney failure
epoetin alfa	Procrit	Bone marrow stimulating agent	Anemia from kidney failure
etanercept	Enbrel	TNF* antagonist	Inflammatory disorders
filgrastim	Neupogen	Stimulates white blood cell production	Prevent infection
infliximab	Remicade, Remsima, Inflextr	TNF blocking agent	Inflammatory disorders
pegfilgrastim	Neulasta	Stimulates more white blood cell production	Prevent infection

* Note: TNF (Tumor Necrosis Factor)

TAKE NOTE

There are FDA-mandated black box warning statements for several inject-able biotechnology drugs, including Enbrel, Remicade, and Humira. These drugs work by suppressing the immune system, thus increasing patient susceptibility to two rare but serious bacterial and fungal infections.

Miscellaneous Drugs

Other common prescription drugs fit in less anatomically based areas. A sample is offered in Table 1.19. Skin conditions like eczema, psoriasis, allergic reactions from bug bites, and dermatitis from poison ivy are often treated with topical corticosteroids (those applied on the skin). Triamcinolone (Kenalog) is a topical corticosteroid and is the most frequently prescribed topical drug, available in different strengths in both a cream and an ointment. Triamcinolone is more potent than the topical OTC hydro-cortisone.

TABLE 1.19 Miscellaneous Agents

Generic Name	Brand Name	Classification	Indication
cholecalciferol	Vitamin D	Fat-soluble vitamin	Deficiency, osteoporosis
folic acid	Many generics	B vitamin	Heart disease, with MTX
potassium chloride	K-Dur, Klor-Con	Mineral	K^+ replacement
triamcinolone	Kenalog	Topical steroid	Inflammatory skin disease, eczema

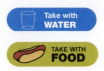

Potassium chloride (K-Dur, Klor-Con) can be prescribed alongside diuretic drugs as one daily dose or two in tablet, capsule, or liquid form. This potassium medication *should be taken with food and a glass of water so that it does not irritate the esophagus.*

Vitamin D and folic acid are commonly prescribed vitamins. Though both are available as an OTC drug, the higher prescribed dosages must be carefully monitored. For example, vitamin D is available as an OTC drug in dosages of 400 to 2,000 international units (IU) per day; a common prescription dose is 50,000 IU once a week. Vitamin D improves the absorption of calcium and is usually prescribed or recommended for patients who have or are at risk for osteoporosis.

Folic acid reduces the toxicity of methotrexate (MTX), a potent drug commonly prescribed for rheumatoid arthritis. Folic acid is also recommended for patients who are or may become pregnant to decrease the risk of spina bifida (a birth deformity) in the child. High doses are found in all prenatal vitamins. Some cardiologists recommend taking folic acid to reduce blood levels of homocysteine, which is thought to be a risk factor for heart disease.

TAKE NOTE

A number of new drugs have just been approved that technicians will be seeing:

- Addyi for enhancing women's sexual drive
- OxyContin extended release for chronic pain treatment; also approved for youth ages 11 to 16 (a new indication for an existing drug)
- Procysbi delayed release for kidney buildup of cysteine, now also approved for children ages 2 to 6
- Repatha (injectable evolocumab) for diet and statin therapy for those needing additional reduction of LDL cholesterol
- Spritam (3-D printed levetiracetam with a porous pill structure for quick dissolving) for treatment of epileptic seizures without swallowing
- Synjardy for glucose control for type 2 diabetes
- Zubsolv for transition off of opioids for those who are dependent

Over-the-Counter Drugs

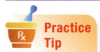

Practice Tip

You should remind customers that most OTC drugs should typically only be used for seven days or less.

Customers often seek counsel to help them select the appropriate OTC product for a special condition. You cannot just show them the right OTC aisle. You need to direct them to a pharmacist's counsel. *Pharmacists are the only ones who can legally address questions about the right medication for a medical purpose or indication, the right dosage and administration, expected therapeutic effects, side effects, contraindications, and interactions—even for OTC drugs and vitamins!* However, you can and should help customers find the brands and types of medications they are looking for. Technicians can also help customers understand the OTC product labels, which include the following: product name and therapeutic purpose, directions for dosage and frequency of administration for different age groups, active and inactive ingredients (such as dyes), expiration dates, any precautions or warnings, and any special storage requirements.

Commonly requested OTC drugs are listed in Table 1.20. Many popular OTC drugs, such as hydrocortisone and ibuprofen, once required a prescription. The active ingredients are the same as those found in the higher-strength prescription formulations but are simply present in lower strengths and dosages. For example, OTC ibuprofen is available in a strength of 200 mg, whereas the prescription strengths are 400 mg, 600 mg, and 800 mg.

Safety Alert

OTC cough and cold products are generally not suitable for children under age six.

TABLE 1.20 Common OTC Drugs and Their Indications

Brand Name	Generic Name	Indication(s)
Advil/Motrin	ibuprofen	Headache, pain
Afrin	oxymetazoline	Nasal decongestant
Aleve	naproxen	Headache, pain
Align	bifidobacterium	Probiotic
Allegra	fexofenadine	Allergy
Benadryl	diphenhydramine	Allergy
Claritin	loratadine	Allergy
Colace	docusate sodium	Stool softener
Cortizone-10	hydrocortisone	Itching, inflammation
Culturelle	lactobacillus	Probiotic
Dulcolax	bisacodyl	Constipation
Flonase	fluticasone	Allergy
Imodium	loperamide	Diarrhea, irritable bowel syndrome
Lotrimin	clotrimazole	Topical antifungal
Miralax	polyethylene glycol	Constipation
Monistat	miconazole	Vaginal antifungal
Mucinex	guaifenesin	Expectorant
Nasacort	triamcinolone	Allergy
Neosporin	triple antibiotic	Topical anti-infective
Nexium	esomeprazole	Heartburn
Pepcid	famotidine	Heartburn
Prevacid	lansoprazole	Heartburn
Prilosec	omeprazole	Heartburn
Senokot	senna	Constipation
Zantac	ranitidine	Heartburn
Zyrtec	cetirizine	Allergy

Note: Drugs in table are listed by brand name first, as these are the names more often requested by customers at the pharmacy.

Pharmacy technicians should also be aware that a few significant OTC drugs are located in the refrigerated area of the pharmacy—in particular, the fast-acting regular insulins including Novolin and Humulin.

Manufacturers typically provide a toll free number in the event that consumers have additional questions or concerns when they get home. You can point this out.

Consumer Cautions Technicians may remind patients that when the dosages recommended by the manufacturer are exceeded, OTC medications can be very dangerous. For instance, products containing the cough suppressant dextromethorphan (DM) can cause auditory and visual hallucinations in high doses. Because DM products have a history of abuse among adolescents, consumers must be *age 18 or older to buy these products and must present an ID to purchase them*.

In addition, technicians can make patients aware that *the FDA discourages giving any child under the age of six OTC cough and cold products* because the risk of adverse reactions is greater than the potential benefits.

Consumers should be reminded that OTC products should be used for a restricted period—usually less than seven days—unless otherwise directed by a physician. (For example, a physician may direct an adult patient to take a low-dose aspirin on a long-term, daily basis in order to lower a patient's risk of heart disease.) If a patient has self-medicated with an OTC drug for seven or more days without resolution, the patient should be referred by the pharmacist to the appropriate healthcare professional.

Holistic Health Medications and Dietary Supplements

Qualified holistic practitioners can prescribe conventional treatments combined with alternative medicine, such as recommending acupuncture to a cancer patient receiving chemotherapy. This is called **integrative medicine**. **Alternative medicine** is when patients treat themselves or are treated with only nonconventional treatments, such as natural products (homeopathic medications, herbals, vitamins, minerals, and other dietary supplements), specialized diets, acupuncture, deep breathing and relaxation techniques, guided imagery, exercise movements like yoga and Pilates, meditation, massage therapy, and chiropractic manipulations.

Some consumers associate "natural" with "safe," *yet many of these drugs have side effects or problematic interactions with prescription drugs even when used appropriately.*

Pharm Facts

Because many homeopathic medications are diluted so much, even to 1,000 times, only trace amounts of the desired ingredients remain. Skeptics say these traces are not enough to provoke any medicinal effect.

Homeopathic Medications

Homeopathy is based on the philosophy that the body can heal itself if the immune system can be stimulated in targeted ways through the concept of "like cures like." Introducing highly diluted natural substances that create minor symptoms can activate an immune system response to help overcome illnesses with the same symptoms. The trigger substances can be plant and animal substances (or diseased tissues) or from metal, chemical, and mineral substances.

Homeopathics, due to their highly diluted forms, do not usually interact with prescription or OTC drugs, and generally do not mask symptoms of underlying illness.

In the United States, homeopathic medications for humans are sold mostly without a prescription for common short-lived illnesses, such as flu, cough, cold, allergies, dermatitis, arthritis, and stomach disorders. For instance, sulfur is used for acne of very oily skin and *Pulsatilla* (pasque flower) for acne associated in puberty in young girls. *Colchicum* (crocus) is recommended for arthritis caused by changes with weather. Veterinary medicine integrates far more homeopathy. For dogs pacing back and forth with anxiety, *Arsenicum album* (made from arsenous acid) in highly diluted form is recommended.

The active ingredients in homeopathics are diluted and shaken, then diluted and shaken again, with the cycle repeating in a series of progressions called **succussion** for different dosage levels. Homeopathics are available in low dilutions (with higher concentrations) for immediate, direct symptoms progressing to high dilutions (with lower concentrations) for more general symptoms.

Homeopathic medications are available in many different formulations, such as tablets (often sublingual, or under the tongue), liquids, syrups, gels, creams, ointments, eye drops, and suppositories. Most homeopathics do not have extensive labeling and dosing information, often listing only the active ingredient, dilution, and most common use. Sugar is sometimes added to improve the taste, or the dilution is present in a sugar-coated tablet. As with OTC products, you should refer customers to the pharmacist for treatment advice.

Dietary Supplements

A **dietary supplement** can be a vitamin, mineral, or an herbal product that is considered useful for healthy nutrition, the prevention of an illness, or the alleviation or reduction of an illness's symptoms. The typical uses, or indications, for some common dietary supplements are listed in Table 1.21.

The Dietary Supplement Health and Education Act (DSHEA) states that supplements must be *safe and accurately labeled*. As with other food products, the label of a supplement indicates the recommended "serving size" rather than a dose. The label provides far less product information than an OTC drug label.

If a label contains a promise of a medical cure or effective treatment, the FDA can act to remove the drug from the market for the reason of false advertising since no proof of the label's claims has been submitted to the FDA. The FDA can also remove any dietary supplement that is deemed dangerous. It's best to steer consumers toward products with the seal of USP Verified on them. The pharmacy technician should, of course, not counsel customers regarding the therapeutic uses of dietary supplements but refer patients to the pharmacist.

Vitamins and Minerals

There are many OTC vitamin and mineral products on the market that range from multivitamins to the doses of specific minerals and vitamins like the B complex, A, C, D, and E. Listed on the label of each is the proportion of active substance contained as compared to the **recommended daily allowance (RDA)**. The RDA is the average intake level needed to meet the daily nutrient requirements of nearly all (97% to 98%) healthy people. Children or adults may need this type of daily vitamin just to reach the minimum daily allowance standards. Pregnant women are encouraged to consume a daily prenatal vitamin (prescription or OTC) to promote the health of their unborn children and prevent birth defects. A technician can be helpful in directing patients to both brand name and generic vitamins, including those in chewable, gummy, and liquid formulations for children and elderly consumers.

Some consumers take short-term high doses of individual vitamins for different indications, such as vitamin C to build one's immunity and fight the common cold,

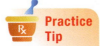

Practice Tip

Most consumers do not realize that dietary supplements, including vitamins and minerals, are not regulated by the FDA in the same manner as are OTC drugs.

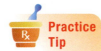

Practice Tip

Most vitamins lose potency when exposed to heat and light. Advise customers to keep their vitamins on dimly lit, cool shelves.

Pharm Facts

Vitamin E is not just one vitamin. It is actually a collection of eight fat-soluble vitamins with specific antioxidant properties.

TABLE 1.21 Common Dietary Supplements

Dietary Supplement	Indication(s)
calcium and vitamin D	Improves bone strength
echinacea	Boosts the immune system
ferrous sulfate	Anemia
garlic	Has an antibacterial and antiviral action; maintains healthy cholesterol
ginger	Treats nausea, motion sickness, and morning sickness
ginkgo	Improves memory; treats tinnitus and peripheral vascular disease
glucosamine/chondroitin	Lessens joint pain
lactobacillus (a bacterium)	Improves digestion, helps prevent diarrhea
lutein	Maintains eye health
melatonin	Treats insomnia, especially in shift workers or time-zone travelers
omega-3 fatty acids (fish oil)	Lowers triglyceride levels
policosanol	Maintains healthy cholesterol levels
red yeast rice	Maintains healthy cholesterol levels
saw palmetto	Treats benign prostatic hypertrophy (BPH)
St. John's wort	Treats mild depression
tea tree oil	Alleviates skin ailments, such as acne, athlete's foot, and boils
turmeric	Anti-inflammatory
vitamin C	Treats the common cold
zinc	Boosts the immune system; helps in the treatment of the common cold and wound healing

vitamin E for heart health, and lutein for eye health. However, research has found that habitual megadoses of certain vitamins can be harmful to health. For instance, doses of vitamin E in excess of 800 IU per day may interfere with blood clotting or increase the risk of heart disease. High supplement doses of Vitamin A and other vitamins absorbed by fat *can build up in the body and cause toxicity, liver damage, birth defects, and problems in the central nervous system.*

Popular mineral supplements include iron and calcium. In many cases, these may be prescribed or recommended by the physician. Vegans and vegetarians, menstruating and pregnant females, and postsurgical patients may require extra iron to prevent anemia. Calcium combined with magnesium and vitamin D is recommended to keep bones strong and prevent osteoporosis (a weakening of the bones). Since the salt combinations of iron and calcium in different products contain variable amounts of "active minerals," questions should be referred to the pharmacist for proper product selection.

Herbal and Medicinal Plants

Though considered "natural" drugs, **herbals** are also regulated as dietary supplements rather than as drugs by the FDA. The most popular herbals are echinacea, ginger, garlic, ginkgo, St. John's wort, and soy. Their indications were also listed in Table 1.21. Herbals are also dosed in serving sizes like food.

Herbals have powerful components that are metabolized by the liver as with other drug substances. That is why they *can cause drug interactions* or affect the absorption, distribution, and elimination of prescription and OTC drugs and other supplements. Like OTC drugs, herbal medications *do have side effects and can cause allergic reactions*—not just the first time they are used but even after sustained use. Some herbal substances can accumulate in the body or cause an immune response to build up gradually.

Goldenseal has a high potential for herb-drug adverse interactions. Concentrated and prolonged ingestion of ginger, garlic, and ginkgo should not occur with blood thinners and must be discontinued a week prior to surgery. *St. John's wort should not be used with a wide range of prescription drugs*, such as antidepressants, birth control medications, antiseizure drugs, cyclosporine (an organ-rejection prevention drug), digoxin (a heart medication), and warfarin (along with other anticoagulants).

Protein Shakes and Nutritional Supplements

Physicians often recommend protein shakes and nutritional supplements to patients who do not eat well and are losing weight, such as seniors or patients undergoing cancer treatments who need to replenish or build up their systems. Protein sources include milk, whey, casein, egg, rice, and soy (plant proteins). Some processed supplements are high in sugar, *so caution must be exercised with diabetic patients*. Ensure is a brand of nutritional supplement that is available in various flavors. Like other brands, it supplies needed calories containing protein, minerals, and vitamins without fat, and it can be used as a meal supplement or replacement. Thick-It is a supplement requested by many elderly customers. When added to water, juices, tea, milk, or protein shakes, Thick-It assists in swallowing and digestion.

Probiotics

Probiotics work to build up the "good" or "friendly" microorganisms in one's body, especially the positive-acting bacteria in the digestive system. Since antibiotics often destroy the bacteria causing the infection as well as the positive bacteria in the gastrointestinal (GI) tract (stomach and intestines), common side effects of antibiotic therapy include diarrhea and vaginal yeast infections. Physicians often advise patients taking antibiotics to eat yogurt that contains live bacteria cultures of *Lactobacillus acidophilus* or ingest a probiotic sold in the pharmacy. Patients who are lactose (milk sugar) intolerant often use probiotic supplements in order to combat digestive issues when they drink milk or eat cheese and other dairy products.

Common probiotics contain various strains of *Lactobacillus* and *Bifidobacterium*, which can restore the balance of microorganisms in the GI tract. Some brand name probiotics include Culturelle, Align, and Lactinex (the latter is found in the refrigerator). Probiotics may also be used to treat the abdominal pain, cramping, and bloating of irritable bowel syndrome. Some scientific research is now finding that probiotics can help heal skin conditions, such as eczema, prevent allergies and colds, and improve oral health.

Reviewing Pharmacology

Throughout the chapter, you have seen drug name endings highlighted. To learn the many drug families and their similarities, it is helpful to memorize these suffixes for quick recognition. To help you study, use Table 1.22.

TABLE 1.22 **Drug Suffixes and Prefixes**

Suffix or Prefix	Classification	Generic Drug Examples
-prazole	Proton pump inhibitor	omeprazole, lansoprazole
-tidine	Histamine-2 antagonist	ranitidine, famotidine
-statin	HMG CoA reductase inhibitor	lovastatin, simvastatin
-ine	Opiate analgesic	codeine, morphine
-one	Opioid analgesic or corticosteroid	Hydrocodone, hydromorphone or prednisone, triamcinolone
-pam or -lam	Benzodiazepine	diazepam, alprazolam
-triptan	Serotonin agonist for migraine headaches	sumatriptan, zolmitriptan
-olol	Beta-adrenergic blocker	propranolol, metoprolol
-pril	ACE inhibitor	lisinopril, quinapril
-sartan	Angiotensin receptor blocker	losartan, olmesartan
-dipine	Dihydropyridine calcium channel blocker	nifedipine, amlodipine
-cillin	Penicillin antibiotics	ampicillin, ticarcillin
Ceph- or cef-	Cephalosporin antibiotic	cephalexin, ceftazidime
-oxacin	Fluoroquinolone antibiotic	ciprofloxacin, levofloxacin
Sulf-	Sulfonamide antibiotic	sulfamethoxazole, sulfasalazine
-penem	Beta-lactam antibiotic	meropenem, imipenem
-omycin	Macrolide antibiotic	erythromycin, clarithromycin
-cycline	Tetracycline antibiotic	doxycycline, minocycline
-vir	Antiviral, may be flu, herpes, or HIV infection	acyclovir, ritonavir
-azole	Antifungal	fluconazole, miconazole
-caine	Topical anesthetic	lidocaine, prilocaine
-gliptin	DPP-4 inhibitor	sitagliptin, saxagliptin
-ide	Sulfonylurea	glipizide, glyburide
-glitazone	Thiazolidinediones	pioglitazone, rosiglitazone
-dronate	Bisphosphonates	alendronate, risedronate
-terol	Beta-2 agonist for respiratory disease	albuterol, salmeterol
-tropium	Anticholinergic for respiratory disease	ipratropium, tiotropium
-parin	Thrombin inhibitors	heparin, enoxaparin
-mab	Monoclonal antibody-biotech drug	infliximab, rituximab

Throughout the chapter, you have also seen pictures of auxiliary labels in the margins. It is important for technicians to be aware of which labels are important to medications. Auxiliary labels help the patient to understand how to take their medication and prevent side effects. The computer may print off more labels than may fit on the prescription vial, check with the pharmacist to identify which are more important and must be on the vial prior to dispensing to the patient. Table 1.23 lists the most used auxiliary labels and common drugs that need them.

TABLE 1.23 Auxiliary Labels

Auxiliary Label	Common Drugs Requiring Label
Avoid exposure to sunlight	Antibiotics, antifungals, amiodarone, carbamazepine, doxycycline, fluoroquinolones, ibuprofen, isotretinoin, loop diuretics, naproxen, spironolactone, sulfa drugs, sulfonylureas, thiazide diuretics, trazodone
Discolors urine or feces	Cefdinir, ferrous sulfate, phenazopyridine, nitrofurantoin, rifampin
Do not drink alcohol when taking medication	Antidepressants, antipsychotics, depressants, disulfiram, metronidazole, narcotics, NSAIDs, oral contraceptives, phenytoin, sulfonylureas
Do not take if pregnant, nursing, or trying to conceive	isotretinoin, finasteride
Do not take with dairy products, antacids, or iron preparations	Ciprofloxacin, doxycycline, gabapentin, levothyroxine, sucralfate, synthroid
Do not take with grapefruit	Statins
Do not smoke when taking medication	Female contraceptives
Finish all medication as prescribed	All antibiotics, antifungals, and antivirals
Interferes with contraceptives	Antibiotics, doxycycline
May cause dizziness	Anticonvulsants, pregabalin
May cause drowsiness	Antidepressants, antipsychotics, benzodiazepines, hypnotics, muscle relaxants, narcotics, opioid analgesics, tramadol
Take at bedtime	Alpha blockers, nicotinic acid
Take on an empty stomach, 1 hr before meals, or 2 hr after a meal	Bisphosphonates, captopril, sucralfate, penicillin
Take with food	Antibiotics (azithromycin, erythromycin), corticosteroids, metformin, narcotics, nicotinic acid, nonnarcotic analegesics, NSAIDs, oral contraceptives, potassium chloride
Take with a full glass of orange juice or eat a banana daily	Loop diuretics, thiazide diuretics
Take with water	Potassium chloride, sulfa drugs, phenazopyridine, bisphosphonates, NSAIDs

STUDY SUMMARY

The study of pharmacology requires a great deal of memorization. Remember that you can do it. Think of all the products and brands you know in a grocery or clothes store without even thinking about it. So study the drugs in families of products to get to know them well. With study, flashcards, and practice, you will get to know this pharmacological knowledge and be able to put it to use.

- Know the names of the pharmacological fields and their descriptions.
- Memorize different kinds of drug agents based on bodily systems and the drug families based on chemical composition and action.
- Use flashcards to study generic to brand and brand to generic names.
- Get to know the common indications, contraindications, side effects, warnings, and typical auxiliary labels.

ADDITIONAL RESOURCES

For more in-depth explanations, check out *Pharmacology for Technicians* 6e, from Paradigm Education Solutions. To master and extend the material presented in this chapter, take advantage of the resources available through the eBook resources links. These include digital supplements, study resources, and a practice exam generator with 1,000+ exam-style questions. End-of-chapter tests are accessible through the eBook for individuals using the self-study course and through Navigator+ for individuals enrolled in the instructor-guided course.

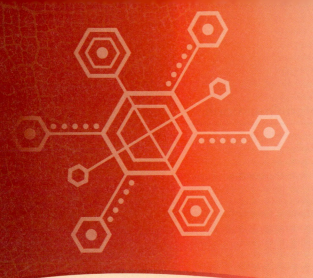

2

Pharmacy Conversions and Calculations

Learning Objectives

1 Develop consistent methods for answering calculations questions for a certification exam.

2 Convert temperatures between the Fahrenheit and Celsius systems.

3 Convert standard time into military time.

4 Understand the concepts for solving problems using ratio and proportion techniques.

5 Convert common systems of measurement into the metric system.

6 Apply dimensional analysis in solving pharmacy dosage calculations that also include conversions.

7 Calculate oral drug dosages using proportions.

8 Calculate the dose of a drug based on the patient's weight.

9 Compute concentration percentages and the amounts of diluents needed to make desired dosage concentrations.

Access eBook links for resources and an exam generator, with 1,000+ questions.

Pharmacy conversions and dosage calculations are a major component of any pharmacy technician certification exam. Although some students express apprehension about this part of the exam, with the right preparation and sufficient study, this challenge can become a source of confidence and satisfaction. Conversions and pharmacy calculations are covered in domain 6 of the PTCE and topic area 3 in the ExCPT. This chapter and its examples as well as the end-of-chapter "Sample the Exam" practice problems and the exam generator accessed through the eBook or Navigator+ provide excellent preparation for your certification exam and career as a pharmacy technician.

Although there are often numerous ways to approach a pharmacy calculation problem, developing consistent approaches to the different types of problems will help you develop assurance in finding accurate solutions. Being precise in your conversions and calculations as a pharmacy technician will mean safety for your patients and trust from the pharmacists. That is why math questions are so significant a part of the PTCE and ExCPT. Table 2.1 offers helpful tips for answering calculation questions on a certification exam.

TABLE 2.1 Tips for Calculation Questions

- Read each problem carefully. The difficulty with word problems is usually found in the words rather than in the math.
- Make certain you understand exactly what the question is asking.
- Approach each problem in a methodical way.
- Be aware that some questions contain unnecessary information.
- Review the answer choices, and eliminate those that do not make logical sense—those too far out of the range of possibility or having the wrong measurement units.
- Understand that there may be multiple ways to solve the problem. Choose one method and stick with it.
- Take time to write out the applicable units of measurement when setting up a problem, and calculate the answer in the appropriate unit of measurement.
- Do not panic. If you are stumped, take a moment to review. The approach will likely become clear. If not, pick an answer in the range of possibility, flag the question, and come back after finishing other questions.
- Make certain the answer is in the correct unit(s) of measure. If the units do not correlate, rework the problem.
- Double-check the placement of the decimal in the final answer.

Reviewing Conversion Formulas and Measurements

Practice Tip

The refrigerator should be maintained between 2°C and 8°C and freezers between -25°C and -10°C.

To help you answer the calculation questions in a timely manner in a certification exam, memorize the common conversion formulas and amounts, and practice using them.

Temperature Conversions

When converting temperatures between Celsius and Fahrenheit, you have to apply formulaic equations. Table 2.2 lists the options, which are important for pharmacy technicians to know. For instance, technicians are often asked to monitor refrigerator and freezer temperatures to ensure that the pharmaceuticals are properly stored. If a frozen nafcillin IV solution needs to be kept at -15°C, what would that be on the freezer's Fahrenheit thermometer? You would calculate $(-15 \times 1.8) + 32 = 5°F$. Example 2.1 shows the reverse processes.

Study Idea

Memorize your favorite temperature conversion equations.

TABLE 2.2 Conversion Formulas for Temperature

From Celsius to Fahrenheit	$(°C \times \frac{9}{5}) + 32 = °F$
	$(°C \times 1.8) + 32 = °F$
From Fahrenheit to Celsius	$(°F - 32) \div \frac{9}{5} = °C$
	$(°F - 32) \times 5/9 = °C$
	$(°F - 32) \div 1.8 = °C$

Example 2.1

NuvaRings must be refrigerated at a temperature between 36°F and 45°F before dispensing. Calculate the equivalent temperatures in degrees Celsius. (Two different but equivalent formulas will be applied.)

Calculate the Celsius equivalents of 36°F and 45°F.

$$°C = (36 - 32) \times \frac{5}{9}; \quad °C = 2.2$$

$$°C = (45 - 32) \div 1.8; °C = 7.2°$$

The refrigerator must be kept between Celsius 2.2° and 7.2° for NuvaRings.

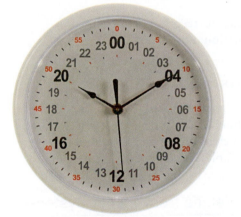

Twenty-four-hour clocks begin at midnight each day, and the first twelve hours until noon are similar to the normal clock. From noon to midnight, the counting continues after 12 instead of starting to count again.

Time Conversions

While the 12-hour clock works for most everyday activities, it has become common internationally in healthcare to use the 24-hour clock, also called **military time**. The military system counts from midnight continuously until 2359 (written in international time as 23:59), to start again at 0000, the next midnight as shown on the clock on the left. This means that all of the p.m. hours in the 12-hour clock are eliminated, in favor of escalating hours up to 24, as shown on Table 2.3.

The pharmacy technician must be able to convert between the two time systems for the correct administration time to be labeled on the medication in a hospital. Review the Example 2.2 on the next page to see the steps of conversion.

💡 **Study Idea**

Some hospitals use international time notation, which uses the 24-hour clock, but inserts the colon between the hours and the minutes, as in 23:59 (11:59 p.m.).

TABLE 2.3 Time Conversions

12-Hour Clock	24-Hour Clock
Midnight – 12:00 a.m.	0000
12:30 a.m.	0030
1:00 a.m.	0100 (the first hour)
2:30 a.m.	0230
6:00 a.m.	0600 (the 6th hour)
8:45 a.m.	0845
Noon – 12:00 p.m.	1200 (the 12th hour)
4:45 p.m.	1645
6:00 p.m.	1800 (the 18th hour)
9:30 p.m.	2130
11:00 p.m.	2300 (the 23rd hour)

Example 2.2

A patient is to receive the intravenous antibiotic penicillin every 6 hours around the clock. If the first dose is taken at 8 a.m., when will the next dose be taken in military time?

Step 1 Calculate what time it would be for the next dose using the familiar 12-hour clock.

$$8 \text{ a.m.} + 6 \text{ hours} = 2 \text{ p.m.}$$

Step 2 Since 2 p.m. is after the noon time, think of the military clock count continuing for the 2 hours after 12 noon from 1200:

$$0200 + 1200 = 1400 \text{ hours (fourteen hundred hours or}$$
$$14:00 \text{ international time).}$$

Earlier Measurement Systems and Conversions

As you know, pharmacy practices over the years have utilized three different measurement systems, avoirdupois, apothecary, and household systems. In health care today, most all products are dosed in metric units, such as milligrams or milliliters. Memorize the common conversion values in Table 2.4 before taking the exam.

TABLE 2.4 Common Conversion Values from Earlier Systems

Volume	Weight
1 gr = 65 mg	1 oz = 30 g
1 tsp = 5 mL	1 lb = 454 g
1 tbsp = 15 mL	2.2 lb = 1 kg
1 fl oz = 30 mL	
1 cup = 240 mL	
1 pt = 480 mL	
1 qt = 960 mL	
1 gal = 3,840 mL	

The avoirdupois, apothecary, and household systems have survived. However, with very few exceptions, these measurements are not used in general pharmacy practice today and can lead to medication errors if put into practice. The only apothecary unit still sometimes used in prescription stock labels is the grain (gr), a dry weight measure. A common example can be seen in aspirin, acetaminophen, and ferrous sulfate products, which are sometimes labeled as 5 grains (5 gr), an amount approximately equivalent to 325 mg (since 1 gr = 65 mg).

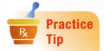
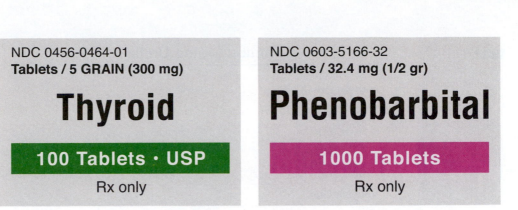

NDC 0456-0464-01
Tablets / 5 GRAIN (300 mg)

Thyroid

100 Tablets · USP

Rx only

NDC 0603-5166-32
Tablets / 32.4 mg (1/2 gr)

Phenobarbital

1000 Tablets

Rx only

But there are problems: 1 grain can also be equal to 60 mg (as in Armour Thyroid) and 64.8 mg (as in phenobarbital). Often the differences depend on whether the drug is synthetic, semisynthetic, or naturally sourced. Some drug stock labels reflect both units of measurement (see phenobarbital image). Because of such confusion, the grain (gr) is not a safe measurement to use and is being phased out.

The household system is based on the apothecary system and was used for cooking and helping patients take their medications at home. Because some OTC medications still use the household system of teaspoons and tablespoons for dosages, it is essential to memorize how they compare to the metric system.

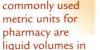
Knowing the Metric System

As you are well aware, the metric system is based on multiples of ten, one hundred, and one thousand. The advantages of the metric system include the following:

- consistent measurement values across the world and fields of use, especially science
- consistent decimal notation in which units are based on multiples of ten
- consistent escalation and de-escalation in value for easy memory and use
- same correlations of value proportion in units of measurement across the dimensions of length, volume, and weight

The metric system of measurements is considered universal, so it is necessary to memorize the units of measurement in Table 2.5 on the next page.

Prefixes, or syllables placed at the beginnings of words, are added to the names of the basic metric units to specify a particular size of unit measure, such that *milli-* (meaning 1/1,000) can be added to *liter* to form a new unit milliliter, or one-thousandth of a liter. The set of standardized metric prefixes based on powers of 10 is called the Système International (SI)—see Table 2.6 on the next page.

Converting to Proportionally Larger or Smaller Metric Units

The most common calculations in pharmacy involve conversions up to higher metric proportional amounts and down to lower ones using milligrams, grams, and kilograms, or milliliters and liters. Multiplying or dividing by 1,000 takes you up and down the unit steps. After properly doing your calculations, you end up moving the decimal point positions to the left to convert to larger units; or you move the decimal point to the right to convert to smaller units. Table 2.7 and Figure 2.1 show how these conversions work.

TABLE 2.5 Common Metric Units

Measurement Unit	Equivalent
Length: Meter	
1 meter (m)	100 centimeters (cm)
1 centimeter (cm)	0.01 meter (m); 10 millimeters (mm)
1 millimeter (mm)	0.001 meter (m); 1,000 micrometers or microns (mcm)
Volume: Liter	
1 liter (L)	1,000 milliliters (mL); 1,000 cubic centimeters (cc)
1 milliliter (mL)	0.001 liter (L); 1,000 microliters (mcL)
Weight: Gram	
1 gram (g)	1,000 milligrams (mg)
1 milligram (mg)	0.001 grams (g); 1,000 micrograms (mcg)
1 kilogram (kg)	1,000 grams (g)

TABLE 2.6 Système International Prefixes

Prefix	Symbol	Meaning
kilo-	k	one thousand times (basic unit $\times\ 10^3$, or unit $\times$ 1,000)
*hecto-**	h	one hundred times (basic unit $\times\ 10^2$, or unit $\times$ 100)
*deca-**	da	ten times (basic unit $\times$ 10)
no prefix (*liter, gram,* or *meter*)	L, g, or m	base unit
*deci-**	d	one-tenth (basic unit $\times\ 10^{-1}$, or unit $\times$ 0.1)
*centi-**	c	one-hundredth (basic unit $\times\ 10^{-2}$, or unit $\times$ 0.01)
milli-	m	one-thousandth (basic unit $\times\ 10^{-3}$, or unit $\times$ 0.001)
micro-	mc or μ	one-millionth (basic unit $\times\ 10^{-6}$, or unit $\times$ 0.000001)

* These units are generally not used in pharmacy.

TABLE 2.7 Common Metric Conversions

Conversion	Instruction	Example
kilograms (kg) to grams (g)	multiply by 1,000 (*move decimal point three places to the right*)	6.25 kg = 6,250 g
grams (g) to milligrams (mg)	multiply by 1,000 (*move decimal point three places to the right*)	3.56 g = 3,560 mg
milligrams (mg) to grams (g)	multiply by 0.001 (*move decimal point three places to the left*)	120 mg = 0.120 g
liters (L) to milliliters (mL)	multiply by 1,000 (*move decimal point three places to the right*)	2.5 L = 2,500 mL
milliliters (mL) to liters (L)	multiply by 0.001 (*move decimal point three places to the left*)	238 mL = 0.238 L
microliters (μL or mcL) to milliliters (mL)	multiply by 1,000 (*move decimal point three places to the left*)	1,000 μL or mcL = 1 mL

FIGURE 2.1
Steps Worth a Thousand

Metric units of measurement go up and down by steps of 1,000. Remember each step is separated by three decimal places, by a power of one thousand. To go to smaller measurements, move from left to right. For larger measurements, move from right to left.

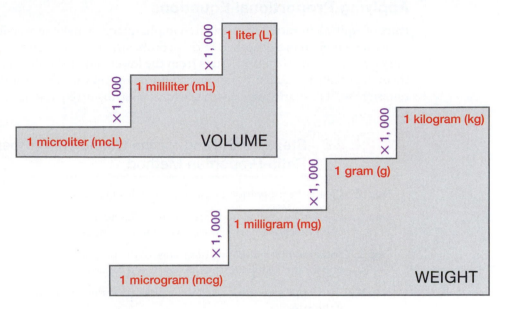

Reviewing Ratio-Proportion Equations

Perhaps no mathematical technique is used more frequently in pharmacy practice than that of ratios and proportions. Ratios and proportion equations are used in converting measurement units, determining dosages, and in compounding formulas.

Proportions with Means and Extremes

Study Idea

Pharmacy technicians should always double-check the units in a proportion, the setup of their ratio equations, and their calculations. The pharmacist needs to check them as well.

Two ratios that have the same value when simplified are different ways of saying the same ratio, such as 1/2 and 4/8. They are called equivalent ratios. A pair of equivalent ratios together is called a **proportion**. Because the ratios are equivalent, you can multiply the numerator of the first ratio by the denominator of the second; and it will equal the denominator of the first ratio multiplied by the numerator of the second ratio. The first and fourth numbers, or outside numbers, are called the **extremes**, and the second and third numbers, or inside numbers, are called the **means**.

For instance, $\dfrac{3}{4} = \dfrac{15}{20}$ is the same as:

$$3{:}4 \quad = \quad 15{:}20$$

means

extremes

$3 \times 20 = 60$ and $4 \times 15 = 60$; or $3 \times 20 = 4 \times 15$

When you see it with the colors above, you can see why some people call this cross multiplication the "butterfly technique" or butterfly multiplying.

This cross multiplying can be stated as a rule:

If $a/b = c/d$, then $\mathbf{a} \times \mathbf{d} = \mathbf{b} \times \mathbf{c}$

extremes = means

Applying Proportional Equations

Pairs of equivalent ratios are used often in pharmacy to make conversions from one measurement system to another. In these problems, it is common to express the unknown quantities by using letters from the lower end of the alphabet to represent them, especially x, y, and z. Because x can get mixed up with the x for the multiplication sign, we'll primarily use y and z. See tips on setting up equations in Table 2.8.

TABLE 2.8	Steps for Solving for the Unknown Number in the Ratio-Proportion Method
Step 1.	Create the proportion by placing the ratios in fraction form.
Step 2.	Check that the unit of measurement in the numerators is the same and the unit of measurement in the denominators is the same.
Step 3.	Solve for y by multiplying both sides of the proportion by the denominator of the ratio containing the unknown, and cancel.
Step 4.	Check your answer by seeing if the product of the means equals the product of the extremes.

Pharm Facts

Remember, when calculating with rounded off conversion measurements, the margin of error becomes much larger when larger volumes are multiplied. In general, use more precise amounts for larger calculations, such as for IVs, and round down for pediatric calculations.

Using Ratio-Proportion Equations to Convert Measurements to Metrics

To convert any other system to metrics, first convert the units into decimals and then apply the conversion amount ratios listed on Table 2.4 on page 62 in ratio-proportion equations. Most conversion amounts have been rounded to whole numbers for ease of use. For example, when converting from fluid ounces to milliliters, it is common practice to round 29.57 mL to 30 mL.

Rounding off, though, introduces a margin of error that increases in bigger volumes or weights. Consider converting a household pint (16 fl oz) to metric units, which is a common bottle size for bulk solutions. When you multiply the rounded off 30 mL by 16, it equals 480 mL. Yet when calculating with the more exact 29.57 mL, the answer is equal to only 473.12 mL—a difference of almost 7 mL! However, pharmacy solutions bottled in 8 or 16 fluid ounce containers are usually dosed out in 30 mL increments. So you may use the rounded 30 mL value for a fluid ounce and the rounded 480 mL for a pint when performing pharmacy calculations for this chapter, but it is important to be aware of this issue of precision.

Practice the ratio-proportion method for calculating conversions, going through the steps outlined in Example 2.3.

Example 2.3

A patient weighs 66 pounds (lb). What is her weight in kilograms?
You are seeking to find out: 66 lb = y kg. The conversion rate is: 1 kg = 2.2 lb.

Step 1 Convert the problem into fractions: $\dfrac{y \text{ kg}}{66 \text{ lb}} = \dfrac{1 \text{ kg}}{2.2 \text{ lb}}$

Step 2 Set up the proportional ratio equation:

$$y \text{ kg} \times 2.2 \text{ lb} = 66 \text{ lb} \times 1 \text{ kg}; \quad \text{or } 2.2 \text{ (lb) } y \text{ kg} = 66 \text{ lb};$$

$$\text{So } y \text{ kg} = \frac{66 \cancel{\text{lb}}}{2.2 \cancel{\text{lb}}} = 30 \text{ kg}$$

Since the pounds are equally distributed, you can cancel them as they balance each other out.

$$y \text{ kg} = 30 \text{ kg}. \text{ The patient weighs 30 kg.}$$

Using Dimensional Analysis to Calculate Conversions

Another way to do many conversion is a process known as **dimensional analysis calculation**. This is a very intimidating term for a very simple process that uses techniques *you already know*: multiplying by fractions that equal "1" and canceling out elements that balance each other. In fact, dimensional analysis is often considered an accurate shortcut, cutting out extra steps to get to the same end by combining numerous steps into one equation.

You already know that if you multiply anything by 1, the amount stays the same. So if you are trying to convert from pounds to kilograms, you multiply the pounds by a fraction of different measurements that equal the value of one, as in 1 kg/2.2 lb.

When working out the equation, the known units on the top and bottom of the multiplication equation cancel, or balance, each other out, leaving a clean equation with the answer being in the new unit of measurement (as shown in the following instance). That is why dimensional analysis is also known as "unit cancellation" or "calculation by cancellation". Review the steps in Example 2.4.

Example 2.4

Consider you have a prescription for:

> ℞   **Acetaminophen 400 mg tablets**

However, the stock bottle only measures the drug in grains. How many grains of acetaminophen are prescribed?

Step 1 Look up the conversion rate for grains to mg. Table 2.4 shows the conversion rate is 1 gr = 65 mg, which means 1 gr/65 mg equals 1. Set up the equation with the unknown factor on one side and the known information multiplied by the conversion rate on the other (the unit of measurement you are seeking should be on the top of the conversion fraction).

$$y = 400 \text{ } \cancel{\text{mg}} \times \frac{1 \text{ gr}}{65 \text{ } \cancel{\text{mg}}} ;$$

$$\text{So } y = \frac{400 \text{ gr}}{65} ; \text{ then } y = 6.153846 \text{ gr}$$

Step 2 Round the answer to an amount that can be measured with the pharmacy balance or down to the nearest whole number. This means 6 gr should be measured and used in the prescription. If you have tablets of 3 gr each, you will need two tablets per dose.

Alternative Method and Ratio-Proportion Checking System: To double-check, the conversion can also have been done as a ratio proportion equation using the butterfly technique of multiplying the ends and means and then cancelling measurement units to come up with the same end equation and answer. This is why some people see dimensional analysis as a short cut.

$$\frac{y\text{ gr}}{400\text{ mg}} = \frac{1\text{ gr}}{65\text{ mg}} \quad \text{so } y \times 65\text{ mg} = 400\text{ mg} \times 1\text{ gr}; \quad 65\text{ mg } y = 400\text{ mg}$$

$$y = 400\text{ mg} \times \frac{1\text{ gr}}{65\text{ mg}} = 6.153846....\text{ gr}; \quad \text{rounded to 6 gr.}$$

Calculating Dosages

A common use of ratios in dosage calculations is to express the number of parts of one substance contained in another substance of known parts. For example, suppose that there are 3 mL of an ophthalmic solution dissolved in a total of 60 mL sterile saline solution. Thus it would be expressed as the ratio 3:60 or 3/60, which reduces to 1/20. In other words, the ratio of the active ingredient to the sterile saline solution is 1 to 20, or 1 part in 20 parts.

Drug Ratio Strengths

Drug stock is generally labeled with the concentration ratio of an active ingredient in the carrying vehicle: w/v (weight/volume) and v/v (volume/volume) for solutions and suspensions, and w/w (weight in weight) for solid formulations. The term **ratio strength** in pharmacy refers to this concentration level of active ingredient to the completed product or substance that holds it—the first number being the number of parts (numerator) of active ingredient compared to the total, which is the second number (denominator).

$$\frac{active\ ingredient\ (by\ weight\ or\ volume)}{final\ product\ (weight\ or\ volume)}$$

You will use the ratio strengths of stock medications versus prescribed/ordered medications in proportion equations to determine the missing information—both in practice and in your certification exam.

A crucial step is arranging the equation properly with y for the missing information. Because a proportion is a mathematical comparison of similar things, it is essential that the units of measurement are the same in the numerators and are the same in denominators. On the one side of the equation, write out the strength/concentration of the available drug and on the other, the prescribed strength/concentration. (Or you can do vice versa, with the prescription on one side and the in-stock on the other.) You can review how this is done in Example 2.5.

Example 2.5

You need to make 35 mL of a distilled water solution with a concentration 2 grams sodium chloride (salt) to each 7 mL of distilled water (or 2 g: 7 mL). How many grams of sodium chloride are needed?

Step 1 2 g: 7 mL = y g: 35 mL; put into fractional form: $\dfrac{2\text{ g}}{7\text{ mL}} = \dfrac{y\text{ g}}{35\text{ mL}}$

Step 2 By the proportional rule, $2 \times 35 = 7y$, which equals $7y = 70$;

Step 3 That means that y alone is equal to 70 divided by 7   or $y = 70 \div 7$
or $y = 10$.   This leaves $y = 10$ grams of sodium chloride.

Converting a Strength Ratio to a Percent

Study Idea

When ratio strengths are given, it is often easiest to convert them into percentages for calculation: liquid v/v percents are usually % mL/100 mL as in 70% isopropyl alcohol (IPA); solid w/w percents are % g/100 g.

Prescription strengths can also be expressed in a ratio not of specific measurements to each other but of percentages of the whole. For instance, the percent strength of a volume/volume ratio would be y mL/100 mL and a weight/weight ratio would be z g/100 g.

To express a strength ratio as a percent, designate the first number of the ratio as the numerator and the second number as the denominator. Multiply the fraction by 100 ($^{100}/_1$) and add a percent sign after the product.

To turn 1:20 into a percent, you take $\dfrac{1}{20} \times \dfrac{100}{1} = 5\%$

For 5:1, you do the same: $\dfrac{5}{1} \times \dfrac{100}{1} = 5 \times 100 = 500\%$

For 1:2.5, you take $\dfrac{1}{2.5} \times \dfrac{100}{1} = \dfrac{100}{2.5}$;   then $100 \div 2.5 = 40\%$

To see how this is applied, see Example 2.6.

Example 2.6

If the ratio of dexamethasone in a 100 mL oral suspension is 1:3, what is the percent of dexamethasone in the suspension?

$$\frac{1}{3} \times \frac{100}{1} = \frac{100}{3}; \quad \text{then } 100 \div 3 = 33\%.$$

Concentrations with Weight-in-Volume Percentage Strength

Put Down Roots

Remember the word *percent* literally means per hundred.

When the strength or concentration of a solution is expressed as a weight-volume percentage, the notation is g/mL. For example, as noted earlier, the intravenous fluid D_5W is a shorthand notation for a solution of 5% dextrose in water, or 5% of the 100 mL volume of final solution of dextrose dissolved in water. Therefore, a D_5W solution can be expressed mathematically as:

$$\frac{5 \text{ g dextrose}}{\text{to every 100 mL solution}}$$

Remembering this, you can use this fractional form to solve a problem with weight-to-volume solution (g/mL) concentrations, as in Example 2.7.

Example 2.7

How many milligrams of dextrose are in 75 mL of D_5W? Express D_5W as a percentage fraction, and then determine the amount of dextrose in grams required to create this concentration in 75 mL. Convert that amount to milligrams in the final answer.

Step 1 Put into an equivalent ratio and proportion equation, and do the calculations:

$$\frac{5\text{ g}}{100\text{ mL}} = \frac{y\text{ g}}{75\text{ mL}}; \quad \text{then } 100\,y = 5 \times 75;$$

$$100\,y = 375\text{ g}; \quad \text{so } y = 3.7\text{ g}$$

Step 2 According to the original proportion, this is 3.7 g of dextrose. This is not the final answer, however. The question asked how many *milligrams*, not how many *grams*. Certification exams may offer this as an answer for a distractor choice. *Be careful not to jump at an attractive wrong answer.*

For the correct answer, convert 3.7 g into milligrams.

$3.7\text{ g} \times 1000 = 3{,}750\text{ mg}$. There are 3,750 mg of dextrose in 75 mL of D_5W.

Alternative Method with Dimensional Analysis To simplify, you can make this into one dimensional analysis equation:

$$y = \frac{5\;\cancel{g}}{100\;\cancel{mL}} \times 75\;\cancel{mL} \times \frac{1000\text{ mg}}{1\;\cancel{g}}; \quad y = 3{,}750\text{ mg}$$

Converting a Percent to a Strength Ratio

Study Idea

If you move decimal places to change a decimal to a percent, always double-check by multiplying by 100.

To convert a percent to a ratio, you reverse the process by dividing the percent by 100 and expressing the fraction as a ratio by making the numerator the first number and the denominator the second number.

$$2\% = 2 \div 100 = \frac{2}{100}; \quad \text{then } 2{:}100$$

You can simplify this ratio by reducing the original fraction—dividing both the numerator and denominator by 2 to get:

$$\frac{1}{50} = 1{:}50$$

To see how this is applied, see Example 2.8.

Example 2.8

The pharmacy receives a prescription for:

℞ 100 mL IV bag of 4% lidocaine to treat arrhythmia

The active ingredient of lidocaine solution comes in grams. What is the ratio of grams to mL of sterile water solution?

$$4\% = 4\text{ g} \div 100\text{ mL} = \frac{4\text{ g}}{100\text{ mL}} \text{ means 4 grams of lidocaine in 100 mL.}$$

$$\frac{4\text{ g}}{100\text{ mL}} \text{ simplifies to } \frac{1}{25}; \quad \text{or 1:25 ratio—or } \frac{1\text{g}}{25\text{ mL}}.$$

Calculating Tablet Dosages

For solid oral formulations, the drug strength of the medication stock supply is displayed on the container's label as drug weight per tablet or capsule. Pharmacy technicians need to know how to use an equal proportion equation to calculate the proper dosage amount to fulfill the prescription strength per dosage form. You can see these steps done one at a time in Example 2.9.

Example 2.9

The prescriber ordered:

> ℞ **Lamotrigine 87.5 mg PO twice a day, every 12 h**

On hand, you have a drug stock of lamotrigine 25 mg scored tablets. So how would many tablets would you dispense?

Step 1 Set up the equation:

$$strength\ on\ hand = amount\ to\ be\ dispensed$$

$$\frac{25\ mg}{1\ tablet} = \frac{87.5\ mg}{y\ tablets}$$

Step 2 Cross multiply.

$$25\,y = 87.5 \times 1;\ \ so\ 25\,y = 87.5\ tablets$$

Step 3 Divide both sides of the equation by 25, so $y = 87.5 \div 25$;

So $y = 3.5$ tablets   3.5 tablets equal an 87.5 mg dose.

Keep in mind that not all tablets are scored, so you may have to split some before dispensing. Scored tablets usually have a line down the middle with an equivalent amount of drug distributed on each side of the line. This scoring will help the patient cut the tablet in half as is needed for the dosage.

Calculating Dosages Using Body-Weight Ratios

The prescribed or ordered dosage for a specific patient may be calculated based on the patient's body weight in metric kilograms rather than pounds. So these dosage calculations have to include calculating the weight conversions from pounds. During a certification exam, be careful to remember this step and that 1 kg = 2.2 lb. Example 2.10 shows the process.

Example 2.10

Sally S., a 50-year-old patient who weighs 140 pounds, has a seizure disorder. She has been prescribed the following:

> ℞ **Levetiracetam 15 mg/kg po BID**

What is the dosage that Sally has been prescribed per day?

Step 1 Calculate Sally's weight in kilograms.

$$\frac{y \text{ kg}}{140 \text{ lb}} = \frac{1 \text{ kg}}{2.2 \text{ lb}}; \quad \text{So } \mathbf{2.2}\,y = \mathbf{140}\,\text{kg};$$

$$y = \frac{1 \times 140}{2.2}; \quad \text{so } y = 63.6363... \text{ rounded down to } 63.64 \text{ kg}$$

Step 2 Calculate the dose Sally could receive per day:

$$\frac{z \text{ mg}}{63.64 \text{ kg}} = \frac{15 \text{ mg}}{1 \text{ kg}}; \quad \text{so } z = 15 \times \frac{63.64}{1} \quad z = 954.6 \text{ mg twice a day.}$$

Two doses of 954.6 mg equals 1,909.2 mg, converted to 1.9 g. (Remember this, because the answer may need to be converted into grams.)

Alternative Method: Dimensional Analysis You could also have figured out this example with a dimensional analysis equation that included all steps in one:

$$y = 140 \text{ lb} \times \frac{1 \text{ kg}}{2.2 \text{ lb}} \times \frac{15 \text{ mg}}{1 \text{ kg}} \times 2 \times \frac{1 \text{ g}}{1000 \text{ mg}}; \quad y = \frac{420 \text{ g}}{220} \text{ or } 1.9 \text{ g}$$

Calculating Dosages for Children

Safety Alert

Always remember to round down the dosage for pediatric and neonatal patients rather than up for safety reasons.

Many medications have a wide range for recommended dosages because people don't come in one size. Patients' body shapes, sizes, bodily responses, and adverse reactions vary extensively, even among adults. Children are particularly vulnerable to problems in dosing because they vary even more as they go through their developmental stages. Since their cells, systems, and bodies are still in formation, wrong doses, particularly higher doses than are healthy for them, can do even more harm than to an adult.

Most pediatric prescribers favor those medications that have been specifically formulated by the manufacturer for pediatric doses rather than strict body weight ratios. However, there are times when a medical order comes in for calculating a child's portion of an adult-use drug. The prescriber or pharmacist will determine the proper calculation approach, which is often based on body surface area.

Applying Body Surface Area for Dosages

A dosing formula that considers both metric height and weight is called **body surface area (BSA)**. This formulation is calculated in square meters. Dosage prescriptions are then written as mg/m². The prescriber's or pharmacist's software determines this number and then the technician applies it. Physicians prescribing cancer chemotherapy drugs particularly use BSA dosing formulas so their dosages of these toxic drugs can be more precise. See Table 2.9 for US averages for BSA. As can be seen, these are very general averages since female adults of different ages would have different subcategory averages, as would males of different ages. Males and females who are 12 to 13 years old have different averages. Each of these categories could have very different averages for subcategories within them, so it is best to use the patient's BSA formula for dosages.

After the patient's BSA in m² has been determined, the technician uses the BSA dosing prescription in an equal proportion equation, which is something that will be tested in the PTCE. The process is shown step by step in Example 2.11:

$$\frac{y \text{ mg}}{patient's \text{ m}^2} = \frac{average\ adult\ dose \text{ mg}}{1 \text{ m}^2}$$

TABLE 2.9   Average US Pharmacy BSAs

General Body Type	Average BSA
Male adult	1.9 m^2
Female adult	1.6 m^2
12–13-year-olds	1.33 m^2
10 years	1.14 m^2
9 years	1.07 m^2
2 years	0.5 m^2
newborn	0.25 m^2

Example 2.11

To treat the breast cancer of Jenny, a 20 year-old patient with a BSA of 1.6 m^2, the oncologist writes a prescription for

> ℞   **Doxorubicin at a dose of 40 mg/1 m²**

Doxorubicin is toxic to the blood cells and heart in excessive doses. What is the proper dose?

$$\frac{y \text{ mg}}{1.6 \text{ m}^2} = \frac{40 \text{ mg}}{1 \text{ m}^2}$$

$$y \text{ mg} = 40 \text{ mg} \times 1.6; \quad y \text{ mg} = 64 \text{ mg}$$

The prescribed dose of doxorubicin is thus 64 mg.

Calculating Liquid Dosage Amounts

Practice Tip

First rule of thumb when substituting one drug concentration for another to fulfill a prescribed drug strength: follow the drug's directions for use, and set up your ratios based on the recommended ratios and prescribed strength.

When a drug is put into a solution, whether for oral use or a parenteral injection, the drug generally loses its properties as a solid and becomes one with the liquid. Even so, it is important to know how much of a given drug is contained in the liquid drug solution. For example, an amoxicillin oral suspension is manufactured in different strengths expressed as follows:

$$\frac{200 \text{ mg}}{5 \text{ mL}}; \quad \frac{400 \text{ mg}}{5 \text{ mL}}$$

These show two different milligram amounts of amoxicillin, both contained in 5 mL of oral drug solution. As explained earlier, this information is essential when setting up equations properly for determining the correct dosage amounts for a prescribed drug strength using an available stock of a different concentration.

Keep in mind that if the amount of active drug prescribed is larger or smaller than in the stock concentration, the medication volume dispensed of the stock medication must be proportionally larger or smaller. By setting up a proportion or using dimensional analysis, problems of calculating the right dosage using a stock concentration can be easily solved. You would follow the steps shown in Example 2.12.

Example 2.12

A prescriber orders:

R̸ **Amoxicillin 350 mg PO q12h**

You have on hand amoxicillin 400 mg/5 mL

Step 1 Begin by setting up the proportion equation

$$strength\ on\ hand = amount\ to\ be\ dispensed$$

$$\frac{400\ mg}{5\ mL} = \frac{350\ mg}{y\ mL}$$

Step 2 Cross-multiply.

$$400\,y = 350 \times 5; \quad 400\,y = 1{,}750$$

$$y = 4.375\ mL\ \ of\ \ \frac{400\ mg}{5\ mL}\ \ every\ 12\ hours$$

Step 3 Quick check: is this answer available in the proper unit of measurement and does it make sense? If the patient needs a dose of 350 mg of amoxicillin, and the pharmacy has 400 mg/5 mL in stock, the volume of antibiotic must be less than 5 mL, which 4.375 mL is. You could also do this calculation in one dimensional analysis equation:

$$y = 350\ \cancel{mg} \times \frac{5\ mL}{400\ \cancel{mg}}; \quad y = \frac{175}{40}; \quad y = 4.375\ mL;\ \text{reduced to } 4.4\ mL$$

Example 2.13

A prescription for a sick child is received from the emergency room on Saturday night for:

R̸ **Cephalexin 125 mg/5 mL for 4 mL *po* twice daily**

No other pharmacies are open in town. The pharmacy technician discovers that the pharmacy is out of stock on the 125 mg/5 mL concentration of the prescribed suspension, but has 250 mg/5 mL concentration in stock. The prescribed concentration could be ordered, but the child would be without medication until Monday at noon. Since the child needs 4 mL of a 125 mg/5 mL concentration, what is the amount of cephalexin per dose? How much of the 250 mg/5 mL stock concentration would be needed for this individual dose?

Step 1 Calculate the original prescribed dose for a child:

$$\frac{y\,\text{mg}}{4\,\text{mL}} = \frac{125\,\text{mg}}{5\,\text{mL}}$$

$$5y = 4 \times 125; \quad \text{so} \quad y = 500\,\text{mg} \div 5; \quad y = 100\,\text{mg}$$

This is the amount of cephalexin needed to be taken two times each day according to the prescription. How many mL of a 250 mg/5 mL suspension would be required to fill the prescription?

Step 2 Calculate the volume (mL) of the available concentration of $\frac{250\,\text{mg}}{5\,\text{mL}}$:

$$\frac{250\,\text{mg (stock)}}{5\,\text{mL}} = \frac{100\,\text{mg (prescribed)}}{y\,\text{mL}}$$

$$250\,y\,\text{mL} = 100 \times 5\,\text{mL}; \quad y\,\text{mL} = \frac{500}{250}; \quad y = 2\,\text{mL}$$

The 2 mL dosage of the stock 250 mg/5 mL concentration of cephalexin suspension is equal to the prescribed 4 mL dosage of the 125 mg/5 mL suspension. Consequently, the pharmacy fills the prescription and allows the sick child to begin treatment right away. The child will take this 2 mL twice a day.

Calculating Dilution Amounts

A pharmacy technician is often required to take a stock solution of a liquid and dilute it to a less concentrated solution. Though the pharmacist usually calculates the dilution amounts, the technicians double check the answers to ensure accuracy. If there is a discrepancy, the technician queries the pharmacist to recalculate. Dilution questions are common in the certification exams.

The first step in calculating dilutions is to determine the sufficient volume needed to decrease the drug concentration to the prescribed/ordered percentage. The amount you decrease in the concentration will be in inverse proportion to the amount you need to increase in volume for the diluted solution. That is why the following simple formula for figuring out the end volume or end strength works:

Study Idea

Always use the same units of measure on both sides of the dilution proportion equation. If needed, perform any necessary conversions (e.g., liters to milliliters, ratio to decimals) before inserting numerical values into the equation.

initial strength $\times$ *initial volume* = *final strength* $\times$ *final volume;* or *is* $\times$ *iv* = *fs* $\times$ *fv*

When solving a dilution problem, there are four variables—three from the problem statement and one missing that needs to be determined. It is advisable to write down the basic formula above, and plug in the terms from the word problem as shown in Example 2.14. There are two important things to remember about a dilution:

- The final volume will always be larger than the initial volume because water (or some other solvent) has been added.
- The final strength will always be less than the initial strength because this is a dilution.

Example 2.14

**You have 30 mL of a 20% *N*-acetylcysteine solution. How many milliliters of
10% solution can be made if sterile water is added?**

Step 1 Begin by identifying the known values given in the problem statement
and the value to be determined.

$$
\begin{aligned}
\textit{initial strength (is)} &= \text{20\% (or 0.2)} \\
\textit{initial volume (iv)} &= \text{30 mL} \\
\textit{final strength (fs)} &= \text{10\% (or 0.1)} \\
\textit{final volume (fv)} &= \text{to be determined}
\end{aligned}
$$

Step 2 After identifying the known values, enter them into the equation:

$$0.2 \times 30 \text{ mL} = 0.1 \times fv$$
$$6 \text{ mL} = 0.1 \, fv$$

Step 3 Calculate the value for the final volume by dividing 6 mL by 0.1.

$$\frac{6 \text{ mL}}{0.1} = fv; \quad 60 \text{ mL} = fv$$

It is clear that 60 mL of 10% *N*-acetylcysteine solution can be made 30 mL of 20%
solution. *N*-Acetylcysteine (Mucomyst) is an oral antidote for acetaminophen
overdose. It has the smell of rotten eggs.

Calculating Amounts of Diluent to Add for Proper Dilution Concentration

A pharmacy technician may also be asked to calculate the volume of diluent that must
be added to reach the prescriber/ordered volume. For these problems, remember the
following equation.

final volume – initial volume = diluent volume

Although this second step uses subtraction to determine the amount of diluent needed, you will actually be adding the diluent to the original concentration.
Questions of this sort are also common on a certification exam. Example 2.15 builds
on the previous example but requires one additional step.

Example 2.15

**Now that you have determined your final volume of the 10%
N-acetylcyteine solution will be 60 mL, how much water will be added to
the 20% solution to make the required product?**

Step 1 Begin by identifying the known values given in the problem statement
and the value to be determined.

$$
\begin{aligned}
\textit{final volume} &= \textit{60 mL;} \\
\textit{initial volume} &= \textit{30 mL}
\end{aligned}
$$

Step 2 Enter the known values into the equation:

$$60 \text{ mL} - 30 \text{ mL} = 30 \text{ mL needs to be added.}$$

Study Idea

In dilutions, the volume increases from the initial solution to final solution as the strength or concentration decreases. Always make sure the answer makes sense in this context. If it does not, re-examine the question and insert the correct values into the equation.

On your certification exam, always read the dilution questions very carefully. They could be a two-part question (such as Examples 2.14 and 2.15 together), where you have to first calculate the final volume and then determine how much liquid is needed to to be added to reach this dilution. They almost certainly will offer the answer to the first part of the question as a distractor. So watch out and make sure you know what they are asking for!

Compounding-related dilution equations and examples will be covered in Chapter 5 on Nonsterile Compounding and Chapter 6 on Sterile and Hazardous Compounding.

Calculations for inventory and other retail math will be covered in Chapter 9, while calculations of days supply for insurance coverage will be covered in Chapter 10. In all calculations and conversions, the most important thing is practice, practice, practice to build up confidence!

STUDY SUMMARY

Calculations are an important component in the certification exams. Memorize the formulas for converting temperatures between Fahrenheit and Celsius systems. It is also important to be confident in converting times from the 12-hour clock to the 24-hour clock and back.

You also need to memorize the amounts for converting the most common apothecary, avoirdupois, and household measurements into the metric system. Practice converting between proportionally larger or smaller units of metric measurement.

Most pharmacy calculations for dosages and concentrations can be easily set up in ratio and proportion or dimensional analysis equations. Practice both calculating techniques, and utilize them to solve and check your answers. Dilution and other complex calculations add some more steps of simple math. For practice, start with the end of chapter "Sample the Exam" questions through the eBook link or Navigator+. Carefully read each test question to identify what is being asked and in what units. Be prepared to interpret concentration percentages, and utilize them in your calculations.

ADDITIONAL RESOURCES

For more in-depth explanations, check out *Pharmacy Calculations for Technicians*, 6e from Paradigm Education Solutions. To master and extend the material presented in this chapter, take advantage of the resources available through the eBook resources links. These include digital supplements, study resources, and a practice exam generator with 1,000+ exam-style questions. End-of-chapter tests are accessible through the eBook for individuals using the self-study course and through Navigator+ for individuals enrolled in the instructor-guided course.

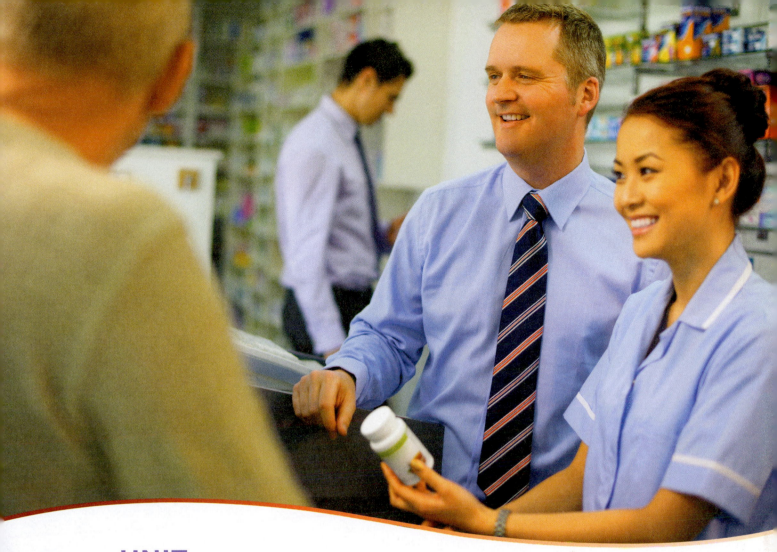

Chapter 3   Pharmacy Law and Regulations   83

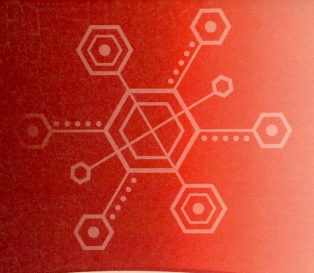

3

Pharmacy Law and Regulations

Learning Objectives

1 Be familiar with landmark legislation pertinent to the practice of pharmacy.

2 Identify legislation that affects patient counseling and confidentiality of health records as required by HIPAA, and sale of pseudoephedrine products.

3 Know the definition of a controlled drug and schedule of restricted classes.

4 Identify the classes of controlled drugs.

5 Identify three characteristics that differentiate a Schedule II prescription from other prescriptions.

6 Recognize situations that may indicate potential abuse or forged prescriptions and how to verify a prescriber's DEA number.

7 Understand the fill, refill, and transfer restrictions and legal record-keeping requirements for Schedule II through V medications.

8 Know DEA-mandated ordering, inventory, disposal, and recordkeeping requirements for Schedule II, III, and IV medications.

9 Be familiar with nationally recognized professional standards that affect pharmacy operations.

10 Define standard of care and ethics, and apply examples to pharmacy practice.

Access eBook links for resources and an exam generator, with 1,000+ questions.

The practice of pharmacy is governed by numerous laws and regulations. The pharmacy technician needs to be familiar with these laws and regulations and their effect on various issues, such as patient privacy and counseling, product and ingredient safety, and controlled substances. This chapter covers these topics and discusses special requirements for handling controlled drugs, including storage, recordkeeping, inventory control, safety, and abuse potential. It also outlines the professional standards for products, services, and personal behavior. These are topics addressed in domain 2 of the PTCE and topic area 1 of the ExCPT.

Pharmacy Oversight

Pharmacy technicians must practice within federal laws and the laws of their state, as recommended by their state's board of pharmacy and passed by their state and municipal lawmakers. *The strictest law always applies when state and federal laws conflict.*

A timeline of the key federal laws affecting pharmacy that may be mentioned in a certification exam can be seen in Table 3.1.

Some of these laws require specific actions on the part of the technician, such as the laws and regulations governing the dispensing, ordering, inventory, disposal, and documentation of controlled drugs (covered in depth later in the chapter). Other key federal laws that affect pharmacy procedures that could be mentioned in a certification exam are described in more depth below.

Poison Prevention Packaging Act To prevent accidental childhood drug poisonings, the Poison Prevention Packaging Act was passed in 1970. This act, enforced by the Consumer Product Safety Commission, required that most OTC and prescription drugs be packaged in child-resistant containers that cannot be opened by 80% of children under age 5 but can be opened by 90% of adults. Upon request from a patient, a drug may be dispensed in a non-childproof container. In fact, the patient—not the prescriber—can make a blanket request that all their drugs be dispensed without child-resistant containers.

> **Study Idea**
>
> Remember that certain drugs are exempt from the Poison Prevention Packaging Act, such as nitroglycerine SL and oral birth control tablets in memory packs. More information can be found at the Consumer Product Safety Commission website.

TABLE 3.1 Timeline of Pharmacy-Related Federal Laws

Law	Year Passed	Significance to Pharmacy Practice
Pure Food and Drug Act	1906	First law to regulate the development, compounding, distribution, storage, and dispensing of drugs. It prohibited any false or misleading information on labels about drug strength or purity, and interstate transport or sale of adulterated or misbranded food or drugs.
Food, Drug, and Cosmetic Act (FDCA)	1938	Clearly defined adulteration and misbranding; created the US Food and Drug Administration (FDA); required that products be safe for human use and that manufacturers include product package inserts
Durham-Humphrey Amendments to FDCA	1951	Distinguished between prescription and nonprescription drugs; required that all drug products have adequate usage directions or bear the legend "Caution: Federal Law Prohibits without Prescription" and a label on OTC drugs that includes a list of active ingredients; allowed verbal prescription and refill requests to pharmacies by telephone
Kefauver-Harris Amendment to FDCA	1962	Required that drugs be safe and effective, and that pharmaceutical manufacturers file an Investigational New Drug Application (INDA) before starting clinical trials on human subjects to win FDA approval (amendment resulted from thalidomide case)
Comprehensive Drug Abuse Prevention and Control Act (Controlled Substances Act)	1970	Established the federal Drug Enforcement Administration (DEA); created a schedule of drugs that have the potential for abuse and/or addiction and categorized them into five classes
Poison Prevention Packaging Act	1970	Required child-resistant containers for most prescription and OTC drugs to prevent accidental ingestion and poisoning

Drug Listing Act	1972	Required National Drug Code (NDC) numbers be assigned to every marketed drug
Orphan Drug Act	1983	Provided tax incentives for developing and marketing drugs used to treat rare conditions (orphan drugs); established lifelong exclusive license for manufacturers that develop orphan drugs
Drug Price Competition and Patent Term Restoration Act	1984	Streamlined the FDA approval process for marketing generic drugs; extended the term of patents for companies that develop new drugs
Prescription Drug Marketing Act	1987	Prohibits the reimportation of drugs to the United States, except by the manufacturer
Anabolic Steroids Control Act	1990	Redefined anabolic steroids as Schedule III controlled substances
Omnibus Budget Reconciliation Act (OBRA)	1990	Required pharmacists to engage in drug utilization reviews (DURs) and offer Medicaid patients the option of free prescription counseling
Dietary Supplement Health and Education Act (DSHEA)	1994	Classified herbal supplements as food products rather than drugs; prohibited manufacturers of herbs and dietary supplements from making claims that their products treat or cure any specific disease or illness
Health Insurance Portability and Accountability Act (HIPAA)	1996	Addressed patient privacy concerns by requiring signing of a confidential annual HIPAA form outlining who has access to patient information; allowed employees to easily move their health insurance from one job to another; resulted in privacy-protection practices for the communicating, collecting storing, disclosing, and disposing of patient data
Comprehensive Methamphetamine Control Act	1996	Established methamphetamine as a dangerous addictive drug requiring legislative oversight, and control of the exportation, importation, and manufacturing of methamphetamine substances and its ingredient chemicals
Medicare Modernization Act	2003	Provided a voluntary prescription drug plan for Medicare patients for additional cost; created the health savings account (HSA); allowed pharmacists to get reimbursed for medication counseling and therapy management
FDA Modernization Act	2004	Changed federal legend to "Rx Only"; allowed pharmacists to compound for individual patients any product not commercially available
Combat Methamphetamine Epidemic Act (CMEA)	2005	Restricted sales of OTC drugs used in making methamphetamines (pseudoephedrine, ephedrine, and phenylpropanolamine), to limited amounts; stored behind counter with monitored sales (in some states, only by PharmD)
Patient Safety and Quality Improvement Act (PSQI)	2005	Promoted mechanisms for patient safety and continuous quality improvement; encouraged creation of Patient Safety Organizations (PSOs) to collect confidential information on medical errors to develop systematic changes for safety
Patient Protection and Affordable Care Act (ACA)	2010	Mandated universal health care coverage availability for US citizens; established health insurance exchanges; provided catastrophic coverage for high-cost illnesses; prohibited insurers from refusing coverage to those with preexisting conditions
Best Pharmaceuticals for Children Act (BPCA) and the Pediatric Research Equity Act (PREA)	2012	Passed to improve drug safety for children
Drug Quality and Security Act (DQSA)	2013	Established a national database to "track and trace" drug products through the supply chain from the manufacturer to the pharmacy or compounder to dispensing; must be implemented by 2023; required all compounding be overseen by licensed pharmacists and encouraged registration of all facilities

Omnibus Budget Reconciliation Act of 1990 This act, known as OBRA-90, mandated that pharmacies complete a drug utilization review (DUR) for medication dispensing to identify potential drug or supplement interaction or allergy warnings. The pharmacy technician should not override an interaction warning. The pharmacist must evaluate the warning and decide on the correct action. OBRA-90 required that free counseling with a pharmacist be offered to each Medicaid patient. State boards of pharmacy and private insurers adopted this policy as well, and it has now become the "standard of care" in all US community pharmacies.

Health Insurance Portability and Accountability Act Established in 1996, the Health Insurance Portability and Accountability Act (HIPAA) is responsible for ensuring the confidentiality of all health records, under penalty of law. All new patients to the pharmacy must be given a copy of the pharmacy's HIPAA privacy practices, and the patient must sign an acknowledement of receipt of the information. This document needs to be scanned into the patient's profile and stored for six years after the last affiliation with the patient. Technicians must be careful when dispensing and discussing patient's prescriptions so that the patient's confidential information is not overheard by other patients or staff. Patient cases cannot be shared or discussed with others not directly involved with their care because this breaks the confidentiality. All labels and printed documents must have the patient information marked out or be shredded before disposal. Violators of HIPAA can be fined and likely let go by their employers. For an overview of pertinent HIPAA guidelines for pharmacy, refer to the online course supplements accessed at the end of this chapter in the eBook.

Combat Methamphetamine Epidemic Act Established in 2005, the Combat Methamphetamine Epidemic Act (CMEA) limits and tracks the sale of OTC products that contain pseudoephedrine, ephedrine, and phenylpropanolamine, which can be used in the production of methamphetamine. OTC products with these active ingredients must be stored behind the counter and sales are *restricted to 3.6 grams total per week and 9 grams per 30 days*. Pharmacy technicians working under the direction of the pharmacist may handle the sale of pseudoephedrine but must make sure all required purchaser information is documented in an electronic or paper log that must be kept for two years. The electronic or hard copy log must contain the drug name and quantity, customer name and home address, date purchased and time, and customer's signature, completed with presentation of a legal photo ID with signature.

Medicare Modernization Act Pharmacy technicians must be aware of several prescription drug plans developed because of the Medicare Modernization Act of 2003. This act created the use of health savings accounts for patients. The Centers for Medicare & Medicaid Services regulates Medicare Part D prescriptions and dictates the documentation and patient counseling opportunities with the pharmacist that technicians have to provide in order for the claims of the Medicare prescriptions to be reimbursed (addressed in Chapter 10).

Patient Protection and Affordable Care Act The Affordable Care Act of 2010 established pathways to provide universal health care coverage access for all US citizens and provides catastrophic coverage for high-cost illnesses; it prohibits insurers from refusing coverage to those with pre-existing conditions. Technicians need to know how to direct patients without coverage to the state healthcare insurance exchanges.

Drug Quality and Security Act The Drug Quality and Security Act (DQSA) came about because of an incident where the New England Compounding Center produced an injectable steroid product contaminated with meningitis that harmed patients in 19 states, and the distribution was hard to trace to stop further harm. It has two parts: the Compounding Act and the Drug Supply Chain Security Act. The DQSA aims to decrease the number of counterfeit drugs and provide more safety oversight for compounding facilities. It requires the establishment of a national database to "track and trace" drug products through the supply chain from the manufacturer or compounding facility to the patient. This means DQSA documentation is required at the delivery of a manufactured or compounded product to a wholesaler and again when a product is delivered by the wholesaler to the pharmacy for dispensing or healthcare facility for administration. Technicians involved in inventory management need to understand the pharmacy documentation requirements (see Chapter 9).

Oversight Agencies and Organizations

Study Idea

Review how each of the agencies and organizations affect the practice of pharmacy.

National and state agencies and governing bodies were established to oversee the laws. Here are some of the key federal agencies that provide oversight:

- Food and Drug Administration (FDA)
- Drug Enforcement Administration (DEA)
- Centers for Disease Control and Prevention (CDC)
- Occupational Safety and Health Administration (OSHA)
- Health Care Financing Administration (HCFA) of the Department of Health & Human Services (HHS) and Centers for Medicare & Medicaid Services (CMS), which has authority over reimbursement under the Medicare and Medicaid government drug insurance programs
- Federal Trade Commission (FTC), which has authority over business practices like direct-to-consumer drug advertising
- Individual state boards of pharmacy.

Pharmacy practice is also overseen/guided by professional organizations, including the following:

- US Pharmacopeial Convention (USP)
- The Joint Commission (TJC), which is a professional hospital and healthcare system accreditation organization
- National Association of Boards of Pharmacy (NABP)
- American Pharmacists Association (APhA)
- American Society of Health-System Pharmacists (ASHP) International Pharmaceutical Federation
- National Pharmacy Technician Association, American Association of Pharmacy Technicians, and the Pharmacy Technician Educators Council.

Based on all the laws, rules, and guidelines from these sources, each community and institutional pharmacy *creates a policy and procedures manual that the technicians and pharmacists must follow.*

FDA Drug Labels and Recalls

Since the creation of the FDA, this agency has had the power to make manufacturers adhere to labeling and other regulations or have its products pulled from the shelves. A summation of the major labeling requirements can be found in Table 3.2.

TABLE 3.2 Drug Label Requirements (Legal and USP Standards)

Label Type	Description
Prescription Drug Label	Name/address/phone # of dispensing pharmacy, patient's name, prescriber's name, prescription number and Rx, date filled, drug name/strength/quantity/directions for use, name/initials of dispensing pharmacist or technician, patient address, expiration date, refill information, precautions, the statement "federal law prohibits dispensing without a prescription," and package insert on selected drugs; if it is a controlled drug substance, it needs the C-II, C-III, C-IV, or C-V designation clearly displayed.
OTC Label	Product name, manufacturer name and address, all ingredients (active or inactive), net contents, directions for use (drug's purpose, dosage amount and frequency, symptoms, route of administration), caution/warning labels, including if habit-forming drugs contained within
Unit Dose Label	Drug name, dose, strength, manufacturer's name, lot number, expiration date, barcode
Repackaged Medication Label	Patient's name (and room often) drug name, strength, dose, administration time, lot number, expiration date, barcode
Patient Package Insert	Name and description of the drug, indications and usage, dosage/administration information, contraindications, precautions, warnings, adverse reactions, drug abuse information (habit forming, tolerance dependence, addiction) overdose information, date of the most recent label revision. Patient package inserts must be distributed with the following drug classes: oral contraceptives and other hormone products containing estrogen, intrauterine contraceptive devices, diethylstilbestrol products, and metered-dose inhalers; for medications with REMS, MedGuides are required.
Nonsterile Compounded Products Label	Patient and physician names, name of preparation and date of compounding, internal ID or lot number, direction for use, storage requirements, pharmacist initials, and BUD
Compounded Sterile Product Label	Patient and room number, prescriber, solution and volume, drug name, strength, dosage, administration time and/or directions, storage requirements, BUD; infusion rate may also be needed.
Hazardous Drug Label	All drugs containing hazardous agents must include the proper labeling appropriate to the product, as noted previously, but also the yellow caution label. A safety sheet on administration instructions and cleanup must also be included.
National Drug Code (NDC)	Each drug produced by a manufacturer is identified with a specific NDC number. The FDA requests but does not require the NDC on each label, but the NDC makes the product trackable for community and hospital uses, so manufacturers include it. The NDC number is composed of three sets of numbers, which identify the manufacturer, drug, and package size.
• NDC first 5 #s	Manufacturer
• NDC second 4 #s	Specific drug and strength
• NDC last 2 #s	Package size

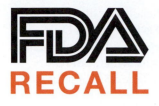

Drug Recall Classifications and Procedures

When an official alert for the drug is released by the manufacturer and/or FDA, known as a **drug recall**, the wholesaler will typically email or mail the drug recall information to the pharmacy, which includes: drug name, dose, NDC, lot number, expiration date, as well as the date and type of recall. The FDA can either mandate the recall if the threat to the public is severe enough or request a voluntary recall by the manufacturer, wholesaler, and pharmacy. Three classes of response levels of recalls exist, with Class I being the most urgent and dangerous. The FDA staff determines the class based on the healthcare situation, manufacturer actions, and customer data from MedWatch and other sources. Table 3.3 describes the levels of drug recalls.

TABLE 3.3 Recall Classes for Drugs

Class	Risk	Action Response
I	**Urgent, immediate danger**—A reasonable probability exists that the product will cause or lead to serious harm or even death.	All patients who have received or purchased this product should be notified.
II	**Moderate danger**—A probability exists that the product could cause adverse health events, but the events would be medically reversible or temporary.	Pharmacists and/or physicians must decide the best practice about notifying patients.
III	**Least danger**—The product will probably not cause an adverse health event, but there is a product quality problem.	Pharmacists and/or physicians must decide the best practice about notifying patients.
	Market withdrawl—The manufacturer chooses to take a drug product off the market because of minor problems until they are corrected. Pharmacies can follow suit with their drug inventory.	Pharmacists and/or physicians must decide the best practice about notifying patients.
	Medical device alert—If there is an unreasonable risk of harm, the FDA can mandate a manufacturer recall or request voluntary recall if less serious	All patients who have received or purchased this product should be notified or pharmacists decide depending on FDA mandates.

Study Idea

Memorize the difference beween Class I, II, and III drug recalls.

For all drug recalls, the technician must check the drug inventory and the retail shelves for each recalled item, pull it from inventory right away "to protect the patient," and notify the pharmacist, who signs a recall form. This form is then returned to the wholesaler with any recalled drug stock items. The pharmacist should also designate the appropriate plan to notify the patients who have received recalled drugs: notification in Class I is required; notification in the cases of Class II, III, and manufacturer withdrawl are up to the pharmacist's/physician's judgment. Cash register and insurance transaction reports are essential for tracking down the customers who purchased the recalled items. If patients have specific questions about what to do to counteract any medication problems from the recalled drug, the technician must connect them with the pharmacist.

After a recall is complete, the FDA makes sure that the product is destroyed or suitably "reconditioned" (recategorized with new conditions for sale). It also investigates why the product was defective and what actions should be taken. The FDA posts weekly reports on drug recalls that pharmacists should read. These are posted at http://PharmPractice6e.ParadigmCollege.net/SafetyReport1.

Web

Web

In an effort to prevent problems even before drugs are officially classified, the FDA also posts two pages of drugs pending recall classification. One is for Human Drug Product Recalls Pending Classification at http://PharmPractice6e.ParadigmCollege.net/SafetyReport2. The other is Non-Blood Product On-Going Recalls, which can be accessed at http://PharmPractice6e.ParadigmCollege.net/SafetyReport3. These sites should also be checked regularly to keep patients informed.

At times, pharmacists and technicians may see that the drug has been recalled or is pending classification. When a product has been identified on either list, it should be immediately pulled from the shelves, and the manufacturer should be notified that a return and credit are desired. Consumers can also return a recalled drug for refund or credit, per pharmacy or drug wholesaler policy.

Controlled Substances Regulations

The Drug Enforcement Administration (DEA) is the federal agency responsible for supervising and enforcing laws related to the use and sale of legal (and illegal) controlled substances. A controlled drug is defined as a substance that has the potential for abuse and physical or psychological dependence. The DEA monitors and tracks the flow of controlled drugs from manufacturer to wholesaler to pharmacy to patient.

Pharmacies, physicians and other prescribers, manufacturers, and wholesalers are required to register with the DEA to dispense, prescribe, produce, or distribute controlled drugs. Pharmacy technicians assist in pharmacies maintaining their legal dispensing status by following the dispensing and documentation regulations. The DEA, working with state drug agencies, investigates unauthorized prescribing and dispensing and conducts unannounced inspections of pharmacies.

Study Idea

Methadone for opioid detoxification and maintenance may only be administered at specially licensed clinics and hospitals.

Pharmacies that dispense narcotic drugs that are used in the treatment of substance abuse (e.g., methadone clinics) must complete a separate DEA registration annually. Suboxone (buprenorphine-naloxone) and Subutex (buprenorphine), which are *alternatives to methadone used in the treatment of narcotic-addicted patients, require a special X DEA number to dispense* at the local community pharmacy. *Methadone for opioid maintenance treatment may be dispensed only at properly licensed clinics.* The hospital or community pharmacy is allowed to dispense methadone if it is prescribed for pain management.

Drug Classifications

The 1970 Controlled Substances Act (CSA), as part of the Comprehensive Drug Abuse Prevention and Control Act, established the classification system for drugs with great potential for abuse. It categorized them into schedules denoted by Roman numerals. The lower the schedule number, the higher the risk of abuse. (See Table 3.4.) For a list of the classifications of commonly prescribed controlled substances, see Appendix B. Schedule I drugs, such as heroin, have the highest risk of abuse and dependence, and are therefore illegal.

Stock bottles of all controlled substances must be clearly marked with an uppercase Roman numeral with the uppercase letter C.

- CII or C-II
- CIII or C-III
- CIV or C-IV
- CV or C-V

TABLE 3.4 Controlled Drug Schedule Restrictions

Schedule	Manufacturer's Label	Abuse Potential	Accepted Medical Use	Examples
Schedule I	C-I	Highest potential for abuse—illegal	For research only; must have license to obtain; no accepted medical use in the United States	heroin, lysergic acid diethylamide (LSD), marijuana
Schedule II	C-II	High possibility of abuse, which can lead to severe psychological or physical dependence	Dispensing severely restricted; cannot be prescribed by telephone except in an emergency or hospice; no refills on prescriptions	morphine, oxycodone, meperidine, hydromorphone, fentanyl, methylphenidate, dextroamphetamine, hydrocodone with aspirin or acetaminophen
Schedule III	C-III	Less potential for abuse and addiction than C-II	Prescriptions can be refilled up to five times within six months if authorized by physician	testosterone or other anabolic steroids, buprenorphine/naloxone, buprenorphine, acetaminophen with codeine
Schedule IV	C-IV	Lower abuse potential than C-II and C-III; associated with limited physical or psychological dependence	Same as for Schedule III	benzodiazepines, zolpidem, eszopiclone (Lunesta), phenobarbital, carisoprodol, tramadol
Schedule V	C-V	Lowest abuse potential	Some sold without a prescription depending on state law; if so, purchaser must be over 18 and is required to sign log and show driver's license	liquid codeine combination cough preparations, diphenoxylate/atropine

Controlled substances must be prescribed for legitimate medical needs, and any controlled drug dispensed must include a transfer warning label that reads, "Caution: Federal law prohibits the transfer of this drug to any person other than the patient for whom it was prescribed."

Based on the public use and abuse of drugs on the market, the DEA and individual states have the option to re-evaluate and reclassify any drug. As noted, when there is a disparity between state and federal regulation of a drug, the strictest regulation is applied. For example, many states classified carisoprodol (Soma) as a Schedule IV drug (or C-IV) before the DEA approved the change to C-IV in 2011.

Marijuana, which is a Schedule I drug, has been made legal for specific purposes in certain states. However, the strictest law still applies in pharmacy, so DEA licensed pharmacies cannot dispense marijuana even if the state laws allow it.

Schedule II

Schedule II (C-II) drugs are legally prescribed and dispensed but are carefully regulated because of the high risk for abuse and dependence. Many of the top 200 prescribed drugs are in this category, including morphine, Percocet (oxycodone-acetaminophen),

Study Idea

When there is a disparity between federal, state and local laws, the strictest rule must be applied to your practice.

FIGURE 3.1
DEA 222 Form

When ordering
Schedule II
controlled
substances, the
pharmacist must
complete and sign
this form.

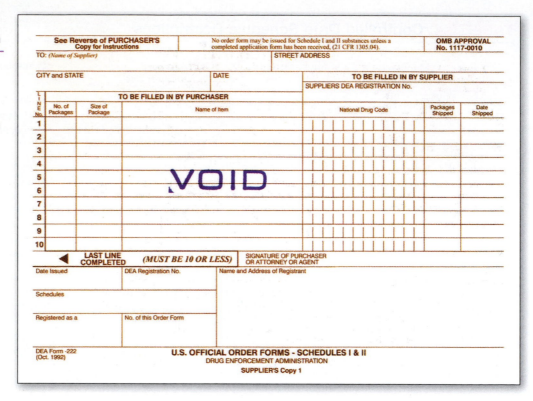

Study Idea

Pharmacist may reorder Schedule II drugs with either a paper DEA Form 222 or electronically using CSOS.

OxyContin (oxycodone), Adderall (dextroamphetamine-amphetamine), and Ritalin (methylphenidate). The most dispensed Schedule II drug in community pharmacy is a hydrocodone with acetaminophen combination (Lortab, Lorcet, and Vicodin).

Unlike other drugs that technicians can order for stock inventory, Schedule II drugs must be ordered and purchased by the pharmacist. *The order must be submitted in triplicate on a DEA 222 form* (see Figure 3.1—a list of other required DEA forms comes later in the chapter in Table 3.8). Some states permit electronic ordering online of these drugs through a specially encrypted system, the Controlled Substance Ordering System (CSOS), administered by the DEA. Controlled substance prescriptions from a foreign physician (such as from Canada or Mexico) cannot be filled because they do not have a DEA license and number. Some pharmacies are not licensed to fill Schedule II prescriptions from out-of-state providers.

The pharmacist must verify the inventory receipt of all Schedule II drugs, including type and quantity. Schedule II drugs must be stored in a safe or locked cabinet. Dispensing of Schedule II drugs is tightly regulated. In most pharmacies, the pharmacist is also the only person allowed to dispense a Schedule II drug. In the hospital, narcotics are stored in a locked unit at the nursing station. Access is limited to a nurse with the appropriate key or lock code.

In community and hospital pharmacies, each dosage unit of a Schedule II drug must be accounted for by a computerized or manual inventory record (see Figure 3.2). A shortage of a Schedule II drug triggers an immediate investigation. In hospitals and institutions, secure dispensing machine stations (e.g., Pyxis) automatically update inventory anytime a drug is dispensed. Technicians, pharmacists, and nurses must continually check that the amounts documented as being filled and dispensed match with the quantities in the automated station. Nurses also do periodic blind counts of the contents in secure dispensing cabinets to verify the quantity totals match those the cabinet is tracked to store.

Although most pharmacies today have a computer system that verifies a physician's DEA number, it is possible to verify the number by hand using the DEA verification formula known as the **DEA Checksum Formula**.

Step 1: Add the first, third, and fifth digits of the DEA number.
Step 2: Add the second, fourth, and sixth digits of the DEA number.
Step 3: Double the sum obtained in Step 2.
Step 4: Add the results of Steps 1 and 3. The last digit of the sum should match the last digit of the DEA number.

Example 1
Check the validity of Dr. Jones' DEA number: **BJ2243551**.

Step 1: $2 + 4 + 5 = 11$
Step 2: $2 + 3 + 5 = 10$
Step 3: $10 \times 2 = 20$
Step 4: $11 + 20 + 31$

The last digit of the sum in Step 4 matches the last digit of the DEA number. The number is valid.

FIGURE 3.2
Perpetual Inventory Record

A perpetual inventory record accounts for each unit of a Schedule II drug dispensed or received. This should match the information that is tracked electronically during prescription filling.

The Corner Drug Store – C-II Perpetual Log

Drug Name: _Methylphenidate 5mg Tabs_   NDC: _0123-4567-10_

Prescription No.	Dispense Date	QTY Dispensed	Inventory	RPh Initials
Starting	_Inventory_	– – – – –	380	– – – – –
2001415	01/22/20XX	−30	350	JPS
2001423	02/07/20XX	−90	260	RJA
INV. 55874	02/08/20XX	+200	460	RJA
2001439	02/10/20XX	−120	340	CA
2001445	02/15/20XX	−30		

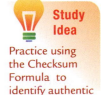

Study Idea

Practice using the Checksum Formula to identify authentic DEA numbers.

The technician must review every prescription carefully for completeness and authenticity, and especially prescriptions for Schedule II drugs (discussed in Chapter 4). They must be able to check the authenticity of the DEA number by using the DEA Checksum Formula as described in the Take Note above.

Electronic prescriptions for controlled substances are allowed by the DEA as long as the prescriber and pharmacy meet strict electronic security requirements. The prescriber identity must be authenticated and double protected by at least two of the following:

- a password or response to a security question
- a biometric, such as a fingerprint or eye scan
- a hard token that serves as a cryptographic or one-time password device

A hard-copy prescription for a Schedule II drug must be complete, written in indelible black ink, and signed by the prescribing physician. There may be no alterations. The pharmacist should recognize the prescriber's signature. The date on the prescription is important; some states limit the amount of time a Schedule II prescription is valid (e.g., from 72 hours to 30 days). *No refills are allowed on Schedule II drugs, and most pharmacies are not allowed to file these prescriptions for future use.*

However, since many children (and some adults) take methylphenidate (Ritalin, Concerta) and other stimulants like dextroamphetamine-amphetamine salts (Adderall) daily to control attention-deficit hyperactivity disorder (ADHD), the DEA and most states allow the prescriber to provide prescriptions for future use with the notation, "Do not fill until XX/XX/20XX" with the correct date. The fill date cannot be more than 90 days from the date the prescription was written.

All prescriptions for Schedule II drugs must be filed separately from other prescriptions and must be readily retrievable. *Each prescription must be signed and dated by the pharmacist.* Federal law requires pharmacies to keep Schedule II prescriptions for a minimum of two years; state laws may require such prescriptions be kept on file for up to five years. In practice, most pharmacies keep all prescription records indefinitely for legal reasons.

Individual states may have additional regulations for Schedule II drugs. Some states allow a Schedule II prescription to be submitted by phone in an emergency, provided the prescriber mails a hard copy to the pharmacy within a specified amount of time (usually 72 hours to one week). The pharmacist must verify the authenticity of the prescriber's DEA number, reduce the verbal order to writing, and document the nature of the emergency on the back of the prescription. Some states also allow prescribers to order a Schedule II prescription for a hospice patient via fax or phone; most pharmacies treat this situation as an emergency and require the prescriber to mail a hard copy of the prescription within a week.

Schedule III–IV

Schedule III and Schedule IV (C-III and C-IV) medications have less risk for abuse and dependence, but the risk is clearly present, especially if these medications are used in high doses over a long period of time. Prescriptions for Schedule III and Schedule IV drugs can be *refilled a maximum of five times, and refills must be dispensed within six months from the original date of the prescription.*

The DEA also limits the transfer of Schedule III and Schedule IV medications between pharmacies. Patients may request the transfer of a prescription to another pharmacy for convenience, during a vacation, or if the patient has a second home in another community. In most states, only the pharmacist can legally transfer a prescription for a controlled drug. A patient may request that the receiving pharmacy call to request the transfer from the pharmacy that holds the hard copy of the prescription.

However, a prescription for a *Schedule III or Schedule IV drug can only be transferred one time.* The patient cannot then refill the prescription again at the original pharmacy; instead, a new prescription must be requested from the prescriber. In transferring the prescription, the originating pharmacy must close the prescription for the transferred drug so that no additional refills can be obtained from that location. Documentation must include the name and phone number of the receiving pharmacy and the receiving pharmacist, as well as the DEA numbers of both pharmacies.

Prescriptions for Schedule III and Schedule IV drugs are less likely to be forged than Schedule II drugs, *but are more likely to be refilled early*. The pharmacy technician must review the date of the last refill and the days supply. For example, a prescription for "Acetaminophen with Codeine 300 mg/30 mg #90 with Sig: 1 tab PO t.i.d. p.r.n." written on November 1, should last until around December 1. If the patient tries to refill the prescription on November 20th, the technician may have to tell the patient that the prescription cannot be refilled early. Each pharmacy has a policy regarding how far in advance (usually 24–48 hours) it will provide refills of Schedule III and Schedule IV drugs.

Most physicians have started writing Schedule II–IV controlled substance prescriptions for a 28-day supply. This allows the patient exactly four weeks of medication so they can return on the same day of the week four weeks later for the refill. This way, patients do not run out on the weekend when their physician is not in the office.

Most Schedule III and Schedule IV drugs *do not have to be kept in a safe or locked cabinet* and are generally stored with the inventory of nonscheduled drugs. No special DEA forms are needed to order or dispose of Schedule III and Schedule IV drugs, and a senior pharmacy technician may be responsible for ordering them. The pharmacist is often responsible for verifying and signing for the receipt of all Schedule III and Schedule IV drugs; these signed inventory receipts are kept on file.

C Prescriptions must be readily accessible for inspection. If not separated from other prescriptions, Schedule III and Schedule IV prescriptions must be marked for easy identification with a large (at least one inch high) red C for control in the lower right corner.

Schedule V

The Schedule V (C-V) drugs have the lowest potential for abuse and dependence and include prescription cough syrups that contain codeine (such as Cheracol or Robitussin A-C) as well as diphenoxylate (Lomotil) for diarrhea, and pregabalin (Lyrica) for neuropathic pain.

Some states—and many pharmacies—require a prescription to dispense these medications. *Insurance companies will not cover the cost of these medications without a prescription.* Schedule V prescriptions are generally filed with the prescriptions for Schedule III and Schedule IV drugs for easy retrieval.

Federal law and many states allow pharmacists to dispense a Schedule V drug without a prescription if certain restrictions and recordkeeping requirements are met. Restrictions for the sale of Schedule V medications include:

- Drugs must be stored behind the counter in the prescription area (or can be locked with other controlled substances).
- The amount of cough syrup sold to a single customer is generally limited to a specific volume (such as 120 mL or 4 fl oz) within a 48-hour period.
- Only the pharmacist (or the pharmacy technician under direct supervision) can make the sale.
- The purchaser must be 18 years of age or older and have proof of identity.

If the state allows sale of Schedule V drugs without a prescription, the pharmacy technician or pharmacist must legally record all sales in a record book or computerized database and include the following information:

- name and address of the purchaser
- date of birth of the purchaser
- date of purchase
- name of the drug and quantity sold
- name and initials of the pharmacist handling or approving the sale

To apply these Schedule II–V regulations properly, one needs to get to know and remember the most commonly prescribed controlled substances, as shown in Appendix B.

Restricted Sale of Certain Over-the-Counter Products

Certain OTC products also have specific restrictions and procedures that must be followed during consumer purchases. These products include OTC Schedule V drugs, such as the OTC cough medications containing codeine and products containing ephedrine and pseudoephedrine. These OTC products must be stored behind the counter, and technicians must follow the same sales restrictions and documentation procedures as mentioned previously for C-V prescriptions. These drugs are often referred to as behind-the-counter medications.

Study Idea

Memorize the protocols to follow regarding OTC drugs that contain pseudo-ephedrine and ephedrine.

Over-the-Counter Drugs with Pseudoephedrine and Ephedrine Because of the Combat Methamphetamine Epidemic Act (CMEA), the amount of products containing pseudoephedrine and ephedrine that can be purchased at one time or within one month is limited, as has been noted. The restricted OTC products include cold and sinus medications, ephedrine-containing tablets, and metered-dose inhalers (MDIs). Some states limit the purchase of these products to "prescription only," and several states require that only pharmacists conduct the sales. Violations of the state or federal laws may result in the loss of the pharmacist's license or the pharmacy's business license.

Technicians must legally document the purchases and purchasers of pseudo-ephedrine or ephedrine in a software program or manual logbook similar to that for Schedule V drugs and have the individuals sign for the purchases. This documentation must be kept for a minimum of two years to allow for DEA and FDA tracking.

In addition, to continue offering these drugs for sale, all pharmacies must electronically submit an annual self-certification to the DEA. This certification confirms that:

- all employees have been trained in how to handle these products,
- training records are being maintained,
- sales limits are being enforced (3.6 grams per day, 9 grams per 30 days),
- products are being stored behind the counter or in a locked cabinet,
- an electronic or written logbook is being maintained.

For an example of a hard-copy log and the information, see Figure 3.3. Many pharmacies are now using the online, real-time National Precursor Log Exchange (NPLEx), which tracks and consolidates the data on these sales and helps law enforcement see trends in areas and overlapping sales.

To calculate the limits for these sales, you must take the weight of each tablet in a package and multiply it by the number of tablets to find the total in the package. For ease in calculations, the DEA supplies tables for restricted amounts per packages, as shown in Tables 3.5 and 3.6. It is useful to know how to use these tables but not

FIGURE 3.3
Sales Log of Restricted Products Containing Pseudoephedrine and Ephedrine

Pseudoephedrine Products Dispensing Record

Purchaser's Name	Driver's License Number	Purchaser's Address	Date of Purchase	Product Name	Quantity Purchased	Dispensed by (Initials)	Purchaser's Signature

TABLE 3.5 Number of Tablets That Equal Retail Sales Limits

Drug and Form	Limits	Number per Package = 3.6	* Number per Package = 7.5 g	Number per Package at Retail = 9 g
Epherdrine				
Ephedrine HCl 25 mg	3.6 g per day; 9 g per month	175 tablets	366	439 tablets
Ephedrine Sulfate 25 mg		186 tablets	389	466 tablets
Pseudoephedrine (as HCl)				
Pseudoephedrine HCl 30 mg	3.6 g per day; 9 g per month	146 tablets	305	366 tablets
Pseudoephedrine HCl 60 mg		73 tablets	152	183 tablets
Pseudoephedrine HCl 120 mg		36 tablets	76	91 tablets
Pseudoephedrine (as Sulfate)				
Pseudoephedrine Sulfate 30 mg	3.6 g per day; 9 g per month	155 tablets	324	389 tablets
Pseudoephedrine Sulfate 60 mg		77 tablets	162	194 tablets
Pseudoephedrine Sulfate 120 mg		38 tablets	81	97 tablets
Pseudoephedrine Sulfate 240 mg		19 tablets	40	48 tablets

*The monthly limit for mail-order pharmacies is less, at 7.5 grams.

Note: The DEA also supplies a table listing the limits of milliliters of liquid base of products containing ephedrine and pseudoephedrine to guide sales of liquid OTC products.

Source: DEA website

TABLE 3.6 Sales Limit of Milliliters of Liquid Base Containing Restricted Substances

Drug and Form	mL Limits per Day	mL Limits per Month
Ephedrine		
Ephedrine HCl 6.25 mg/5 mL	3,515 mL	8,788 mL
Pseudoephedrine (as HCl)		
Pseudoephedrine HCl 15 mg/1.6 mL	468 mL	1,171 mL
Pseudoephedrine HCl 7.5 mg/5 mL	2,929 mL	7,323 mL
Pseudoephedrine HCl 15 mg/5 mL	1,464 mL	3,661 mL
Pseudoephedrine HCl 15 mg/2.5 mL	732 mL	1,830 mL
Pseudoephedrine HCl 30 mg/5 mL	732 mL	1,830 mL
Pseudoephedrine HCl 30 mg/2.5 mL	366 mL	915 mL
Pseudoephedrine HCl 60 mg/5 mL	366 mL	915 mL

memorize them. Instead, memorize the general limits per day and month. Be aware that states may have even more or tighter restrictions.

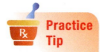

Practice Tip

The DEA launched a texting tip line in some areas to anonymously report suspicious prescription drug activity. Type TIP411 (847-411) for the phone number, then type DEADRUGS or PILLTIP. Text description of the suspicion or send an image. The DEA cannot see the texter's phone number (100% anonymous) but can assign an investigator to respond. Various cities and states are encouraging its use in their area.

Preventing Forgeries and Diversion

The pharmacy technician must be vigilant in reviewing narcotics prescriptions. It is not uncommon for a forged prescription to be presented by a new, supposedly out-of-state patient on a weekend or evening when the prescription cannot be authenticated. A patient who requests a brand name narcotic and offers to pay cash (instead of providing insurance information) should raise a red flag. Cash payment does not create a paper trail that could alert other pharmacies that receive a similar prescription. Table 3.7 (on the following page) provides a list of indicators that should alert the technician to check with the pharmacist.

Most pharmacies have a computerized physician database containing DEA, National Provider Identifier, and state license numbers, and contact information. However, pharmacy technicians should learn to recognize the names and legal signatures of the local prescribers who send prescriptions to the pharmacy, especially for controlled substances, to help prevent forgeries on the spot. Insurance plans require a pharmacy to have a physician's DEA number on file to be reimbursed for prescriptions for all controlled medications. Some pharmacies fill controlled substances only for patients residing in their immediate geographical area and for prescribers who practice in their community and write their prescriptions with tamper-proof paper.

Controlled Drug Inventory

The DEA requires that all pharmacies *complete a biennial (every two years) inventory* that includes an exact count of all Schedule II drugs and an estimate of other controlled drugs. If a C-II container designed to hold 1,000 doses or more has been opened, an exact count is necessary. The inventory record must contain the following information for each controlled medication:

- name of the drug
- dosage form and strength
- number of dosage units or volume in each container
- number of containers

Many community pharmacies have a policy or are subject to state law that requires them also to perform an exact inventory of all Schedule II drugs monthly or by some other regular schedule. In the hospital, inventories of narcotics are conducted at the start of each nursing shift, typically three times per day, or perpetually if an automated drug dispensing system is in use. Inventories of Schedule III and Schedule IV drugs are checked at least annually in most community and hospital pharmacies. Upon discovery of loss or theft, DEA Form 106 must be completed. For a list of commonly required DEA forms, see Table 3.8 (on the following page).

TABLE 3.7 Indicators of a Potentially Forged Prescription or Drug-Seeking Behavior

- The prescription is altered (for example, a change in quantity).
- Prescription pads have been reported missing from local doctors' offices.
- The prescription is presented as a clever computerized fax and is not on tamper-proof safety paper.
- There are misspellings on the prescription.
- A refill is indicated for a Schedule II drug.
- A prescription from the emergency department is written for more than a #30 count or 7-day supply.
- A prescription is cut and pasted from a preprinted, signed prescription.
- A second or third prescription is added to a legal prescription written by a physician. More than one handwriting style is used.
- A patient presents a prescription containing several medications but wants the pharmacy to fill only the narcotic prescription.
- The prescription is signed with different handwriting or in different ink, or the prescription is not signed by the physician.
- The DEA number is missing, illegible, or incorrect.
- The prescription is written by an out-of-state physician or a physician practicing in an area far from the pharmacy. This event is particularly suspicious if the prescription is received at night or on the weekend, when it would be difficult to confirm the prescription.
- An individual other than the patient drops off the prescription. Pharmacy personnel should require a driver's license or other photo ID and document this information.
- A new patient specifies a brand name narcotic.
- A new patient wants to pay for the prescription with cash, even though he or she has insurance. Doing so prevents a paper trail.

Disposal of Controlled Substances

Disposal or destruction of any Schedule II drug must be recorded on a DEA 41 form and witnessed and signed by another pharmacist. Expired drugs and broken dosage units are generally saved until the next visit by a state drug inspector or until the pharmacist travels to a licensed destruction center. Disposal records must contain the following information:

- pharmacy DEA number, name, and address
- reverse distributor's DEA number, name, and address
- number of units (in finished forms and/or commercial containers) disposed of and the manner of disposal

The records must be electronically sent to the local DEA branch (or two hard copies sent by mail) and a copy stored by the pharmacy for at least two years. The disposal record must be dated to reflect when the product was sent for destruction. Besides the DEA 41 form, the reverse distributor will fill out a DEA 222 form as the "purchaser" of the outdated Schedule II drugs even if no value is assigned to them. This helps close the loop on the products distribution trail. (See Table 3.8 for a more complete list of common DEA forms.)

TABLE 3.8 Commonly Used DEA Forms for Pharmacies

DEA Form	Description
DEA 224	Application form for a pharmacy to dispense controlled substances or a prescriber to prescribe them
DEA 222	Controlled substance order form
DEA 41	Destruction of controlled substances report and witness form
DEA 106	Theft/loss of controlled substance form (required when there is a "significant loss")
Automation of Reports and Consolidated Orders System (ARCOS)	The DEA's Electronic Data Interchange (EDI) to make it easier for ordering, tracking, and submitting monthly, annual, and biannual reports
Controlled Substance Ordering System (CSOS)	DEA-run system that allows for secure electronic transmission of Schedule I–V controlled substance orders without the supporting paper Form 222

State Laws

In addition to knowledge of federal laws affecting pharmacy practice, the technician must be cognizant of state laws and regulations. The pharmacy technician may be responsible for registering annually with the state board of pharmacy (required in most states) and fulfilling all continuing education (CE) requirements. The state board of pharmacy may also require technicians to pass a certification exam within a certain period of time. If the technician is practicing in a specialty area, such as a sterile or nonsterile compounding pharmacy or facility or a nuclear pharmacy, additional training and certification may be required. In most states, the pharmacy technician may legally perform the following duties:

- dispensing medication, recordkeeping, pricing, and billing
- preparing doses of a premanufactured product
- compounding sterile and nonsterile medications according to protocol
- customer service for prescriptions
- transporting medications to patient care units in the hospital
- checking and replenishing drug inventory

In all practice locations, however, all duties must be carried out under the direct supervision of a licensed pharmacist. Some states may allow the technician to perform additional responsibilities, such as taking telephone refill requests from prescribers or assisting in drawing up medications for vaccine administration. It is important that you know what the state board of pharmacy allows. In some states, certified pharmacy technicians are allowed to check the work of other technicians, called "tech-check-tech."

The Courts and Professional Standards

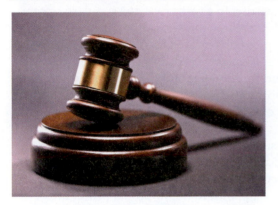

Serious violations of laws, regulations, or ethics by pharmacy technicians may result in loss of job, suspension or revocation of professional ability to practice, or criminal or civil penalties.

In addition to federal and state laws and regulations, the pharmacy technician is expected to observe accepted professional and ethical standards. A standard is a criterion established to measure product quality or professional performance against a norm. Standards exist for both drug products and professional behavior, including an accepted standard of care. The federal government and state boards of pharmacy use these concepts in forming their regulations, and they are applied in the courts. The United States Pharmacopeial Convention (USP) sets standards for compounding sterile and nonsterile products as well as standards for drug manufacturing. The Joint Commission establishes standards for pharmacists and pharmacy technicians in the hospital and other institutional settings for accreditation.

Criminal and Civil Court Cases

When a legal problem arises involving a pharmacy practice, the courts often become involved. The courts are separated between those established to resolve issues between the government and offending parties—**criminal law** cases—and those between citizens—**civil law** cases. In the criminal cases, a prosecutor argues the government's case against the person or organization accused of breaking the law, and these cases can result in jail time for the perpetrator if a case is won. Civil law handles the wrongs US citizens commit against one another, resulting in monetary damages being awarded when the injured party wins, but not jail time for the perpetrator.

When pharmacy violations occur under any level of law—federal, state, or local—a government prosecutor or public representative often brings cases against the suspected parties. Before court, the state board of pharmacy reviews each pharmacy case, and lesser cases are generally settled out of court. The board applies varying levels of consequences based on the offenses, such as suspending or not renewing the person's professional license or putting the practitioner on probation.

If the violation is serious or damage done merits going to court, the case is filed using phrases like *State v. Diana Jones, PharmD*. Consequences can include jail and/or monetary sanctions. In cases where a pharmacy offense resulted in personal injury or damages, the victim or victim's family may sue the offending party in civil court and provide the burden of proof. (A violator may be tried in two different courts, criminal and civil.)

There are two main types of civil court actions pertinent to pharmacy: torts and contracts. **Torts** address personal injuries and wrongs that one citizen commits against another, including negligence, malpractice, slander (using spoken words to speak falsely of another), libel (using written words to falsely represent another), assault (threatening another with bodily harm), and battery (causing bodily harm to another). The most common tort in the medical/pharmacy arena is **negligence**, or carelessness—not acting as a reasonably prudent person would in the same situation. **Malpractice** is the form of negligence where a professional fails to offer the minimum standard of care that results in injury.

Standard of Care

Standard of care is the legal term for the accepted level of care healthcare providers are expected to provide in each field of expertise. In a court case, the standard of care is measured against the actions of other healthcare professionals in the same situation; existing written guidelines, training programs, protocols, or policies and procedures; and expert testimony of health professionals provided by the plaintiff or the defense. If the standard of care was not met and a patient was harmed as a result, a medical negligence lawsuit may result. OBRA-90, the federal law that required all community pharmacies to offer patient counseling on prescriptions is an example of a standard of care.

When determining the appropriate standard of care, two criteria are considered: the healthcare provider's level of training, and what is considered normal practice for the provider's geographic area. A pharmacy technician would not be held to the same standard as a pharmacist unless the technician failed to follow proper procedure or have the work verified by the pharmacist. If a technician knowingly oversteps his or her role without the knowledge of the supervising pharmacist, the technician could be held liable. For example, if a technician performed a function not permitted under state or federal regulation—overriding an allergy or drug interaction alert or counseling a patient—that resulted in direct harm to the patient, the technician could be subject to a lawsuit and possible termination.

Ethics

Ethics are the standards of right conduct and moral judgment. Ethics provide a structure for reflection and analysis of behavior and decision making when the proper course of action is unclear.

Many ethical dilemmas confront pharmacy professionals in their daily activities. For example, some pharmacists and technicians have reservations about dispensing birth control, the "morning-after pill," or other medications to terminate a pregnancy. If a pharmacist or technician is not comfortable dispensing a medication to terminate a pregnancy (or a potential pregnancy), another staff member may dispense the drug and counsel the patient, or the patient may be referred to another local pharmacy.

To guide technicians, the PTCB and NHA both have published ethical codes that those desiring certification must promise to uphold (see page 8). Pharmacy technician and pharmacist professional organizations also have their codes of ethics.

STUDY SUMMARY

Knowing the key laws and standards that affect your practice as a technician is essential. For taking the certification exam, study the tables in this chapter, especially those that list the laws, controlled substance levels, and types of recalls. You will need to also review the supplement on HIPAA regulations, accessed with the eBook link. The flash cards that are also linked in the eBook will be helpful in your studies. It is particularly important to know the pharmacy procedures and expectations that resulted from the laws so you can do things legally and safely. The exam will ask questions about how to apply of these laws and when. That is why it is important to recognize the common controlled substances and their schedules, which are listed in Appendix B, to know how to properly dispense them.

ADDITIONAL RESOURCES

For more in-depth explanations, check out *Pharmacy Practice for Technicians*, 6e from Paradigm Education Solutions. To master and extend the material presented in this chapter, take advantage of the resources available through the eBook resources links. These include digital supplements, study resources, and a practice exam generator with 1,000+ exam-style questions. End-of-chapter tests are accessible through the eBook for individuals using the self-study course and through Navigator+ for individuals enrolled in the instructor-guided course.

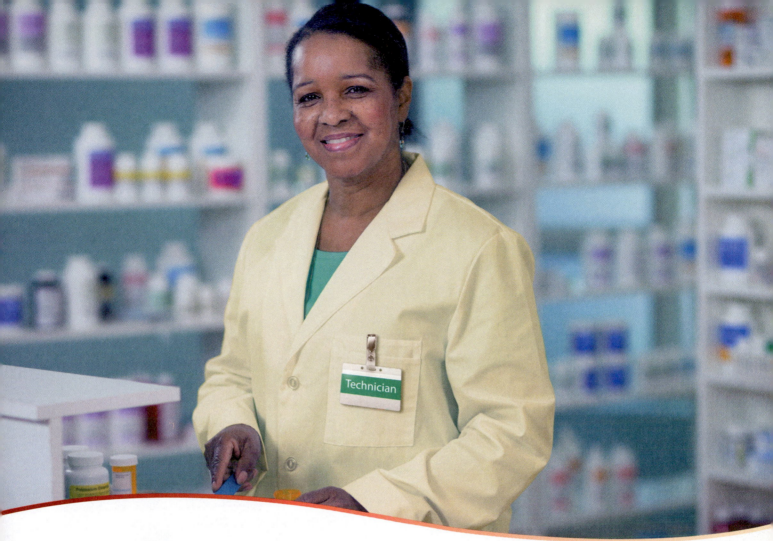

UNIT
3
Dispensing Processes

Chapter 4   Prescription and Medication Order Dispensing   107

Chapter 5   Nonsterile Compounding   133

Chapter 6   Sterile and Hazardous Compounding   151

Chapter 7   Medication Safety and Quality Assurance   181

Chapter 8   Pharmacy Information Systems and Automation   203

Chapter 9   Pharmacy Inventory Management   215

Chapter 10 Pharmacy Reimbursement and Claims Processing   233

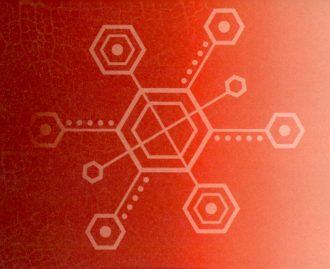

Prescription and Medication Order Dispensing

Learning Objectives

1. Know when generic drugs can be legally substituted for prescribed brand drugs and the references for identifying a generic equivalent.

2. Interpret common notations and abbreviations used by prescribers in community and hospital settings.

3. Understand the importance of the patient profile and continuously updating it. Know the implications of HIPAA and the information in the patient profile.

4. Explain the similarities and differences between a prescription and a medication order.

5. Identify the components of a prescription and how to check it for completeness, accuracy, legality, and authenticity.

6. Identify the components of a medication order and how to check it.

7. Review the differing processes for filling, labeling, and verifying a prescription and a medication order.

8. Calculate the quantity of medication to be dispensed in a q.s. medication order.

9. Identify legally required parts of a label.

10. Know the parts of the National Drug Code (NDC) and its importance in filling orders.

11. Identify five mechanisms for transferring medication information to a patient.

12. Understand the various types of prescription refills and the legality of each type. Know when a prescription is not refillable.

13. Know techniques to prevent forgeries and to identify authentic prescriptions.

14. Explain the reasons for repackaging and the repackaging control log.

15. Know the additional information needed on a parenteral medication order.

16. Understand the role of the pharmacist in the many steps of the dispensing processes.

 Access eBook links for resources and an exam generator, with 1,000+ questions.

I n both community and hospital pharmacies, the pharmacy technician is responsible for assessing the prescription or hospital medication order for completeness and accuracy. In the community pharmacy, the technician has the added responsibility of checking the prescription for legality and authenticity. This chapter reviews the components of a prescription and a medical order, and the common notations and abbreviations used by prescribers. It also discusses the patient profile, medication history, the drug utilization review, and the process of filling, packaging, labeling prescriptions, gathering patient education resources, and the final check by the pharmacist. In both exams, a large percentage of the questions relate to this knowledge base: domain 6 of the PTCE is 17.5% of the exam, and topic area 3 of the ExCPT is 54% of the exam.

Reviewing Common Dosage Forms and Routes of Administration

For safe and efficient dispensing practice, technicians need to know well all the dosage and release delivery forms, because patients will be harmed if you mix them up and the pharmacist does not notice. That is why the exam may include questions on them. Study Tables 4.1 and 4.2 to review them.

TABLE 4.1 Common Dosage Formulations and Routes of Administration

Dosage Form or Route of Administration	Dispensing Description and Tip
Oral	
Tablet	Comes as compression, multiple compression, chewable, oral disintegrating, and caplet with possible coatings: sugar coated, film coated, enteric coated, and buffered for different purposes and release delivery modes. Make sure to type in the direction "By mouth." A delayed release tablet should not be crushed for administration. A tablet should not be divided unless scored.
Capsule	Available in hard and soft gelatin and is transparent, semitransparent, or opaque. Label oral capsules with "By mouth." Hard gelatin capsules may be opened and mixed with food or liquid.
Oral liquid	Comes as solution, syrup, suspension, elixir, emulsion, magma, colloid, aromatic water, fluidextract, solid extract, tincture, or spirit. Dispense with dosing cups or oral syringes for infants and young children. Label oral liquids with "By mouth." Label suspensions, magma, and colloids with "Shake well" auxiliary label.
Powders for reconstitution, effervescent tablets, or powders.	Due to short expiration dates for some drugs, such as liquids, the active ingredient is supplied as a powder or effervescent tablet with instructions on how much water or other suitable liquid is to be mixed with the drug for a given concentration. Check manufacturer label for the beyond-use date for the reconstituted product. Label oral liquids with "By mouth" and apply "Shake well" auxiliary label. Dispense with appropriate measuring spoon/cup or oral syringe.
Buccal	Transmucosal route of administration for gum, tablet, lozenge (troche), and lollipop. Label directions should include "Place between gum and inner lining of cheek..." Always label with "Keep out of reach of children" and dispense in child-resistant packaging, since these dosage forms may look like candy to a child. Nicotine gum should be dispensed with direction for how to chew it to prevent nicotine overdose.
Sublingual	Available usually as tablets and sprays, though compounding pharmacies and homeopathic practitioners may have solutions in which a given number of drops are placed under the tongue. Label with "Dissolve 1 tablet under the tongue..." Nitroglycerin sublingual tablets must be dispensed in their original glass bottles and be replace every 6 months.

Dosage Form or Route of Administration	Dispensing Description and Tip
Transmucosal	
Ophthalmic	Available as solution, suspension, ointment, and inserts. Solutions and suspensions are not interchangeable. Calculate the days supply by assuming 15 drops per mL. Label in which eye or both eyes the drop is to be placed. Label suspensions with "Shake well." Ophthalmic drops may be used in the ear.
Otic	Available as solutions and suspensions, which are not interchangeable. Label with "With affected ear facing up, place X drops in ear canal, keep head tilted for 2–5 min. May insert cotton plug to prevent leakage. Repeat..." Suspensions should be labeled with "Shake well" label. Never use otic drops in the eye.
Nasal	Comes as a liquid solution or suspension in an atomizer that is sprayed up the nose. Older nasal formulations were liquids with droppers and the patient had to tilt the head back and place the given number of drops up the nostril—these are rarely seen today. The nasal spray should be labeled with directions to "Tilt head back, insert nasal sprayer into nostril and spray prescribed number of sprays. Repeat in other nostril if ordered. Repeat...." Suspensions should have a "Shake well" label.
Rectal	Available as suppositories, enemas, creams, and ointments. Suppositories may be for systemic or local indications. Label suppositories with "Wear gloves. Remove wrap, insert into rectum small tapered end first..." Most suppositories are stored at room temperature but some should be labeled with "Keep refrigerated" and stored accordingly until pickup. Enemas should have directions telling patient to lie on side with knees bent, insert nozzle in rectum, squeeze bottle to release enema into rectum, remain in position for as long as directed. Creams and ointments may come with an applicator, which is inserted rectally, and the tube is squeezed to administer the topical preparation.
Vaginal	Available as creams, ointments, tablets, foams, films, gels, and inserts. Hormone replacement therapy would be for systemic indication. Anti-infective/antifungals would be for local infection. Label directions should include "Insert 1 applicatorful (or tablet) into vagina...."
Topical	
Dermal	Available as ointments, creams, lotions, pastes, plasters, gels, collodions, jellies, or irrigation solutions. Usually for local indication. Instructions should include "Apply sparingly to affected area..." "For external use only" auxiliary label should be attached to the container.
Transdermal adhesives	Patches and discs consist of adhesive fabric with a drug reservoir and a rate-controlling membrane. Provides slow, controlled release of drug to be absorbed systemically through the skin. Directions should include "Apply topically to hair-free, scar-free skin. Rotate sites to prevent skin irritation. Discard used patches safely." Apply "For external use only" auxiliary label.
Transdermal gel, lotion, or spray	Gels, lotions, and sprays in which the drug is used for a systemic indication. Potent active ingredients are absorbed through the skin. Patients should be directed to wear gloves for application. A specific dose is premeasured or a tool to measure doses must be provided. The product should be allowed to dry after application. Use auxiliary label "For external use only."
Inhalation	
Aerosols and metered dose inhalers	Aerosol devices (such as the spray Respimat and HFA) that dispense a measured dose per "puff." If patient has difficulty coordinating the device, a spacer may be used to facilitate administration. Instructions should include "Inhale X puffs by mouth..." Label each container with a "Shake well" auxiliary label. Patients should be advised to rinse their mouth after use and to clean plastic dispensers regularly.

Dosage Form or Route of Administration	Dispensing Description and Tip
Micronized powders and nonaerosolized inhalers	Common inhalers include Accuhaler, Turbohaler, Diskhaler, Diskus, and HandiHaler. Patient labeling must instruct the patient to activate dose and to breathe in deeply and strongly to pull the powder into the lungs. Labeling should say "Inhale 1 puff by mouth X times a day. Rinse mouth after use."
Inhalation solutions and nebulizers	This is a liquid drug solution that must be administered using a nebulizer. Solutions may be premixed and ready to use or in a concentrated solution that must be mixed with sterile saline. Multiple drugs may be mixed together in one treatment for patient convenience. Directions should include "Inhale X mL (or packets) with nebulizer ..."
Volatiles	Volatile medications are liquids that can be used with a vaporizer to help relieve breathing problems. Directions should clearly direct the patient not to take internally or apply externally.
Parenteral	
Intravenous	Sterile solutions for administration into a vein. Usually for systemic use. Must be particulate free and administered by a healthcare professional. May be a small volume for a piggyback or bolus dose, or a large volume parenteral for continuous intravenous infusion.
Intramuscular	Sterile solutions and suspensions designed to be injected into the muscle. Depending on drug salt and diluent, the intramuscular route can provide immediate or delayed effect. Depot-injection drugs are designed to have effects lasting weeks to months. Usually administered by a healthcare professional.
Subcutaneous	Sterile suspensions or solutions that are injected through the skin into the subcutaneous tissue for systemic effect. Includes many vaccinations and insulin. Patients should be directed on how to store the drug and how to administer.
Intradermal	Very small volume of sterile solution injected between the skin layers for diagnostic purpose. Administered by a healthcare professional.
Inserts and Implants	
Vaginal rings	Flexible drug-treated plastic ring, inserted vaginally every month as a contraceptive. Should be stored in refrigerator. Some new inserts have microbials and chemotherapy drugs.
Intrauterine devices	T-shaped plastic device, fitted into the uterus through the vagina by a physician as a drug delivery device to prevent pregnancy.
Surgical Implants	Catheters, drug pumps, radioactive seeds, and hormonal pellets that deliver medication either systemically or locally.

TABLE 4.2 Drug Delivery Abbreviations

Abbreviation	Meaning
DR	Delayed release
CR	Controlled release
CD	Controlled delivery
LA	Long acting
TR	Timed release
SR	Sustained release
XT	Extended time release
XL	Extended length/release

The Filling and Dispensing Roles of the Pharmacy Technician

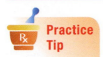
In all settings, the goal of the profession of pharmacy is to get the right drug, right dose form, and right strength by the right route safely to the right patient at the right time with the right patient education and documentation. Though the prescribing and filling processes are different in the community and institutional pharmacy settings, both prescriptions and medication orders depend upon complete patient medication and allergy profiles and the shared language of pharmacy abbreviations, which are described below. (An overview of the general process for both prescriptions and medication orders is shown in Figure 4.1.)

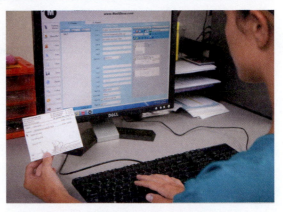

Technicians work hard to make sure prescriptions, medication orders, labels, and the data on the computer match up.

Generic Substitutions for Prescribed Brand Drugs

Pharmacy technicians in all states are permitted (or in some cases required) to substitute without physician approval the appropriate lower-cost generic drug in place of a prescribed brand name drug as long as the generic drug is considered bioequivalent. To be **bioequivalent**, the generic must be *both pharmaceutically and therapeutically equal to the brand*. To be **pharmaceutically equivalent**, the generic drug must contain *the same amount of active ingredient in the same dosage form*. Bioequivalent generic drug products may differ in certain characteristics, including shape, scoring configuration, packaging, inert ingredients (including colorings, flavors, and preservatives), expiration time, and—within certain limits—labeling.

Each generic drug *also* needs to be **therapeutically equivalent**, or *provide the same medicinal benefit at the same dosage with the same degree of safety* under the conditions specified in the labeling. This means that the bioequivalent generic displays the same standards of safety and efficacy as the brand name.

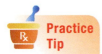
However, since not all patients will respond similarly to a specific drug, the prescriber is permitted by law to write **DAW (dispense as written)** "brand medically necessary" on the prescription. (This often occurs with thyroid prescriptions written by an endocrinologist.) The patient may also specifically request a brand name drug, which would be indicated by "**DAW2**" on the prescription for insurance processing. This generally results in a higher co-pay, so the technician must make sure the patient is aware of this. Conversely, a patient may request a lower-cost generic, even though the physician wrote "brand necessary." A call to the physician's office, however, is necessary to gain approval for the generic drug over the DAW brand drug.

FIGURE 4.1 Overview of Medication Filling and Dispensing Process

Each step in the filling and dispensing processes for prescriptions and medication orders is an opportunity to do things correctly or make an error. At each step, there is also chance to catch and correct any previous errors.

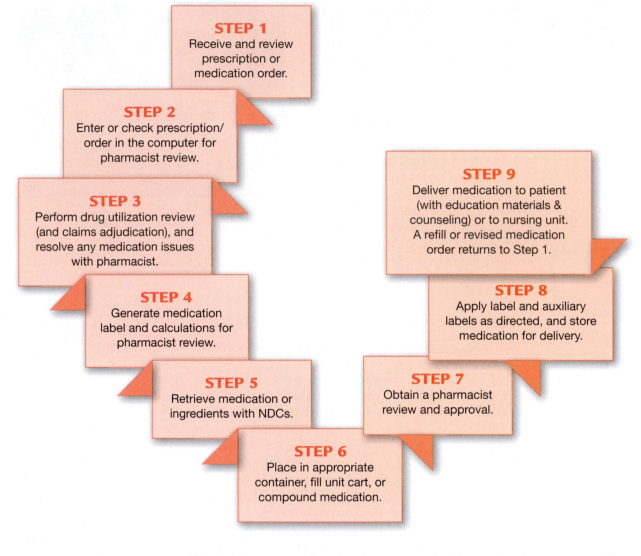

STEP 1
Receive and review prescription or medication order.

STEP 2
Enter or check prescription/order in the computer for pharmacist review.

STEP 3
Perform drug utilization review (and claims adjudication), and resolve any medication issues with pharmacist.

STEP 4
Generate medication label and calculations for pharmacist review.

STEP 5
Retrieve medication or ingredients with NDCs.

STEP 6
Place in appropriate container, fill unit cart, or compound medication.

STEP 7
Obtain a pharmacist review and approval.

STEP 8
Apply label and auxiliary labels as directed, and store medication for delivery.

STEP 9
Deliver medication to patient (with education materials & counseling) or to nursing unit. A refill or revised medication order returns to Step 1.

For refills, it is important that the pharmacy technician review the patient profile to see if a brand or generic product was previously dispensed. Generic drugs do not exist for all brand name drugs because some drug patents have not yet expired. Instead, there are **pharmaceutical alternative drug products** that contain the same active therapeutic ingredients but different salts (for example, hydroxyzine hydrochloride rather than hydroxyzine pamoate) or come in different dosage forms (a tablet rather than a capsule, or an immediate-release tablet rather than an extended-release tablet).

These pharmaceutical alternatives may be recommended by the pharmacist but *cannot be substituted without physician approval*. Thus, for a prescription of 100 mg of metoprolol succinate (an extended-release formulation), a pharmacy technician cannot substitute 100 mg of metoprolol tartrate (an immediate-release formulation). Although the active ingredients and dose are identical, the salts (succinate versus tartrate) and the release characteristics of the drugs differ. For this reason, this type of substitution must not happen unless specifically prescribed.

The FDA Online Orange Book

The first reference for generic-brand substitutions (and pharmaceutical alternatives) is the online FDA Orange Book, officially known as the *Approved Drug Products with Therapeutic Equivalence Evaluations*. The Orange Book lists the drugs and doses that may be safely substituted. For example, two brand name antihypertensive drugs for extended (24 hours) blood pressure control are Adalat CC and Procardia XL. They *cannot be substituted* for each other due to different drug-release characteristics. There are, however, generic manufactured drugs using the active ingredient nifedipine that are compatible with either or both that can be substituted. Each manufacturer's formulation of salts or other ingredients offers different drug characteristics.

Not every generic with the same active ingredient is the same. For example, the Actavis and Watson generic formulations of nifedipine in doses of 30 mg and 60 mg can be substituted for Adalat CC. In contrast, the Mylan generic nifedipine can be used in the place of Procardia XL. The Matrix Labs generic version can be used for either Adalat CC or Procardia XL. In most cases, the pharmacy software will cross-reference the FDA-approved generic equivalents of a given brand name drug.

Biologically Comparable Drug Products

Biological drugs, or biotech drugs (including genetically engineered drugs), come from a variety of live or once-live sources, including animals, humans, and microorganisms, such as yeast, bacteria, and fungi. These drugs include expensive injectable drugs used to treat genetic disorders, various blood disorders related to cancer or chemotherapy, and various inflammatory diseases, such as rheumatoid arthritis. When a brand name biological drug is patented and FDA approved, it becomes the **biological reference product** for all similar biological drug products to come.

Because biological drugs come from living matter or organisms, they *cannot be chemically reproduced with exactitude*, so a generic version cannot be designated as pharmaceutically or therapeutically equivalent. Instead, the FDA has evaluated and approved **biosimilar drugs**, which are "similar" though not "identical" to the parent innovator drugs. They have been proven to address the same indications with the same pharmaceutical mechanisms, or precise ways that the active ingredients exert their influence on the body. The biosimilars must also have the same administration routes, dosage forms, conditions of use, and levels of quality and strength as the originals.

If a biosimilar is tested and *found to be both similar and provide similar levels of therapeutic results*, the FDA can designate it as an **interchangeable biological drug**, which is both biosimilar and likewise therapeutically effective. Once a biosimlar is designated by the FDA as an interchangeable biological drug, *it can legally be substituted for the prescribed biological brand without contacting the physician for approval*, like a generic drug substitution.

As biosimilars and interchangeables move through the FDA approval processes, they are included in the online FDA Purple Book, officially known as the *Lists of Licensed Biological Products with Reference Product Exclusivity and Biosimilarity or Interchangeability Evaluations*.

The FDA also publishes a book on veterinary medications, or the Green Book, officially known as the *Approved Animal Drug Products*. Because some veterinary drugs can be purchased at pharmacies, this is also a valuable reference for pharmacists and technicians.

Additionally, pharmacy technicians should be familiar with other reference books that help identify equivalent drug products. *Facts & Comparisons* is available in paper and online versions and is a good reference for drug products as well as FDA approved and unapproved indications for drugs. *ASHP Drug Information* is commonly used in institutional pharmacies as a drug reference. The *USP-NF* also contains drug monographs.

Many references are available online with a paid subscription, including Lexicomp, Clinical Pharmacology, and Micromedex. Your employer will be required by state law to have available some of these drug references.

Common Pharmacy Abbreviations

To fully review and/or transcribe a prescription or medical order, the pharmacy must recognize all the shorthand abbreviations used. Table 4.3 lists common prescription abbreviations for amounts, dosage forms, time, and site of administration. Most of these abbreviations are derived from Latin. Note that weight and volume amounts borrow heavily from the measurement systems discussed in Chapter 2.

Focus and an attention to detail are critical when reviewing a prescription or medication order. Note that when the units are abbreviated, there is a minimal visual difference between gram (g) and grain (gr), but 1 g is equal to 1000 mg and 1 grain is equal to 65 mg, so there is a potential for a dosage error. That is why metric measurements are the safest ones for prescribers to use.

Arabic numbers are usually used for dosage quantities. Lowercase Roman numerals are generally only seen on prescriptions using apothecary measures, and they follow—rather than precede—the unit of measurement, as in "aspirin gr vi," meaning 5 grains; or "tbsp iii," meaning 3 tablespoons. However, errors have occurred so often that Roman numerals are discouraged. If they are used, *i, ii,* and *iii* are often written with a line above the letters ($\bar{i}, \bar{ii}, \bar{iii}$). The fractions in Roman numerals follow a different notation system (*ss* means ½), which is why Roman numerals are problematic.

In addition, some other traditional pharmacy abbreviations have proven dangerous. For instance, failure to differentiate the directions *q.d.* (daily) from *q.i.d.* (four times a day) can result in serious harm to a patient; often the tail of the *q* in *q.d.* (or a period between the *q* and *d*) may look like an *i* because it loops back. For this reason, the Institute for Safe Medication Practices (ISMP) recommends avoiding the use of the lowercase abbreviation *q.d.*; either use *QDay* or *daily* or *every day*.

In Table 4.3, a red line is drawn through the common abbreviations that the ISMP recommends should NOT be used because of the increased risk of misinterpretation leading to a medication error. For a more a complete list of pharmacy abbreviations, see Appendix A. However, because some prescribers still use these abbreviations, Roman numerals, and nonmetric units, it is very important to still study them and know their uses.

Abbreviations for dosage forms are usually fairly straightforward. Many generic medications are available in both capsule and tablet formulations and can be used interchangeably if they are in the same dosage strength. In some cases, the prescriber may write *tablet*, but if the capsule is in stock, it can generally be substituted if approved by the prescriber. Prescriptions written for the eyes and ears may be solutions or suspensions; there is a subtle difference between these dosage forms, and they should not be interchanged without the approval of the prescriber.

Study Idea

Remember, sterile eye drops can be used in the ear, but ear drops cannot be used in the eye!

Safety Alert

Remember that 1 mL is equal to 1 cc and is used interchangeably. The IMSP recommends not using "cc" as it is easily misread.

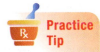
Practice Tip

If a prescription does not clearly state whether the medication is for the left or right eye (or ear), you may type in the sig field of the medication label "instill into the affected eye(s)." The pharmacist can then counsel the patient or parent when the prescription is dispensed.

TABLE 4.3 Common Prescription Abbreviations

Abbreviation	Meaning	Abbreviation	Meaning
Amount/Dosage Form		*Time of Administration—Continued*	
~~cc~~	cubic centimeter (mL)	~~PC~~, p.c.	after meals
cap	capsule	P.M.	evening, after noon
g	gram	PRN, p.r.n.	as needed
~~gr~~	grain	~~QN, qn.~~	every night at bedtime
gtt	drop	~~QD, qd.~~	every day
mg	milligram	QID, q.i.d.	four times a day
mL	milliliter (cc)	~~QOD, qod~~	every other week
QS, q.s.	a sufficient quantity	stat	immediately
tbsp	tablespoonful	t.i.d.	three times a day
tsp	teaspoonful	t.i.w.	three times a week
MDI	metered-dose inhaler	*Site of Administration*	
SOL, sol	solution	~~AD, ad~~	right ear
SUPP, supp	suppository	~~AS, as~~	left ear
SUSP, susp	suspension	~~AU, au~~	each ear
TAB, tab	tablet	NPO, npo	nothing by mouth
UNG, ung	ointment	~~OD, od~~	right eye
#	number of, quantity	~~OS, os~~	left eye
Time of Administration		~~OU, ou~~	each eye
AC, a.c.	before meals	PO, po	oral, by mouth
AM, a.m.	morning, before noon	PR, pr, R	per rectum
BID, b.i.d.	twice a day	SL, sl	sublingual (under the tongue)
hr	hour	TOP, top	topical (skin)
HS, h.s.	at bedtime	VAG, vag	vaginally

Note: The abbreviations with red lines through them are ones that are still in use but are discouraged by the Institute for Safe Medication Practices (ISMP).

Patient Profile

Study Idea

Remember that each prescription must be kept on file on the premises for two years from the date of dispensing.

Each time a patient presents a prescription or refill at the pharmacy or hospital, the technician or admitting nurse must create or update the **patient profile**, including physical address, prescription billing, and allergies (see Table 4.4 for the components of a patient profile). The technician needs to ask the patient questions about allergies, use of alcohol, OTC medications, herbals, and vitamin supplements, because these can also interact poorly with medications, decreasing efficacy or causing adverse medication reactions. The pharmacy software program uses the profile for processing the **drug utilization review (DUR)** to provide alerts about potential adverse reactions, medication conflicts, and allergies, and the pharmacist uses the information in the profile to help in counseling the patient.

The profile contains the patient's medication history, which tracks all the drugs the pharmacy has dispensed to this patient. When a patient requests a refill without the previous medication container or prescription number, the technician can retrieve the prescription information from the patient's medication history. The profile must also include patient requests, such as for containers that are not child-resistant, or for a 90-day supply when possible instead of a month's supply, or for needed accommodations due to foreign language, sign language, or visual impairment.

TABLE 4.4 Components of the Patient Profile

Component	Content
Identifying information	Patient's full name (including middle initial), street address, telephone number, birth date, and gender; increasingly, pharmacy databases enter email addresses so refill notifications and other communications can be made electronically
Insurance information	Information necessary for billing (see Chapter 10 for insurance and billing information)
Medical and allergy history	Information concerning existing conditions (e.g., diabetes, heart disease), known allergies, and adverse drug reactions; pharmacy software reviews patient medical history to make sure the prescription is safe.
Medication and prescription history	Most databases list any prescriptions filled at the individual pharmacy location; some list OTC medications as well. The new prescription is compared to previously filled prescriptions; pharmacy software reviews this information to check for adverse interactions with drugs or food.
Patient requests	Prescription preferences (e.g., child-resistant or non–child-resistant containers, generic substitutions, large-print labels, foreign language preference)
HIPAA and confidentiality	Pharmacies are required by law to provide new patients with a statement outlining patient confidentiality; the action must be documented and included in the profile. (This statement is for the protection of the pharmacy.)

Patient Privacy and HIPAA Regulations

In addition to providing personal and medication information, each new patient or guardian must sign a HIPAA form (outlining the pharmacy's privacy policy) and designate those with whom their medication history information can be shared. This form must be updated annually. A scanned version of this document must be added to the patient profile. Technicians must be on guard to keep the prescriptions, medication history, profile, and other patient information confidential or they are breaking the law. (For an overview of pharmacy-related HIPAA Regulations, refer to the online course supplements accessed at the end of this chapter in the ebook.)

Components of a Prescription

Study Idea

Even e-prescribing can cause medication errors if the prescriber selected the wrong drug or dosage form. Always check to see what the patient has received in the past.

A prescription may be submitted by computer (e-script), paper, phone, or fax. Table 4.5 lists the parts of a prescription, and Figure 4.2 shows a paper version, though most are now delivered as e-prescriptions. Some state Medicaid programs require that if paper is used, it must have a coin-activated security mark or other safety features that prevent copying, erasure or modification, and counterfeiting of the form.

E-prescribing can minimize forgeries and the risk of potential medication errors resulting from failure to understand a prescriber's handwriting, misinterpretation of abbreviations, and illegible faxes. Electronic prescribing of controlled substances must be approved by each state board of pharmacy. Controlled substances require a prescriber's DEA number and can only be done via e-prescribing if the prescriber's transmission is protected with at least two of the following security measures: password or response to security question, a biometric (fingerprint or eye scan), password device, or cryptographic token.

Prescriptions can be phoned in or faxed in to the pharmacist and then transcribed into the patient profile. State laws also determine whether or not technicians can take refill prescriptions over the phone. With all refill prescriptions, technicians must check for accuracy and any changes or additions to the patient profile.

TABLE 4.5   Parts of a Prescription

Prescriber	Name, address, telephone number, and other information identifying the prescriber, including state license number, DEA number, and NPI
Date	Date on which the prescription was written (may not be the same day the prescription was received); prescriptions are valid for one year, unless for a controlled substance (six months)
Patient information	Patient's full name, address, telephone number, and date of birth
℞	Stands for the Latin word *recipe*, meaning *take*
Inscription	Medication prescribed, including generic or brand name, strength, and amount
Subscription	Instructions to the pharmacist on dispensing the medication
Signa	Directions for the patient (commonly called the "sig")
Additional instructions	Any additional instructions that the prescriber deems necessary
Signature	Signature of the prescriber

Checking a Prescription

To be complete, check that the prescription contains all of the necessary information. Figure 4.2 provides an image of how these elements can be assembled in a paper prescription.

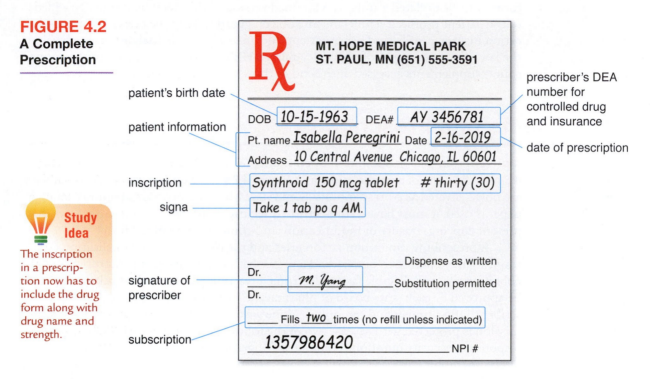

patient's birth date

patient information

inscription

signa

signature of prescriber

subscription

prescriber's DEA number for controlled drug and insurance

date of prescription

MT. HOPE MEDICAL PARK
ST. PAUL, MN (651) 555-3591

DOB *10-15-1963*   DEA# *AY 3456781*
Pt. name *Isabella Peregrini* Date *2-16-2019*
Address *10 Central Avenue Chicago, IL 60601*

Synthroid 150 mcg tablet   # thirty (30)

Take 1 tab po q AM.

Dr. _____ Dispense as written
M. Yang
Dr. _____ Substitution permitted

_____ Fills *two* times (no refill unless indicated)

1357986420   NPI #

Study Idea

The inscription in a prescription now has to include the drug form along with drug name and strength.

Study Idea

The NPI is used for identifying a prescriber for billing purposes. The DEA number, assigned by the DEA, must be present for a prescriber to order controlled substances.

Accuracy

In addition to checking for completeness, the technician must review prescriptions for accuracy. Often the prescriber's name is preprinted on the prescription at the top with address, phone number, and pertinent licensing numbers. If not legible or preprinted, the name may be identified in the computerized database by telephone number, or the **National Provider Identifier (NPI)**. The prescriber's state license number is sometimes required by the state, and the NPI number is usually required by insurance for reimbursement. *The NPI is the 10-digit identifying number established by the HIPAA act of 1996.*

If the prescription is for a controlled drug, such as a narcotic pain medication, nerve medication, sleeping pill, or diet pill, the prescriber *must have a federal DEA number on file* in the pharmacy database and on the prescription (as noted in Chapter 3). This number differs from a state license number and the NPI. If the DEA number is not listed or available, the technician may have to call the prescriber or his/her nurse and request it.

Many prescribers practice in more than one physical location or clinic; in such cases, *it is important to identify both the correct name and phone number of the medical office in which the prescription was written.* This is necessary to clarify prescription information or request future refills on medications. The technician should also compare the signature against the prescriber's known signature to prevent forgeries.

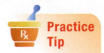
Next, the patient name must be verified. It is not uncommon for two patients to have the same first and last name (e.g., Rhonda Taylor and Rhonda S. Taylor). You may request the patient's date of birth and write it on the prescription. Some patients may prefer their middle names instead of their first names, making locating the record in the database a challenge. *Third-party payers require claims to be submitted under the name listed with the insurer.*

Practice Tip

Remember to check that a general prescription is not older than one year and a controlled substance prescription is not older than six months, or they are invalid.

Check the date the prescription was written. Do not assume that the prescription was written on the same day the pharmacy received it. If the prescription is for a controlled drug, *the prescription cannot be filled without this date.* If missing, a follow-up call to the prescriber is necessary, or the patient may need to get a new prescription. The prescription can be filled up to one year from the date written, unless it is for a controlled substance (which is six months from date written).

In the **inscription**, the technician should verify that the drug name, strength, form, and quantity are correct and legible. There are many drugs with look-alike and sound alike names, so focus and attention to detail are important. Many drugs come in various dosage forms—extended release and sustained release, inhalers and nebulizing solutions, and so on—so it is critical that the correct medication is entered into the patient profile in the computer.

Study Idea

Review techniques to prevent selecting the incorrect drug due to sound alike or look-alike names, such as tall-man lettering and shelf placement.

When the prescriber indicates *"dispense as written" (DAW) or "brand medically necessary,"* then the brand name drug must be entered into the computer and dispensed. Brand name drugs are commonly ordered for Coumadin, Dilantin, and Synthroid because of the narrow therapeutic index of these medications. For insurance billing they would be coded with "DAW1." If the drug name or directions are illegible, or the drug strength or quantity is missing, *a call to the prescriber is necessary.* Depending on the state and pharmacy's regulations, the pharmacist may need to verify any change. It is always good practice to verify information to minimize potential medication errors.

> **R̶x̶**   **Synthroid 225 mcg tablet #30. 1 tablet every day**

If the drug is not available in the prescribed strength, one option is to fill the prescription with a different strength and dosage that equals the original as discussed with calculation examples in Chapter 2. For instance, with a prescription for Synthroid 225 mcg 30 tablets for 1 tablet a day, one could perhaps fill the prescription with 150 mcg tablets and change the directions to "1.5 tablets per day." Another option is to enter two prescriptions of available strengths that can fulfill the prescription—one for 200 mcg and one for 25 mc. But that would result in a higher cost to the patient and the insurer. *For either change, the pharmacy technician must consult with the pharmacists, and any changes to a prescription reviewed and often initialed by the pharmacist,* especially a prescription for controlled drugs.

The quantity to be dispensed is usually stated on the prescription. Sometimes, however, the prescriber may instead simply indicate either a one-month or three-month supply. In such cases, the pharmacy technician must calculate the quantity to be dispensed. For example, the technician would enter *#180* for the quantity of tablets for the following prescription:

> **R̶x̶**   **Glipizide 10 mg tablet PO b.i.d. 90 days supply**

Study Idea

Do not assume refills, always enter the "No Refills" if the prescriber did not indicate whether the prescription should be refilled.

In some states, if a prescription is written for a 30-day supply with two refills, the pharmacy technician/pharmacist is allowed to fill a three-month supply. For example, a prescription for *simvastatin 40 mg #30 2 refills* could be filled (in some states) with simvastatin 40 mg #90. The pharmacy may do this to reduce the patient's out-of-pocket costs. Many insurers charge the equivalent of two monthly copayments for a three-month supply.

Mail order pharmacies, especially those connected to insurance providers, tend to provide 90-day (3-month) supplies of medications of 30-day supply with two refills. In other states, the medical office must be contacted for approval of combining a single prescription with two refills into one dispensing, and the approval must be documented on the prescription.

The **signa (sig)**, or directions for use, should be clear on the prescription so the technician can translate the abbreviations into the proper language for label instructions. The label must be reviewed and approved by the pharmacist before the medication is dispensed to the patient.

Legality

Technicians also need to determine whether or not prescriptions are legal. Legal prescribers include not only doctors but dentists (DMD, DDS), veterinarians (DVM), podiatrists (DPM), optometrists (OD), physician assistants (PA), nurse practitioners (NP), advanced practice nurses (APN), and naturopaths (NP). Physician assistants must practice under the direct supervision (and license) of a practicing physician. Nurse practitioners have prescriptive authority and can write or sign prescriptions according to the defined protocol in their states, even for controlled substances. A registered nurse may write a prescription, *but it must be signed by a licensed prescriber*.

To be legal, each prescriber must also prescribe within his or her specialty. For example, a veterinarian cannot prescribe medications for humans, an optometrist is limited to eye medications, and a dentist is restricted to prescribing appropriate medications, such as antibiotics and pain medications, in quantities limited to the patients' dental needs when prescribing. In some states but not others, physicians can prescribe medications for themselves and for family members, but *this privilege never applies to controlled drugs*.

Study Idea

Review the controlled substance law as it relates to dispensing medications in the retail pharmacy.

Know the regulations in your state. For instance, many states (and pharmacies) require a prescription (or evidence of diabetes) to dispense syringes. Can a physician assistant prescribe narcotics without the signature of his or her supervising physician? Can a nurse practitioner prescribe narcotics? What are the state requirements for tamper-proof prescriptions?

Controlled substance prescriptions must follow all of the federal laws covered in Chapter 3. Check that the prescriptions follow these guidelines:

- Whenever state and federal regulations of controlled drugs conflict, apply the more stringent regulation.

- Prescriptions for Schedule II medications require secure transmissions or a signed hard copy; the prescriber may not fax or phone in such prescriptions unless permitted by state law.

- Most, but not all, states allow the dispensing of Schedule V drugs, such as cough syrups, without a prescription. But the customer must be 18 years old or over, and they must present an ID and sign a tracking log. Limited amounts are allowed for sale at one time, such as 120 mL or 4 fl. oz. of cough syrup within a 48-hour period.

Refills The number of refills prescribed is indicated on the computerized prescription or circled on the hard copy. Generally refills are allowed for prescriptions for up to a year from prescribing date. *If refills are not stated or circled on the prescription, assume that no refills were ordered.* Refill for any prescriptions that are more than 12 months old, for hospital emergency room visits, or for discharge from a healthcare facility usually cannot be filled. Controlled-drug refills are even more limited, as seen in Table 4.6.

Early refills for any prescriptions *are generally only allowed for up to five days in advance*. If a full supply of the drug is not available, the pharmacy can do a **partial fill**, providing a two to five days supply to hold the patient over until the full amount arrives. An **emergency fill** of two to three days supply of medication can be dispensed for essential medications for chronic conditions when it is necessary to bridge a patient over till a doctor's visit for a new prescription. Generally, emergency fills are *not allowed* for controlled substances. However, in extreme circumstances with terminally ill patients, an emergency fill for a controlled substance for pain relief can occur. Emergency fills are at the discretion of the pharmacist.

For maintenance drugs, such as birth control medications, the prescriber may indicate p.r.n. or "as needed" refills for up to a year.

If patients want to transfer a prescription refill from one pharmacy to the other, the pharmacists of the new and the originating pharmacy must converse on the phone or through an online secure system. The new pharmacist can request the "**transfer in**" of the prescription and that the former pharmacist "**transfer out**" and *close the refill account*. For the transfers, the originating pharmacy must verify that the patient's name, birth date, contact information, prescriber, date of prescription, and the details of the prescription (including medication name, strength, form, number of refills remaining, dosage, and sigs) match.

Chain pharmacies that share online patient profiles do refill location changes without the transferring in and out because they share the same database, considering the full chain as a single pharmacy unit. Patients can order a refill online and select the location for pickup.

TABLE 4.6 Controlled Drug Refill Limits

- C-II cannot be refilled or transferred.
- C-III and C-IV may refilled up to 5 times up until 6 months from date written.
- C-V may have up to 11 refills up until 1 year from the prescribing date.
- Controlled substances in any schedule may be subject to even more state restrictions.
- C-III to C-IV drugs can only be transferred once and cannot be refilled early.

Authenticity and Spotting Forgeries

In a community pharmacy setting, the technician as well as the pharmacist must verify the authenticity of the prescription, especially in the case of controlled medications. Technicians need to learn common techniques for spotting forged prescriptions. Has the prescription been altered in any way, especially in quantity or number of refills? No alterations can be made on a Schedule II prescription.

Is the prescription written on tamperproof paper with a visible watermark? Some prescriptions may be photocopies or facsimiles cleverly produced with a laser printer. Prescription blanks are sometimes stolen from doctors' offices and prescriptions forged, especially for narcotics. Be wary of prescriptions written for unusual quantities for new out-of-state patients, especially on weekends and nights when the prescription cannot be verified with the prescriber. Such "patients" often request expensive brand name drugs and pay cash so there is no paper trail.

It is important to know how to verify the prescriber's DEA number. This number consists of two letters (the second letter is the same as the first letter of the last name of the prescriber) plus seven numerals. (To review the steps, see Chapter 3.) Remember, though, even if the DEA number is correct, the prescription still could be forged.

Components of a Medication Order

Pharm Facts

Computerized prescriber order entry is like e-prescribing but done within a hospital or other healthcare institution.

Medication orders are used by prescribers to request pharmaceuticals for patients in hospitals and other institutional settings, including nursing homes, long-term care facilities, and psychiatric hospitals. (Nurse-delivered home health care also uses medical orders.) The order is typically delivered by a **computerized prescriber order entry (CPOE)** from a handheld device or from a computer in the patient's room, surgery, ER, admittance room, or nurses' station. The prescriber will transmit the order to the pharmacy or enter the order into the patient's profile, and the pharmacist will verify the order for accuracy and patient safety before the technician begins the filling process.

The order can also be conveyed via a hard copy. The information on the medication order is then reviewed by the pharmacy technician (or nurse/unit clerk and pharmacist in the hospital) and entered into the patient profile in the computer for pharmacist approval. At the time of administration, nurses reconcile the medication with the order and patient through the **electronic medication administration record (eMAR)** by scanning the barcode on the medication and the patient's wrist band before administering the first dose.

Some institutions do not have a computerized MAR. Physician orders must be transcribed by hand onto a paper MAR to be double-checked by a nurse. Transcription errors may occur with this process. Hospitals are moving toward having pharmacy technicians do the entry of patient medication profiles and medication reconciliation.

Differences from a Prescription

Despite having shared information elements and abbreviations, there are several differences between a medical order and a prescription, including:

- Instead of direct dispensing to the patient, medication orders are filled and delivered to the unit to be administered by nursing personnel in the hospital, nursing home, or other medical facility.

- Medication orders come in the following kinds: **admitting order** (with home medication inclusion order), **daily order** (each day's medications), **continuation order** (periodic review of daily order to continue or modify it), **standing order** (similar order on file for all patient undergoing similar surgery or procedure), **stat order** (emergency order), and **discharge order** (for home therapy upon leaving).

- Depending on state regulations and site policies, hospital medication orders are usually renewed every seven days. Orders for antibiotics and narcotics often have **automatic stop orders (ASOs)** after a given period of time. The ASO requires the physician to continually review medications for each patient.

Study Idea

A formulary is established for an institution by its pharmacy and therapeutics committee.

- Prescriptions are for a defined amount of medication; medication orders, with the exception of narcotics, are *dispensed until the order is changed or discontinued, or the patient is discharged*.

- In the administration of the medication, nurses provide an extra layer of professional review and expertise that helps minimize medication errors.

- Most dispensed medications must be part of the hospital formulary, whereas a community pharmacy does not have a formulary. Specific requests for nonformulary medications must go through a process of approval and special ordering through the Pharmacy and Therapeutics (P &T) committee. If a nonpreferred or nonformulary medication is ordered by a hospital prescriber without DAW, the technician must follow the drug substitution policy outlined in the hospital's **policy and procedures (P&P) manual**. Typically, the hospital pharmacy can automatically substitute the ordered medication with the pharmaceutically equivalent formulary item without specific physician approval (for example, dispensing pantoprazole when omeprazole is ordered). The technician must know the formulary and institutional policies well.

- Increasingly, hospital pharmacies employ robotic devices to assist the pharmacy technician in retrieving and packaging drugs for unit dose use, filling carts, stocking nursing units, and sterile compounding.

- Hospital orders are often for medications administered intravenously (IV), such as parenteral and nutritional solutions, antibiotics, or other medications.

- Medication orders can also be prepared for investigational drugs through studies approved by the hospital's **institutional review board (IRB)**. Often, a technician (or technicians) is dedicated to this task and oversees the inventory, working with the study team to ensure that the investigational drugs are stored and dispensed separately from the general hospital pharmacy.

Checking the Medication Order

Study Idea

Identify the different requirements for a prescription and a medication order.

The pharmacy technician must review the medication order for completion. A hospital medication order must include the following:

- prescriber's name (and identifiers NPI and DEA if needed)
- patient's name, birthdate, and room number
- patient's height and weight
- date and hour the order was written
- drug name, dose form, strength, rationale for use
- site of administration and route
- administration directions, including timing
- prescriber's signature

There is less variety in prescribers in the hospital as compared to the community pharmacy because the prescribers within the hospital are usually doctors (MD, DO), residents, interns in training under direct supervision, or nurse practitioners.

Site of administration is usually *PO* or "per oral" for tablets, capsules, and many liquid solutions or suspensions. A few medications, such as nitroglycerin, work faster if placed sublingually (SL), or under the tongue. If a patient is vomiting continuously, the prescriber may order a drug administered rectally.

In the example below, the dosage form must be part of the prescription and the sig. The suppository (supp) and the *PR* designation indicate that the drug is to be administered per rectum. Creams and suppositories can also be prescribed vaginally or intravaginally (VAG).

> ℞ **Phenergan 25 mg supp. Sig: 1 supp PR every 6h p.r.n.**

Time of administration is important. For instance, if a prescriber writes the following antibiotic prescription, the technician should transcribe it exactly this way in the computer. Entering *b.i.d.* (twice a day) is not quite the same as *q12h* because the patient may take the medication six or eight hours apart in a "twice a day" order.

Some medications, like acid reducers and diabetic medications, are best taken before meals, and this direction will be abbreviated *a.c.* Some medications that can cause stomach ulceration (like ibuprofen) are taken with food. If the prescriber writes *p.c.*, the medication should be taken after meals.

If the amount of medication taken by the patient varies each day, the prescriber may use the abbreviation "q.s." This abbreviation is interpreted as "quantity sufficient" to fill the prescription. The technician will then need to calculate the amount of medication needed, as in Example 4.1 for Orapred. A stock bottle of Orapred is labeled 15 mg/5 mL.

Study Idea

The abbreviation "ac" means before meals, and the abbreviation "pc" means after meals. Review commonly used abbreviations.

> ℞ **Orapred 15 mg/5 mL syringe**
> **Sig: 15 mg PO BID with food on Day 1**
>
> **10 mg BID on Day 2**
>
> **7.5 mg BID on Day 3**
>
> **5 mg BID on Days 4–5**
>
> **Quantity: q.s.**

If a pediatrician writes a medication order as shown in the example, what quantity of medication should the technician dispense?

Example 4.1

Calculate the volume per oral syringe and number of oral syringes to be dispensed for the example above. BID = two times a day. Also, calculate the total q.s. quantity.

Day 1 Dose 15 mg of 15 mg/5 mL, would be 5 mL.

You will need to dispense 2 oral syringes of 5 mL for Day 1.

Day 2 Dose = 10 mg of 15 mg/5 mL

$$\frac{10\ mg}{y\ mL} = \frac{15\ mg}{5\ mL}; \quad 50 = 15\,y; \quad y = 3.3\ mL\ \text{per dose}$$

You will need to dispense 2 syringes of 3.3 mL for Day 2.

Day 3 Dose = 7.5 mg of 15 mg/5 mL

$$\frac{7.5 \text{ mg}}{y \text{ mL}} = \frac{15 \text{ mg}}{5 \text{ mL}}; \quad 385 = 15\,y; \quad y = 2.5 \text{ mL per dose}$$

You will need to dispense 2 syringes of 2.5 mL for Day 3.

Days 4 and 5 Dose = 5 mg of 15 mg/5 mL

$$\frac{5 \text{ mg}}{y \text{ mL}} = \frac{15 \text{ mg}}{5 \text{ mL}}; \quad 25 = 15\,y; \quad y = 1.7 \text{ mL}$$

You will need to dispense 4 syringes of 1.7 mL. Total volume for 5 days is

$$5 + 5 + 3.3 + 3.3 + 2.5 + 2.5 + 1.7 + 1.7 + 1.7 + 1.7 = 28.4 \text{ mL}$$

Filling a Prescription or a Medication Order

For all prescriptions, medication orders, and specialty compounding, drug utilization reviews (DURs) must be run. The DUR will provide alerts for any problems from drug-to-drug, drug-to-allergy, drug-to-medical condition, or dietary supplement interactions. All issues must be resolved by the pharmacist (often with assistance from the technician by contacting the prescriber's office for more information). In the community pharmacy, the technician will also run the insurance and third party claim processing (as will be described in Chapter 10). For many prescriptions, the technician will have to calculate dosage conversion and days supply. In the hospital, the billing department will handle these claims.

For both the prescription and medication order, a patient label or fill list is generated. The technician uses the drug name and strength to select the correct medication, scanning the NDC barcode to aid in identifying the exact drug, dose, and package size. One can see the NDC and the barcodes that accompany them on the stock drug label (Figure 4.3) and unit dose packaging.

Each drug product is also assigned a **lot number**, or control number, by the manufacturer that identifies its manufacturing batch and date. The date of manufacturing determines its expiration date. That is why the lot number is listed on the label in Figure 4.3 as "Expiration Date/Control No." This lot number allows the product to be traced if there needs to be a product recall because of some contamination to this specific batch.

FIGURE 4.3
Parts of a Stock Drug Label

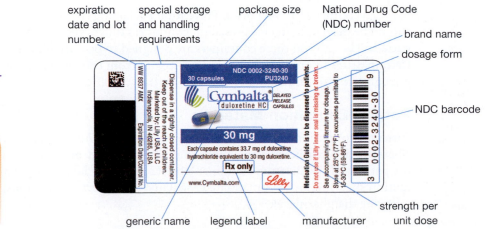

Study Idea

Look at container labels and the NDC codes to identify the various parts.

It is important for a certification exam to know what a lot number is and what the parts of the NDC represent. The first number set is for the manufacturer; the second number set indicates the strength, dosage form, and formula; and the last number set indicates the package code for size and types. (See Figure 4.4).

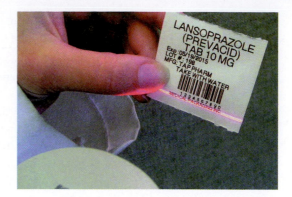

Commercially available unit dose labels contain the drug, dose, and NDC barcode.

Also generated with the medication label or list are the auxiliary labels—the small, colorful labels about warnings and side effects that may be added to supplement the directions on the medication container label (as seen in Chapter 1 on pharmacology). The pharmacist or pharmacy software will choose which auxiliary labels to use.

FIGURE 4.4
Components of the National Drug Code

Source:
www.drugs.com

labeler   product code   package code

NDC 0777 - 3105 - 02

Dista Products   Prozac Capsules 20mg   Total 100

Study Idea

Review Poison Prevention Act for definition of child-resistant container.

Prescription Filling

After the technician confirms the NDC on the stock bottle, the technician may have to reconstitute a solution or suspension product according to manufacturer instructions and then note the expiration date on the label. (Flavorings may also need to be added.) The expiration dates are determined by the manufacturer's guidelines.

Medications must be dispensed in the proper containers. Most pharmacy containers used for tablets, capsules, and liquids are amber-colored plastic or glass to prevent ultraviolet (UV) light exposure and subsequent degradation of the medication. Any product packaging from the manufacturer ensures stability and potency until the listed expiration date.

To comply with the Poison Prevention Packaging Act of 1970, all medications should be dispensed in child-resistant containers unless specifically requested by the patient. The caps on these containers are designed to be difficult for children to open. Certain drugs in original packaging are exempt from this requirement, especially nitroglycerin sublingual tablets.

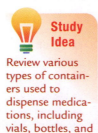

Study Idea

Review various types of containers used to dispense medications, including vials, bottles, and ointment jars.

Patient Education Materials

Patient information about use, warnings, side effects, and storage are very important. There are five distinct ways of communicating necessary medication information to the patient: (1) medication container label, (2) auxiliary labels, (3) medication information sheet, (4) an FDA-mandated MedGuide for select medications, and (5) counseling by the pharmacist.

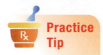
After medication review and verification by the pharmacist, the label is affixed to the container/bottle/box of prescribed medication and includes the following: the date dispensed; name, address, and phone number of the pharmacy; Rx number; patient name; number of refills; prescriber name; drug name; dose; directions; and manufacturer. The label's instructions must read as indicated in the signa on the original prescription. Some pharmacy labels also include a description of the medication.

The storage information on the labels is significant for having patients or nurses maintain medication stability and potency. For instance, most reconstituted antibiotics require refrigeration and expire after 14 days. Vials of insulin at room temperature often have an expiration of 28 days before they lose some potency. Other insulins and many eye drops, suppositories, and injectable medications require refrigeration in the pharmacy and at home. Within the pharmacy, the shingles vaccine (Zostavax) is stored in a freezer and is stable for only 30 minutes after it is reconstituted.

Medication container labels for Schedule II–V drugs must contain a transfer warning that reads, "Caution: Federal law prohibits the transfer of this drug to any person other than the patient for whom it was prescribed."

After the pharmacist conducts a final check of the prescription and medication, the information sheet is printed. It is attached to the prescription bag, which then is ready for patient pickup. Some prescriptions require a MedGuide, which is basically an extended black box warning advising consumers about potential adverse reactions or the proper use of selected high-risk medications. (See pages 185-188.) MedGuides are required for all high-risk drugs with risk evaluation and mitigation strategies (REMS). *Birth control pills must also be packaged with a MedGuide.*

Finally, by law, at the time of prescription pickup, the technician must offer the patient counseling by the pharmacist. At times, the patient may have a question or take advantage of the counseling that the technician offered, but often the patient does not. In some cases, especially with first-time medications or potential drug interactions, the pharmacist will take the initiative to counsel the patient. *The pharmacy technician is never allowed to counsel a patient.*

Patients must sign a document at pickup to verify they were offered counseling, and it will list the prescriptions being picked up by the patient. The document is usually on a computerized signature pad that will store the data in case of future insurance inquiries where proof is required that the patient received the filled medication.

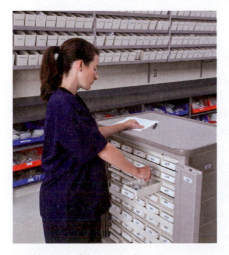

A technician fills a unit dose cart.

Medication Order Filling

Orders in the hospital are filled and delivered through daily unit dose carts, emergency carts, automated dispensing units on the nursing floor, or compounded parenteral medications that are delivered to the patients' rooms as needed. Table 4.7 lists the typical steps for filling a hospital order.

Large hospital pharmacies use a variety of time- and cost-saving devices to assist technicians in medication preparation and repackaging, such as automated pill counting machines and high-speed packaging and dispensing machines for oral medications (for example, PACMED by McKesson). Such automation reduces cart fill times, lowers inventory costs, and improves patient safety. Automated systems can also interface with robotic systems to further increase efficiency and safety in hospital pharmacy operations.

TABLE 4.7 Steps for Filling a Medication Order

The following list outlines the typical steps involved in filling a medication order in the hospital:

- Physician writes the medication order(s) on the patient chart or enters the order(s) in the computerized physician order entry system (CPOE). Home medications, if confirmed for continued use in the hospital, must be added to the patient profile and medication orders.

- The order is transmitted via computer to the patient profile or transported to the pharmacy by a tube system, transportation department, in person, or by pharmacy personnel making regular rounds. The technician or pharmacist would transcribe it into the profile.

- The medication order is reviewed for accuracy and safety by the pharmacist.

- A cart unit fill list per nursing floor or station is generated from the the 24–72 hour medication orders for patients in that unit. The medication order list is checked by the pharmacist for accuracy.

- The technician fills each patient medication drawer in a unit dose cart by selecting the correct medications at a pick station. (Technicians may also manage the robotic pick stations in the pharmacy for filling unit dose carts.) Each unit dose of a medication is labeled by the manufacturer with the generic or brand name of the drug, dosage and strength, administration instructions, manufacturer's name, lot number, expiration date, NDC, and barcode. This information must be matched to the medication cart list.

- The pharmacist reviews the unit dose cart according to the generated list or patient profile.

- Pharmacy technicians are then responsible for delivering the medication cart to the nursing unit. This is usually done once a day in a large acute care hospital, though the cart may carry medications for more than one day in a smaller hospital or long-term care facility.

- Stat orders are processed separately from the unit dose carts. They are given top priority by technicians and delivered immediately for the nurse or doctor to administer immediately.

- Emergency crash carts are checked and refilled by technicians with all the most commonly used emergency medications so they are always at hand. In a Pyxis system, some emergency medications, like nitroglycerin sublingual tablets, can be accessed by the nurse before the pharmacist checks the order.

- A Pyxis or other automated dispensing system may also be used to fill a medication order, especially on nursing floors, with the technicians also checking for and replacing expired medications. The technicians fill the automated dispensing units using the drug names and NDCs, removing expired drugs and reordering those that are low. Once the pharmacist approves a medication order, the nurse may retrieve it from the dispensing station to administer it. Some institutions use a combination of cart-fill and automated dispensing technology.

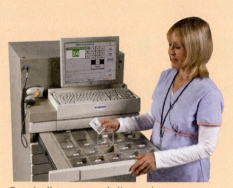

Omnicell automated dispensing system

Practice Tip

Expiration dates and lot numbers must be included on all repackaged medications, which is different from the stock expiration date.

Repackaging Drugs for Unit Doses

Not all drugs are commercially available in unit dose packaging, so the pharmacy technician often needs to repackage medications from bulk containers into unit doses and give them a barcoded label. A **medication special** is a single dose preparation repackaged for a particular patient and checked by the pharmacist.

For solid oral medications, technicians use heat-sealed bags, adhesive-sealed bottles, blister packs, and heat-sealed strip packages. For oral liquids, the medications are measured and sealed into airtight plastic or glass cups, heat-sealable aluminum cups, and plastic syringes labeled "For Oral Use Only."

All repackaged unit doses are placed in an envelope or a plastic bag and labeled with the patient's name, the drug name and dose, the medication administration time, lot number, beyond-use date, and an identifying barcode.

After repackaging, the essential information must be documented in a digital **repackaging control log** (or handwritten repackaging logbook as in Figure 4.5). It must be initialed by the repackaging technician as well as by the pharmacist who checked the medication. Automated repackaging machines can be used that generate and affix the labels.

Any home medications that are to be delivered in the daily dose carts also need to be repackaged as unit doses, affixed with a barcoded label, and portioned out in correct scheduled doses for the cart fill. At discharge, any remaining stock of the home medications will be returned to the patient.

FIGURE 4.5
Repackaging Control Log Information

This information must be entered and filed in the computer or logbook to document and track repackaging.

						Initials	
Date Repackaged	Pharmacy Lot Number	Drug Name, Strength, and Dosage Form	Manufacturer and Lot Number	Expiration Date	Quantity Packaged	Prep. By	Approved By

Repackaging Control Log
Department of Pharmaceutical Services

Parenteral Medication Orders

Patients often depend for survival upon swift administration of individualized sterile drug products, called **compounded sterile preparations (CSPs)**. See Chapter 6 for more information on types of parenteral preparations.

Large volume parenterals (LVPs) usually consist of water with salt (saline, or NaCl) and/or glucose (dextrose). It is not unusual for an LVP to have additional additives, such as potassium chloride (KCl) or multivitamins, depending on the patient's requirements. LVPs may be sent to the nursing unit or may be available at the nursing unit via a Pyxis workstation. Table 4.8 lists the most common IV fluid products and their typical abbreviations.

TABLE 4.8   IV Fluids and Abbreviations

IV Fluid	Abbreviation
Normal saline (0.9% NaCl)	NS
½ Normal saline (0.45% NaCl)	½ NS
5% Dextrose	D_5W
10% Dextrose	$D_{10}W$
5% Dextrose and normal saline	D_5NS
Lactated Ringer's solution	LR or RL

IV medication orders include additional information including fluid and amount, infusion period (such as "infuse over 30 minutes"), flow rate (such as 100mL/hour), and beyond-use date and time. (See Figure 4.6 for examples.)

FIGURE 4.6
Common Physician's Orders for Parenteral Solutions

These are medication orders with sterile compounding sigs and abbreviations. To translate, see Table 4.8.

R℞ cefoxitin 1 g IV every 6 h × 24 hours

R℞ nafcillin 1 g IV every 4 h

R℞ penicillin 2 million units IV every 4 h

R℞ add 100 units Humulin R regular insulin to 500 mL NS @ 20 mL/hour (label ℞ concentration 0.2 units/mL)

R℞ begin magnesium sulfate 5 g in 500 mL NS to run over 5 hours × 1 dose only

R℞ change IV fluids to 0.45 NS with 20 mEq KCl @ 125 mL/hour

Final Check by the Pharmacist

It is extremely important—and required by law—that the pharmacist checks every prescription and medication order to verify its accuracy before it is dispensed to the patient or sent to the nursing unit. Typically in a community pharmacy, the pharmacy technician will present the prescription printout or original hard-copy prescription, the medication information sheet, and the labeled container with the prescribed medication to the pharmacist for final check. The pharmacist reviews the original prescription, compares it with the patient profile, confirms that the medication information sheet has been printed, verifies that the drug selected by the technician (from the stock bottle) is correct, and checks the accuracy of the medication container label.

In the hospital, the medication order, label, compounding procedure, preparation records, and all materials used to prepare or make a compounded sterile product must be inspected by the pharmacist before the medication is sent to the nursing unit. The inspection should include verification of the identity and amount of ingredients, technique for aseptic mixing and sterilization, packaging, labeling, and physical appearance. A pharmacist will also perform a physical check to look for incompatibilities between the additives and an IV solution.

In the case of states and facilities that allow **tech-check-tech (TCT)**, the TCT can do the main checking of specific medications that have been verified and dispensed before. For instance, the University of Wisconsin Hospital and Clinics assigned TCTs to check the filling of unit-dose medication cassettes, and TCTs achieved a greater than >99.8% accuracy rate. The TCT must have advanced training for this responsibility.

STUDY SUMMARY

A major portion of the work done by pharmacy technicians is in the processing of prescriptions and medication orders. To allow the pharmacist more time for medication therapy management and counseling, it is crucial for a technician to understand the steps involved from intake of a prescription or medication order to dispensing. The technician must also be aware of the required attention to detail and accuracy. For the exam, focus on the following:

- the steps in the ordering and filling process
- being able to interpret orders
- reviewing calculations necessary for dosage and quantities to be dispensed
- knowing the labeling requirements for prescriptions and unit-dose packaging
- studying the legality of the order process as it relates to HIPAA
- preventing forgeries and counseling
- knowing the pharmacists role in the final dispensing to the patient or nurse for administration

ADDITIONAL RESOURCES

For more in-depth explanations, check out *Pharmacy Practice for Technicians*, 6e from Paradigm Education Solutions. To master and extend the material presented in this chapter, take advantage of the resources available through the eBook resources links. These include digital supplements, study resources, and a practice exam generator with 1,000+ exam-style questions. End-of-chapter tests are accessible through the eBook for individuals using the self-study course and through Navigator+ for individuals enrolled in the instructor-guided course.

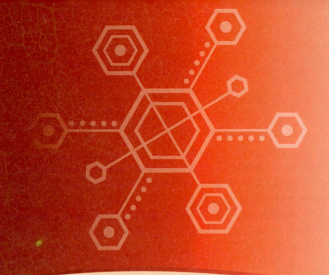

5

Nonsterile Compounding

Learning Objectives

1. Discuss USP guidelines for nonsterile compounding processes in USP Chapter <795>.

2. Know the documentation requirements for nonsterile compounding.

3. Identify the basic components of Good Compounding Practices.

4. Understand the steps in preparing a nonsterile compounded product.

5. Know the commonly compounded nonsterile dosage forms and techniques used in nonsterile compounding.

6. Identify the equipment and supplies for nonsterile compounding.

7. Know how to use and maintain the balances used in compounding, and how to calculate the percentage of error in measurements.

8. Understand how to calculate concentrations for compounding, including using the processes of geometric dilution and alligation.

9. Understand how to determine a product's stability, including beyond-use dating and signs of incompatibility.

10. Identify additional labeling requirements for compounded products.

Access eBook links for resources and an exam generator, with 1,000+ questions.

The purpose of this chapter is to provide the pharmacy technician with study knowledge of the basic skills involved in compounding simple and moderately complex nonsterile pharmaceuticals. Domain 3 of the PTCE includes nonsterile compounding will be described. Aspects of nonsterile compounding questions are also addressed in topical area 3 of the ExCPT. Complex nonsterile compounding is done by specialty pharmacies, and a pharmacy technician would need advanced training and may be required to have compounding certification to work in this environment.

Compounding is defined by the FDA as the *extemporaneous combining, mixing, or altering of ingredients by a pharmacist in response to a physician's prescription to create a medication tailored to the specialized medical needs of an individual patient*. Nonsterile compounding may only legally be done to create a drug preparation *that is not commercially available* to meet a specific medication prescription or order.

A community pharmacy is not allowed to manufacture bulk quantities of product for sale, although the pharmacy *can* prepare an excess amount for refills and similar prescriptions in a short time period. This practice is called **anticipatory compounding**, and it is legal, as long as the excess product is properly labeled with the assigned lot number, ingredients, and a short-term beyond-use date.

Types of Nonsterile Compounding

For a high-grade, nonsterile compounded product, correct professional procedures and policies must be followed with quality control measures, documentation, and recordkeeping. To achieve this, a technician should be familiar with the rules for **Good Compounding Practices (GCP)** outlined in USP Chapter <1075> and summarized briefly in Table 5.1. In addition, compounding technicians must particularly follow **USP Chapter <795>**—Pharmaceutical Compounding: Nonsterile Preparations—for the preparation, dispensing, and administration of these products to humans and animals.

TABLE 5.1 **USP Good Compounding Practices**

Component Standards	
Facility	Designated area with low traffic and adequate space for working and equipment storage
Personnel	Compounding staff trained and proficient in the skills necessary to compound drugs and maintain equipment
Equipment	Must be maintained and calibrated for accurate compounding and adequate for the products being compounded
Ingredient selection	*USP–National Formulary*-quality ingredients stored and used appropriately
Compounding	Periodic and final check by the pharmacist process
Packaging and storage	Appropriate containers that meet the storage requirements for each product
Beyond-use dating	Stability of preparation calculated by ingredients and dosage form, based on the preparation date
Quality assurance	Control programs established to guarantee equipment, staff, and product quality
Labeling of excess product	Ingredients, lot number, compound date, beyond-use date, and compounder information
Records and reports	Records of ingredients, personnel, and equipment for compounding the individual product as well as for all the ingredients and equipment used; the documentation including the Master Formulations Record, label, Compounding Record, and other records
Patient counseling	Patient education by the pharmacist to ensure appropriate use and storage of the medication

Study Idea

Categories of nonsterile compounding are determined by USP Chapter <795> are based on the master formulation and stability data, requirements for special calculations, and need for advanced compounding training.

USP Chapter <795> classifies nonsterile compounding into three categories:

- **Simple Nonsterile Compounding** is for making a preparation from a USP-recommended formulation record or from a peer-reviewed journal article in which the components, procedure, equipment, and stability data are clearly specified. Simple compounding also includes reconstituting or using commercial products that require adding one or more ingredients as directed by the manufacturer. Examples: captopril oral solution, benzoyl peroxide/erythromycin topical gel.

- **Moderate Nonsterile Compounding** requires special calculations or procedures for preparing the individualized product or individual dosage units or for determining the stability data. Examples: morphine sulfate suppositories, diphenhydramine troches, or mixing two manufactured creams together when stability of the mixture must be determined.

- **Complex Nonsterile Compounding** requires special technician training, facilities, equipment, and procedures. Examples: transdermal dosage forms, modified release preparations, and some inserts and suppositories for system effect.

In addition to the guidelines in USP <795>, compounding technicians need to know and apply the guidelines in related USP chapters:

- <1151> Pharmaceutical Dosage Forms
- <1160> Pharmaceutical Calculations in Prescription Compounding
- <1163> Quality Assurance in Pharmaceutical Compounding
- <1176> Prescription Balances and Volumetric Apparatus
- <1191> Stability Considerations in Dispensing Practice
- <1265> Written Prescription Drug Information Guidelines
- <800> Hazardous Drugs—Handling in Healthcare Settings (if using hazardous ingredients)

Web

In addition, technicians need to follow all the guidelines of the facility's policies and procedures (P&P) manual and the Occupational Safety and Health Administration (OSHA). To compound nonsterile drug products with hazardous substances, technicians must have additional training on the storage, handling, and disposal of these chemicals. For animal-oriented preparations, technicians must also follow the rules of the American Veterinary Medical Association's "Guidelines for Veterinary Prescription Drugs," at http://CertExam4e.ParadigmEducate.com/AVMA.

Basic Nonsterile Compounding Steps

It is important for the pharmacy to have a separate, designated compounding area that is removed from excessive traffic and air flow that might interfere with the accuracy of the balance and disturb stock powders. The dedicated area must be well-maintained, neat, clean, and uncluttered with sufficient workspace and storage. If compounded pharmaceuticals are stored in a refrigerator or freezer, the temperature must be recorded at least daily to ensure proper storage conditions are maintained.

Pharm Facts

OSHA is the agency responsible for the safety of workers on the job.

According to the USP Chapter <795>, the compounding pharmacy technicians must wear appropriate clean compounding garb, including hair bonnets, coats, gowns, gloves, face masks, shoes, aprons, or other items depending upon what is needed for protection from chemical exposures and for prevention of drug contamination. Additional PPE can be identified from OSHA and the material safety data sheet. Compounding garb should not be worn outside the compounding area.

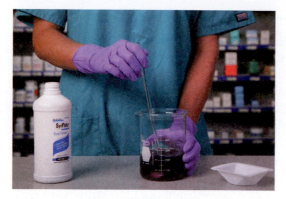

A pharmacy technician often wears scrubs or a lab coat, gloves, and a hairnet when preparing nonsterile products.

Compounding technicians should wash their hands with soap and warm water, rubbing their hands together vigorously for a thorough cleaning before putting on gloves. (For sterile compounding, 30 seconds of hand washing is recommended, with the application of a sanitizing gel just before applying gloves. For nonsterile compounding, the recommendation is to be "thorough" in the washing—the CDC recommends at least 15 seconds and/or the use of a hand sanitizer for healthcare practitioners. Hand gels do not replace the need for hand washing to remove any dirt and particulates before putting on gloves.)

Compounding begins when the prescription is entered into the computer so that it can be checked against the patient profile for the drug utilization review (DUR). The pharmacist then selects the proper **Master Formulation Record** (compounding recipe) to fit the prescription and patient needs. An overview of the full process is provided in Table 5.2. During compounding, only one product should be made at a time, and the equipment and compounding area should be cleaned before starting another preparation.

Once the Master Formulation Record, or recipe, has been determined or approved by the pharmacist, the technician gathers the ingredients according to the record. The pharmacy must use high-grade chemicals and ingredients that meet *USP-National Formulary (NF)*, or *Food Chemicals Codex (FCC)* guidelines for compounding. A **Material Safety Data Sheet (MSDS)**—also known as the **Safety Data Sheet (SDS)**—should be on file for every chemical stored in the pharmacy to facilitate the safe cleanup of any accidental spills or contamination. (More information on MSDSs is in Chapter 6, Sterile and Hazardous Compounding.) An eyewash station should also be readily available.

Water used in compounding preparations must be purified. Sterile water is acceptable because it has been purified. To document the purified water, include the source, lot number, and beyond-use date. Rinse equipment with purified water as required by USP Chapter <795>.

To ensure a high-quality product is produced each time, it is necessary to document that the proper quantities and sequences were used. From the Master Formulation Record, the technician generates the **Compounding Record** (or log), which is filled in with the specific information on the actual process. (See Tables 5.3 and 5.4 for the required components of each type of record.) This documentation occurs each time a product is made, unique for each prescription. A specific prescription and/or extemporaneous compounding lot number must be assigned to each Compounding Record so the compound can always be traced to its date and particular process. The Compounding Record is to be filled in with the calculations, notes on special equipment used, ingredient lot numbers and expiration dates, the initials of the compounding technician, and the pharmacist who checked the technician's work. For an example, see the Magic Mouthwash Compounding Record shown in Figure 5.1. on page 139.

After the product is compounded, a **beyond-use date (BUD)** must be determined. The BUD is the date after which the compounded product should not be used, and *it is calculated from the date the product was compounded.*

Study Idea

Know when a Master Formulation Record, Compounding Record, and MSDS, are needed in nonsterile compounding.

Practice Tip

Lot numbers are used to be able to trace ingredients and compounded prescriptions.

TABLE 5.2 Steps in the Compounding Process

1. The pharmacist judges the suitability of the prescription for appropriateness of dose, safety, and intended use, and accesses the results of the DUR, resolving issues.

2. The pharmacist reviews the technician's selection for the Master Control Record in the computer and approves or modifies the technician's selection. (See Table 5.3 for the components.)

3. The technician generates a Compounding Record (or log sheet) from the formulation record to make the nonsterile preparation. (See Table 5.4 for a description of requirements for a Compounding Record. Figure 5.1 is an example for Magic Mouthwash.)

4. The technician performs all necessary mathematical calculations for ingredient quantities and beyond-use date and identifies the necessary equipment; the pharmacist double-checks all calculations.

5. The technician generates the medication container label with the computer software using information in the compounding log. The label includes the following:

   a. patient name

   b. physician name

   c. date of compounding

   d. name of preparation

   e. prescription and/or extemporaneous compounding ID or lot number

   f. beyond-use date

   g. directions for use, including any special storage conditions

   h. any additional requirements of state or federal law

   i. initials of compounding technician and pharmacist

6. The technician gathers all necessary active and inactive ingredients as well as prepares and calibrates any measuring equipment.

7. The pharmacy technician uses appropriate protective clothing and hand-washing technique.

8. The technician weighs all ingredients for the preparation, initials each step, and adds documentation (such as source and NDC number) to the Compounding Record for the pharmacist to check before ingredients are combined.

9. The technician combines ingredients in the proper order and method according to the Master Formulation Record and stores the medication in a proper container for application, storage, and UV light protection.

10. The technician generates and affixes the medication label and pharmacist recommended auxiliary labels to the proper container.

11. The pharmacist reviews the Compounding Record and labels, and assesses appropriate physical characteristics of the preparation, such as any weight variations, adequacy of mixing, clarity, odor, color, consistency, and pH.

12. The pharmacist signs and dates the compounding log record and/or prescription, and files the records (computer entry and printed copy).

13. The technician places the compounded preparation in proper storage and notifies patient pickup.

14. The technician cleans all equipment thoroughly and promptly, reshelving all active and inactive ingredients, and properly labeling and storing any excess preparation.

15. The technician refers the patient to pharmacist counseling at the time of pickup.

TABLE 5.3 Components of the Master Formulation Record

1. Official or assigned product name, strength, and dosage form
2. Calculations needed to determine and verify quantities of components and doses of active pharmaceutical ingredients (APIs)
3. Description of all ingredients and their quantities
4. Compatibility and stability information, including references when available
5. Equipment needed to prepare the preparation, when appropriate
6. Mixing instructions, which include order of mixing, mixing temperature and other environmental controls, duration of mixing, and other factors relevant to replication of the product
7. Sample labeling information, which shall contain in addition to legally required information: generic name and quantity or concentration of each active ingredient, assigned beyond-use dating, storage conditions, and prescription or control number, whichever is applicable
8. Container used in dispensing
9. Packaging and storage requirements
10. Description of the final preparation
11. Quality control procedures and expected results

Source: USP Chapter <795>

TABLE 5.4 Components of a Compounding Record

1. Official or assigned product name, strength, and dosage form
2. Master Formulation Record reference for the preparation
3. Names and quantities of all components
4. Sources, lot numbers, and expiration dates of components
5. Total quantity compounded
6. Name of person who prepared the preparation, name of the person who performed the quality control procedures, and the name of the pharmacist who approved the preparation
7. Date of the preparation
8. Assigned lot or prescription number
9. Assigned BUD
10. Duplicate label as described in the Master Formulation Record
11. Description of final preparation
12. Results of quality control procedures (e.g., weight range of filled capsules, pH of aqueous liquids)
13. Documentation of any quality control issues and any adverse reactions or preparation problems reported by the patient or caregiver

Source: USP Chapter <795>

FIGURE 5.1
Dispensing Log for Magic Mouthwash

Patient Name _____   Date Prepared 12/2/20XX

Rx # _____   Master Control Record # _____

Compounding Formula for Magic Mouthwash

Ingredient Name	Amount Needed	Manufacturer	NDC #	Lot #	Expiration Date	Prepared By	Checked By
Lidocaine 2% viscous	60 mL	HiTech	50838-0775-04		12/10/20XX		
Diphenhydramine 12.5 mg/5 mL	60 mL	Walgreens	00363-0379-34		07/12/20XX		
Mylanta, generic	60 mL	Qualitest	00603-0712-57		03/12/20XX		
Nystatin suspension	60 mL	Qualitest	00603-1481-58		09/11/20XX		
Total quantity	240 mL						

Prepared by _____

Quality Control checked by _____

Approved by _____

Date and lot number _____

Beyond-use date _____

Directions _____

Auxiliary Labeling: SHAKE WELL

Safety Alert

When compounding drugs with high incidence of allergic reactions, such as penicillin or sulfa drugs, do not use equipment that cannot be cleaned thoroughly. Cross-contamination may harm a patient.

Commonly Compounded Dosage Forms

In compounding different dosage forms, different methods are required.

Tablets A tablet is a solid dosage form made from dry powdered ingredients. The powdered ingredients are mixed together and then pressed together with a single punch tablet press. Compression tablets require expensive equipment and special expertise, and are labor-intensive. They are not commonly made in the community pharmacy.

Capsules A capsule contains the active and inactive ingredients encased in a hard shell made of gelatin, sugar, and water. The capsule shell consists of two parts: (1) the body, which is the longer narrower part; (2) the cap, which is the short part that fits over the body. Capsules come in standard sizes indicated by numbers: 5, 4, 3, 2, 1, 0, 00, and 000. The largest capsule size is 000, and it can contain up to 1,000 mg of medication. The smallest size, 5, can contain up to 100 mg (depending on the substance).

Two methods for filling capsules are the manual **punch method** and the capsule machine. In either method, the body is filled with the compounded powdered ingredients, and the cap is placed over the body and pressed down to seal the capsule.

Solutions A solution is a liquid dosage form in which an active ingredient, the **solute**, is dissolved in a liquid vehicle, the **solvent**. A solution may be the addition of a liquid or powdered solute. The solvent can be aqueous, alcoholic, or hydroalcoholic. Solutions can be for oral administration or topical administration, such as an otic solution for earwax softening. Simple syrup is a common aqueous solution in which 85 g of sucrose is dissolved in 100 mL of purified water.

Suspensions A suspension is a liquid dosage form in which the solute *is not dissolved in the solvent but dispersed throughout the liquid vehicle*. Since the active ingredient may settle in a suspension, the pharmacy technician should always include a "Shake Well" label on the compounded products label.

   The order of mixing ingredients is important to prevent clumping, also known as **agglomeration** (or flocculation), of the active ingredients. The tablet or powder must be vigorously triturated before adding to the suspending agent, and the final liquid vehicle.

Troches, Gummies, and Lolipops A troche, which is also known as a lozenge, is used for buccal administration, or absorption by the mucous membranes into the blood vessels in the cheek or vagina. The active ingredients for the troches and lollipops in powder form is slowly added to a liquid base with other formulated ingredients, heated, and poured into a mold to cool into shape. They are used for pain relief, bioidentical hormones, and the antifungal drug clotrimazole, among other uses.

Ointments An ointment is a **water-in-oil (w/o) emulsion** that is usually greasy and not water washable. An occlusive ointment holds moisture in the skin for hydration. Emollient-based ointments, such as bath oils, are more softening to the skin. It is best to use water-repellant plastic equipment to compound an ointment.

   For ointments, gels, creams, and lotions the goal is not only an accurate, safe, and effective preparation, but also a **pharmaceutically elegant product**, which is smooth and without visible flaws. To create a pharmaceutically elegant ointment, add the active ingredients in small amounts and constantly work the mixture into the ointment base with a spatula on an ointment slab. Automated ointment mills are available that maximize the mixing of ingredients to improve the final preparation.

Creams A cream is generally an **oil-in-water (o/w) emulsion** that is nonocclusive, nongreasy, and water washable. A cream is best prepared using glass equipment. Creams may be made in a glass mortar and pestle.

Lotions A lotion is generally a liquid suspension or an oil-in-water emulsion used topically where lubrication is desired, such as on the skin or scalp. A lotion is similar to a cream but thinner in consistency. Calamine for poison ivy is an example of a commercially available suspension lotion.

Gels Much like a suspension, a gel contains solid particles in a liquid, but the liquid is thickened with gelatin or another agent, and the particles are fine or ultrafine.

Suppositories A suppository is a solid dosage form that has the active ingredient placed in a water-soluble base (like glycerinated gelatin or polyethylene glycol) or oleaginous base (like cocoa butter). Suppositories are inserted into body orifices, such as the rectum, vagina, or urethra, and they melt at body temperature to release the active ingredient. A suppository mold is used to shape the dosage form, or it is molded by hand. The suppository's shape and size is determined by the site of administration. Refrigeration of the final product is usually necessary to maintain shape and stability.

Nonsterile Compounding Equipment

Before each compounding session, *scales and measures should be checked and calibrated for accuracy*. Many state boards of pharmacy list the minimum equipment necessary for a licensed pharmacy, including a scale, spatulas, graduated cylinders, compounding slabs, storage containers, and mortar and pestle.

Measuring and Weighing Instruments

A **digital electronic analytical balance** is the easiest to use and most accurate, but it is expensive and may not be available in some community pharmacies. Most pharmacies have a **Class III prescription balance** (formerly called a Class A Balance), which is a two-pan mechanical balance that uses pharmaceutical weights of various sizes to weigh small amounts of materials, as shown in Figure 5.2.

Typical weight sets include metric and apothecary weights, though the apothecary weights are rarely used. Metric weights vary in size, from 10 mg to 100 g. They should be stored in their original box and *only handled with the forceps* provided to prevent the transfer of hand oil that can result in inaccurate measurements. Pans should always be covered with weighing papers or boats to prevent damage that could cause inaccuracies.

A larger scale, called a **counterbalance**, is used to weigh heavier amounts up to 5 kg.

FIGURE 5.2
Weighing with a Class III Prescription Balance

(a) After the scale is level and locked, transfer weights with forceps to the right pan and ingredients to the left. (b) Make final measurement, and check with the cover down.

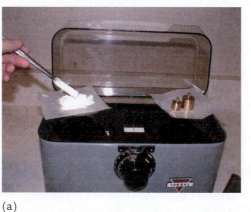
(a)

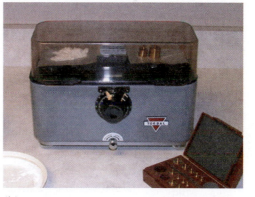
(b)

Percentage of Error

Each type of weighing or measuring device has a different potential range of error, or **sensitivity range (SR)**. The smallest incremental unit of weight that the device uses to measure is how much it can be "off". For instance, a perfectly calibrated Class III balance measures in increments of 6 mg—the smallest amount needed to move the measurement indicator one notch. So each weighed measurement can potentially be off by plus or minus 6 mg ($\pm$ 6 mg), which is this device's sensitivity range.

Each measurement's **percentage of error** is the range of error compared to the measurement quantity. To calculate this, you take the sensitivity range divided by the desired (prescribed or formula) quantity and multiply it by 100%.

$$\frac{sensitivity\ range}{desired\ quantity} \times 100\% = \%\ of\ error\ in\ product$$

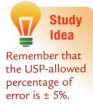
Or if you do not know the sensitivity range but you do know the amount of error, you can use the following formula:

$$\frac{error\ amount}{desired\ quantity} \times 100\% = \%\ of\ error\ in\ product$$

The official USP guidance allows for *a deviation range of plus or minus 5% (± 5%)* in weighted measurements. If the percentage of error is higher, then it is unacceptable.

Example 5.1

The Master Formulation Record asked for 120 mg of a drug powder. Using a Class III balance, the amount was weighed. The amount was double-checked on a digital scale. It showed that the weighed amount was actually 100 mg. What was the amount of error and the percentage of error?

Step 1 Follow the equation to determine the amount of error:

100 mg − 120 mg = −20 mg; the amount was 20 mg underweight.

Step 2 Use the amount of error to determine the percentage of error that occurred:

$$\frac{-20\ mg}{120\ mg} \times 100\% = -16.67\%,\ which\ is\ the\ percent\ of\ error.$$

Since the scale is underweight by 16.67%, it may also be overweight by this much, meaning this scale for 120 mg would have ±16.67% of error. This high percentage of error is unacceptable as it is over the USP limit of ±5%. This scale should be recalibrated or not be used for weighing.

Least Weighable Quantity Per Scale

The lower the quantity being measured and the closer it is to the sensitivity range, the higher the percentage of potential error. Most balances are marked with their degree of accuracy and their **least weighable quantity (LWQ)**.

To calculate an unmarked weighing device's LWQ to check for the 5% or less error percentage, you must divide the device's incremental unit by the highest allowed percentage of error and multiply it by 100:

$$\frac{scale's\ incremental\ unit\ of\ measurement}{maximum\ \%\ of\ error} \times 100 = least\ weighable\ quantity$$

For instance, the LWQ of a Class III balance can be calculated this way:

$$\frac{6\ mg}{5\%} \times 100 = 120\ mg \quad or \quad \frac{6\ mg}{0.05} = 120\ mg$$

(If you use the decimal form of the percentage of error as the denominator, there is no need to multiply by 100; you will get the incorrect answer if you do.)

For the Class III balance, *you may not accurately weigh ingredients for amounts lower than 120 mg.* This is a standard practice, so the calculation does not need to be done each time.

Because inaccuracies are more likely when weighing ingredients for smaller batches, compounding pharmacies like to do anticipatory compounding for a "larger batch" of each small preparation—so the percentage of error in measurement goes down.

Most compounded nonsterile preparations—tablets, capsules, ointments, creams, and gels—are prepared in larger quantities than the original prescription, especially if the prescription will be refilled. For example, instead of preparing 30 capsules of a medication each month, the master formulation record or recipe may call for preparing a minimum quantity of 100 capsules.

Mixing Instruments

A **spatula** is used to transfer solid dosage forms to weighing pans and for other tasks, such as preparing ointments and creams or loosening material from the surface of a mortar and transferring to a container. Spatulas may be made of plastic, rubber, or stainless steel. *Hard rubber is used for corrosive materials like iodine or mercuric salts.*

A **compounding slab**, or ointment slab, is a plate *made of glass, which is smooth, hard, and nonabsorbent.* The slab is used to mix ingredients (spatulation) evenly for an ointment or cream. Ointments and creams are stored in ointment jars that range in size from 1 ounce to 1 pound, or they are put into tubes. Ointment pads, made of parchment paper, are also used in preparing ointments and creams. The paper improves the ease of transferring the compounded product to its dispensing container.

A **mortar and pestle** is used for grinding and mixing pharmaceutical ingredients. Both the mortar and pestle can be made of glass, porcelain, or Wedgwood. The coarser the mortar surface, the finer the triturating (grinding) of the powder or crystal. *The glass variety is used to mix liquids, and the porcelain or Wedgwood type is used to grind crystals, granules, and powders.* High-volume compounding pharmacies may have an electric mortar and pestle for grinding and mixing.

Cylinders, **pipettes**, and **beakers**, which are made of glass or polypropylene, are used to measure liquids. They are calibrated in metric and apothecary units. Graduated cylinders are more accurate and should be read from the bottom of the meniscus. Beakers are used for mixing, *pipettes are used to measure volumes less than 1.5 mL, and cylinders are used for measuring larger volumes.*

Practice Tip

At eye level, read a liquid's measurement from the bottom of the meniscus.

Miscellaneous Equipment Depending on the amount of compounding done on site, the pharmacy may have other equipment, including a convection oven, single-punch tablet press, pellet press, or capsule machine. These facilitate making tablet, pellet, and capsule dosage forms.

Common Techniques for Ingredient Preparation and Blending

Comminution is the act of reducing the particle sizes of ingredients for integration to a smaller one through various methods, including trituration, pulverization by intervention, levigation, and heating and dissolving.

- **Trituration** is the process of rubbing, grinding or pulverizing a substance to create a finer particle. Minimal pressure and rotating of a pestle in a mortar grinds the ingredients into a powder. Trituration can also be used to combine two or more powders to standardize the powder blend.
- **Pulverization by intervention** reduces the size of the particles with the aid of an additional ingredient in which the substance is soluble. A volatile solvent like camphor, alcohol, iodine, or ether is often used in the process. Only a

small amount of the solvent is used, and then it is allowed to evaporate so it is not part of the final product.

- **Levigation** is used to further reduce particle size of a solid during ointment preparation. A levigating agent, such as castor oil, glycerin, propylene glycol, or mineral oil, is slowly added to the large particles of dry ingredients in a glass mortar or on an ointment slab to wet (this does not dissolve) the powder. The resulting paste is triturated with a mortar and pestle, and then added to the ointment base.

- **Heating and dissolving** involves applying gentle heat to dissolve a solid ingredient that is not easily dissolved. This allows for more uniformity and less precipitation.

Blending does not include any particle reduction but is the act of combining two substances. There are many methods of blending, including spatulation, sifting, tumbling, and geometric dilution.

Study Idea

Be able to identify each nonsterile preparation action in terms of the relative particle size being reduced or blended.

- **Spatulation** is a process to blend substances with a spatula. This is useful for fine powder mixing and mixing powders into and ointment base.

- **Sifting** is the mixing of powders using a fine wire mesh sieve. The powder is poured into an appropriate particle size sieve, and a rubber spatula is used to force the powder through the sieve and onto glassine paper.

- **Tumbling** is used to mix or blend powders with a container, such as a resealable plastic bag or glass bottle. After the powders are added, the container is rotated or tumbled to mix the powders.

- **Geometric dilution** is a method for combining two or more ingredients of differing strengths into an ointment or cream base. The ingredients are added a little at a time. The most potent ingredient (often the ingredient in the smallest quantity) is placed into the mortar first, then an equal amount of diluent is added before mixing well. The process is repeated by adding the second ingredient and an equal amount of diluent, and then mixing. This process occurs for each ingredient until all have been integrated effectively. Any small amount of leftover diluent should be added at the end and mixed well. This creates a smooth dispersion of drug(s) in the cream or ointment base.

    To review how this is geometric dilution is calculated and combined, see example 5.2.

Example 5.2

A prescription for 60 grams of an ointment with three active ingredients is to be compounded—hydrocortisone powder, zinc oxide powder, and a hydrophilic ointment—in a ratio of 1:3:6. Calculate how much of each ingredient will be needed, and explain how to use the geometric dilution method for compounding these ingredients into a pharmaceutically elegant product.

Step 1 Find the number of total parts by adding all the elements together.

$1 + 3 + 6 = 10$ parts. Then divide the total weight by the total ratio parts.

$$\frac{60 \text{ g}}{10 \text{ parts}} = 6 \text{ g per part}$$

Step 2 Multiple each ingredient ratio by the weight for one part to find the ingredient content amounts:

hydrocortisone	=	1 parts × 6 g/1 part	=	6 g
zinc oxide	=	3 parts × 6 g/1 part	=	18 g
hydrophilic ointment	=	6 parts × 6 g/1 part	=	36 g
Total weight				60 g

The total amount of preparation is 60 g with 36 g being the diluent of hydrophilic ointment. The method for geometric dilution will be:

- Put 6 g of hydrocortisone powder onto an ointment slab, add 6 g of hydrophilic ointment, and spatulate.
- Put 18 g of zinc oxide on another ointment slab, add 18 g of the hydrophilic ointment, and spatulate.
- Spatulate the two mixtures together.
- Add the remaining 12 g of hydrophilic ointment to the mixture, and spatulate into the final product.

Compounding Calculations

Study Idea

Go back to Chapter 2 and review ratio and proportions calculations.

Pharmacy technicians need to do many calculations when creating nonsterile compounds. They need to convert dosages or ingredients from one measurement system to another, or calculate how to dilute medications or combine ingredients in the correct proportions. In the pharmacy profession, the term **ratio strength** refers to the concentration level of an active ingredient to a completed product. Solutions made of two or more liquids are described as volume-in-volume concentrations, such as mL/mL. (Compounding with solutions and dilutions, with volume-in-volume calculations, are often done in sterile compounding and will be addressed in the next chapter.)

Solutions with powdered ingredients and suspensions are described as **weight-in-volume**, such as mg/mL, and solids and gels are described as **weight-in-weight**, such as mg/g. Proportion equations are often used for these calculations.

Calculating with Concentration Percentage Ratios

Ointments and creams use a percent concentration, which is defined as the percentage weight of the active ingredient per 100 grams of the final drug formulation (cream or ointment). For example, a 2.5% hydrocortisone cream is equal to 2.5 grams of active ingredient (hydrocortisone) per each 100 grams of cream. Percentage concentrations are handled the same as for volume-in-weight percentages, except that the units of measure are all weights, either mg or g (as reviewed in Chapter 2). To see how concentration percentages are applied in nonsterile compounding, study Example 5.3.

Example 5.3

In preparing to dispense a medication lotion of 4 ounces of 10% Menthol, 2% Camphor in Lubriderm Lotion, how many grams of each active ingredient and diluent will you need?

Step 1 Convert the prescribed ounces to grams (1 ounce = 30 grams) to determine how much to dispense, set up the following equation:

$$4 \text{ oz} \times \frac{30 \text{ g}}{1 \text{ oz}} = 120 \text{ g}$$

Then cancel the ounces from the numerator and denominator.

Step 2 Set up and apply a ratio proportion equation:.

$$10\% \text{ menthol: } \frac{10 \text{ g}}{100 \text{ g}} = \frac{y}{120 \text{ g}}; \ 120 \text{ g} = 10 \text{ y}; \quad y = 12 \text{ g}$$

$$2\% \text{ camphor: } \frac{2 \text{ g}}{100 \text{ g}} = \frac{x}{120 \text{ g}}; \ 240 \text{ g} = 100 \text{ x}; \quad x = 2.4 \text{ g}$$

Step 3 Determine the amount of the Lubriderm lotion base needed to make the 120 g preparation by adding the grams of menthol and camphor. 12 g + 2.4 g = 14.4 g of active ingredients need to be added to the Lubriderm.

$$120 \text{ g} - 14.4 \text{ g} = 105.6 \text{ g of Lubriderm base.}$$

To dispense four ounces, the 12 grams of menthol and 2.4 grams of camphor need to be added to the 105.6 grams of Lubriderm. They can be integrated using the geometric dilution method: 12 grams of menthol and 12 of Lubriderm mixed; 2.4 grams of camphor and 2.4 of Lubriderm mixed; then the two mixtures intergrated together before adding the remaining 91.2 grams of Lubriderm.

Using Alligation to Combine More than One Concentration for a New Concentration

Physicians often prescribe concentrations of medications that are not commercially available, and these prescriptions must be prepared by integrating two different concentrations, one higher and one lower, for a midrange concentration. This process, called **alligation**, is used in nonsterile and sterile compounding for mixing varied concentrations of solutions, mixtures, creams, ointments, or other products. The resulting concentration will be greater than the weaker strength but less than the stronger strength.

The principles used to solve alligation problems remain the same regardless of the media combined (e.g., liquid, semisolid, or even solid). An alligation box, demonstrated in the following examples, is a useful tool to help visualize the process. By the end, the boxes look like a tic-tac-toe grid, which is why alligation is sometimes called "tic-tac-toe math." See Example 5.4 for the step-by-step process.

Example 5.4

How much of a 10% and of a 60% urea cream should be mixed to prepare 100 g of a 40% urea cream?

Step 1 To set up an alligation box, place the final concentration (40%) in the middle of the tic-tac-toe grid. Place the higher concentration (60%) in the upper left corner. Place the lower concentration (10%) in the lower left corner.

Step 2 Draw a diagonal line from the upper left higher concentration through the middle with the final concentration to the bottom right. Write the difference between 60% and 40% (20) in the bottom right corner.

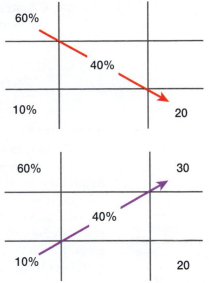

Step 3 Repeat the process for the lower concentration solution, subtracting the lower strength concentration (10%) from the final strength (40%). Write the difference in the top right corner.

Step 4 At this point, read across the lines from left to right to find the relative contributions of each concentration. You will note:

- The 30 at the top right represents how many parts are needed of the 60% urea cream to the final mixture.
- The 20 on the bottom right represents the parts of the 10% cream needed.
- There will always be more parts of the ingredient that is closest to the final concentration than the other. Because 60% is closest to 40%, it will have more parts than that of the 10%. This has been demonstrated, with 30 parts of the 60% and 20 of the 10%.

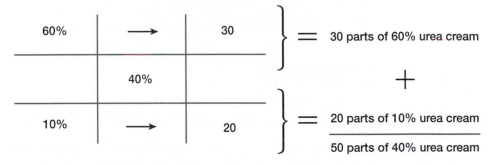

You have worked out the alligation. Now return to the question. It asks to see how much of each concentration is needed for 100 g of the prescribed 40% lotion. Since grams are the measurement unit being used for urea cream, you can convert the parts into grams in the final equation.

Step 5 To calculate the contribution of the 60% concentration, put it in dimensional analysis equation with the first ingredient.

$$y \text{ (of 60\%)} = \frac{30 \text{ parts}}{50 \text{ parts}} \times 100 \text{ g}; y = \frac{300 \text{ g}}{5}; y = 60 \text{ g of 60\%}$$

Step 6 At this point, you can either do another dimensional analysis equation with the second ingredient, or you can subtract the first ingredient from the final weight to determine the amount.

final weight − first ingredient weight = remaining ingredient weight

100 g total − 60 g of 60% = 40 g of 10% urea cream

Study Idea

Remember that in an alligation, the ingredient that is closest to the concentration of the final product will be added in the highest amount. Any answer that doesn't fit this guide can be eliminated.

On the exam, you could also have used logic and the process of elimination to cancel out any impossible answer choices. Eliminating the distractor answers is a helpful way to narrow the choices and improve the likelihood of correctly answering the question. Look at the prescribed concentration (40%). Is 40% closer to the higher concentration (60%) or the lower concentration (10%)? Since the 40% concentration is closer to the 60% prescribed, more of that will be used. Any answer in which the amount of 10% solution is equal to or greater than the amount of 60% solution used could not be correct.

Determining Beyond-Use Dating

After the product is compounded, a BUD date must be determined according to the stability of the compound as determined by USP guidelines and those of the manufacturer for each ingredient. Many compounded products have adequate stability information from the Master Formulation Record to allow for assignment of a BUD based on the expiration dates and stability of the manufactured ingredients.

In the absence of stability data, USP Chapter <795> has established maximum BUD recommendations for nonsterile compounded drug preparations that are packaged in tight, light-resistant containers and stored at controlled room temperatures. The BUD *may never be later than the expiration date on the label of any component of the preparation*. See Table 5.5 for USP <795> BUD guidelines. Example 5.5 shows how to determine the BUD for the nonsterile compounded preparation.

Study Idea

Remember for calculating BUDs, always start counting from the date of compounding, not the date of the prescription.

Example 5.5

On March 24, 2019, the following ingredients are used to compound a topical analgesic. What would be the BUD for the final product?

Drug	Drug Source	Expiration Date
Ketoprofen powder	Bulk chemical	Dec. 2019
Lidocaine powder	Bulk chemical	Aug. 2019
Petrolatum	Bulk chemical	March 2020

Since none of the ingredients are aqueous (water based), we can calculate the BUD as not later than the time remaining on the earliest expiring ingredient or six months from the compounding date, *whichever is earlier*. Six months after the date of compounding, is August 24, 2019. In this scenario six months from compounding and the earliest expiration of an ingredient are the same. The BUD is August 2019.

TABLE 5.5   Beyond-Use Dating by Type of Formulation

- **For nonaqueous formulations:** The BUD is not later than the time remaining until the earliest expiration date of the active ingredient or six months, whichever is earlier.
- **For water-based oral formulations:** The BUD is not later than 14 days when stored at controlled cold temperature.
- **For water-based topical/dermal, and mucosal liquid, and semisolid formulations:** The BUD is not later than 30 days.

Completing Nonsterile Compounding

During the compounding process, the technician must get the pharmacist to check the compounding process and preparation at least three key material points:

- Beginning: prescription, DUR, and Master Formulation Record
- Middle: calculations and measurements before mixing
- End: Compounding Record, label, product integrity, and auxiliary labels

Study Idea

Remember that the pharmacist must legally have a discussion with the patient on the use of the preparation for each compounded product dispensed.

The technician is responsible for accurate and thorough documentation of each step on the Compounding Record. The pharmacist also verifies that the final product looks, smells, and feels correct. If it is a cream, lotion, or gel, it should be pharmaceutically elegant. If it is a solution, it must not have clumps or precipitation.

When the label is applied, it must include the necessary information (as listed in Table 5.6). The pharmacist will choose the proper auxiliary labels and approve of the patient education materials that the technician has printed out. After this, the technician handles the proper product storage and cleanup. At prescription pickup, the technician must also make sure the patient receives counseling on the drug's use and potential side effects and warnings from the pharmacist.

If the nonsterile compounding was completed in a dedicated compounding facility, the facility must have a **continuous quality improvement process** to identify and resolve any problems if it wants to stay accredited. It must perform a monthly or quarterly spot check of each technician's work. A random product is selected and sent to an outside analytical lab for analysis of the exact measurements of the components and its sterile qualities. The product must be ± 2% of the potency of the individual ingredients.

Study Idea

It is the lot number that makes a compounded product traceable for quality control.

TABLE 5.6   Nonsterile Compounding Label

A nonsterile compounding label includes the following:
- patient's name
- physician's name
- date of compounding
- name of preparation
- prescription and/or extemporaneous compounding lot number
- beyond-use date
- initials of compounding technician and pharmacist
- directions for use, including any special storage conditions
- additional requirements of state or federal law

The pharmacist selects appropriate auxiliary labels.

STUDY SUMMARY

Nonsterile compounding is the extemporaneous combining, mixing, or altering of ingredients to create a medication tailored to the specialized medical needs of an individual patient. Pharmacy technicians must be knowledgeable about the requirements in USP Chapters <795>, Nonsterile Compounding, and <1075>, Good Compounding Practices as they relate to nonsterile compounding.

As you study for the exam, review the guidelines for garbing in personal protective equipment, hand washing, correct use and maintenance of equipment, and how to calculate a preparation's beyond-use date. Know the basic steps from prescription receipt to final packaging and storage to patient dispensing. Be able to differentiate between the Master Formulation Record and Compounding Record, and the importance of both. Master the calculations and steps necessary to integrating ingredients with different methods for a pharmaceutically elegant product.

ADDITIONAL RESOURCES

For more in-depth explanations, check out *Pharmacy Practice for Technicians*, 6e and *Pharmacy Labs for Technicians*, 3e from Paradigm Education Solutions. To master and extend the material presented in this chapter, take advantage of the resources available through the eBook resources links. These include digital supplements, study resources, and a practice exam generator with 1,000+ exam-style questions. End-of-chapter tests are accessible through the eBook for individuals using the self-study course and through Navigator+ for individuals enrolled in the instructor-guided course.

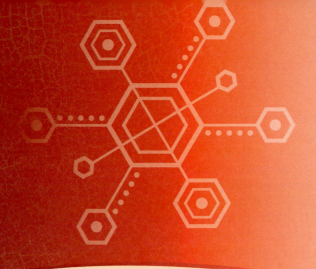

6

Sterile and Hazardous Compounding

Learning Objectives

1. Discuss USP guidelines for sterile and hazardous drug compounding processes.

2. Differentiate between the different types of parenteral administration and common sterile and hazardous products.

3. Know the components of the medication order and the requirements for the label and documentation for sterile and hazardous compounding.

4. Identify the equipment and supplies for sterile compounding.

5. Know the requirements of personal protective equipment and aseptic technique for sterile compounding.

6. Know how to clean, maintain, and use the sterile compounding equipment.

7. Calculate overfill volume, dilution quantities, active ingredient weight, powder volume, flow rate and volume, drip rate, and the time for a replacement IV using the 24-hour clock.

8. Determine product stability including beyond-use dating and signs of incompatibility.

9. Define the role of OSHA, NIOSH, and the NRC in the protection of healthcare workers.

10. Describe some of the key safety requirements and PPE for hazardous and nuclear compounding.

11. Understand the basic requirements for handling and disposing of hazardous and nonhazardous pharmaceuticals.

Access eBook links for resources and an exam generator, with 1,000+ questions.

Though the practice of pharmacy uses mostly manufactured drug products, there are many medical conditions in the hospital and other healthcare facilities that require specially trained pharmacy personnel to prepare both sterile and hazardous products to fill medical orders.

Sterile and hazardous compounding knowledge is assessed in the PTCE's domain 3, exploring the understanding of infection control, compounded sterile and hazardous products, aseptic technique and personal protective equipment, sterile compounding calculations, compounding equipment and facilities, waste disposal, and documentation requirements. The ExCPT's topical area 3 on the dispensing process includes questions on sterile and hazardous compounding.

Sterile Compounding for Parenteral Administration

Study Idea

Review hand washing technique for sterile compounding.

Many drugs ordered for patients in hospitals and other healthcare settings are injected directly into the body, so they must be specially compounded in a strictly controlled environment that is as germfree as possible. Healthcare facilities are particularly concerned about **healthcare-associated infections (HAIs)**—infections that patients contract while receiving care at a medical facility. HAIs can result in lengthy, multi-drug therapies, extended and costly hospitalizations, permanent injuries, and sometimes death. Common organisms causing HAIs include the **methicillin-resistant *Staphylococcus aureus* (MRSA)** bacteria that can cause serious bloodstream infections. MRSA is often passed by contaminated hands.

USP Chapter <797>

To ensure the highest quality and safest possible sterile product, the USP has set out guidelines for sterile compounding in **USP Chapter <797>**. These are more stringent than the USP Chapter <795> guidelines for nonsterile compounding. **Sterile** means the absence of *any* microorganisms, whereas **asepsis** is the absence of any destructive pathogens. Objects can be made sterile but people cannot. **Aseptic technique** is the set of special procedures used to ensure that harmful germs are not passed on, or introduced onto, surfaces and equipment, into the air, or into the compounded drug preparations.

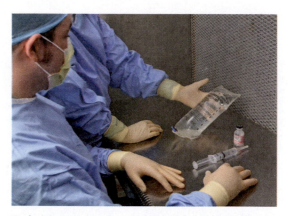

Technicians preparing IVs, injections, and other CSPs must be carefully trained to follow aseptic technique.

According to USP <797>, **compounded sterile preparations (CSPs)** must be prepared in a cleanroom with monitored air quality attained and maintained through primary and secondary engineering controls. Compounding technicians must use sterilized equipment and tools while following strict aseptic technique that includes protocols for hand washing, donning of **personal protective equipment (PPE)**, and careful manipulation of ingredients, containers, and CSPs during the preparation. See Table 6.1 for skills needed.

Pharmacy personnel are evaluated for competency in these skills as required by USP <797>. Based on the compounding risk level (low, medium, or high) of the products the facility prepares, competency evaluations must be completed annually or semiannually.

Study Idea

Parenteral solutions have the advantage of quicker onset of action since they bypass the stomach.

Types of Sterile Parenteral Drug Products

CSPs are generally administered through a **parenteral route of administration**, or one that uses injection to reach its destination in the bloodstream either by direct administration (intravenous) or through intramuscular or subcutaneous injection. A sterile, or microbial-free, solution (with or without medication) is administered by means of a hollow needle or catheter inserted through one or more layers of the skin. Parenteral dosage forms are administered through four paths:

- **intravenous (IV)**—into a vein via an IV line and catheter or syringe
- **intradermal (ID)**—between the layers of skin via a syringe
- **subcutaneous (SUBCUT)**—under the skin into the subcutaneous tissue via a syringe
- **intramuscular (IM)**—into a muscle vial a syringe or injection pen

TABLE 6.1	Sterile Compounding Skills Proficiencies

- Hygiene, garbing, hand washing, gowning, and gloving
- Aseptic manipulation
- Proper cleanroom behavior
- Measuring and mixing technique
- Use of equipment and tools
- Proper use of the primary engineering controls (to be described)
- Understanding of the HEPA-filtered unidirectional airflow within the rooms and equipment
- Understanding of the potential impact of personnel activities, such as moving materials into and out of the compounding area
- Documentation of the compounding process (e.g., Master Formulation Record and Compounding Record)
- Cleaning and disinfection procedures
- Methods of sterilization

Common Types and Sizes of Parenteral Drug Products

There are three basic forms of parenteral IV solutions ordered. The large and small volume parenterals are the most commonly ordered. There are key distinguishing features that affect how each parenteral solution is compounded and administered.

- **Large volume parenteral solutions (LVPs)** are generally administered over a prolonged period that ranges from 8 to 24 hours, available in 250 mL, 500 mL, and 1,000 mL IV bag sizes. They may contain one or more electrolytes that have been added to an IV solution of saline or dextrose.
- **Small volume parenteral solutions (SVPs)** are compounded in a smaller bag containing 25 mL, 50 mL, 100 mL, or 150 mL (and even 250 mL for rapid infusion). Many SVPs are administered as IV piggybacks (IVPBs) with their tubing inserted into the primary lines of LVPs to merge the solutions. SVPs are typically infused over 10 minutes to an hour and are made of a medication dissolved into a sterile **normal saline (NS)**—0.9% sodium chloride—or a D_5W solution.
- **IV bolus injections**, or **push injections (IVPs)**, are small volume medications inserted by syringe into the catheter or port near the catheter.

Medication Orders for Compounded Sterile Products

Once the hospital pharmacy receives the CSP order, a pharmacist (or in certain facilities, a senior technician) enters the order into the pharmacy's computer system, and the software runs the drug utilization review (DUR). This will check the order against the patient's medical history and medication profile to catch any allergies, cross-sensitivities, drug-drug or drug-food interactions, duplicate therapies, or contraindications.

The pharmacist resolves all computer-generated warnings and either modifies the order with the physician or approves it, and the sterile compounding labels are generated. Rather than just issuing a single label for the medication order, a separate label is issued for each individualized dose to be compounded. These are provided to the sterile compounding technician in the cleanroom.

Sterile Compounding Label Components

The label formatting will differ among hospitals and software, but the CSP labels generally include the information in Figure 6.1 and in Table 6.2.

FIGURE 6.1
Small Volume Parenteral Solution Label

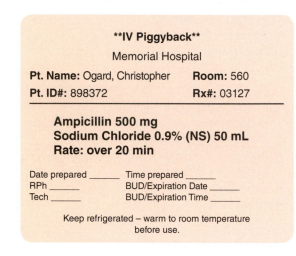

Each IV preparation requires a bag of a base solution to which additive(s) are injected. These additives may include active drug(s), electrolytes, or nutrients. The amount of drug or additive and the volume of the base solution must be listed on the label. See Table 6.3 for a list of common parenteral solutions and additives. The label may also contain the drug dosing interval or the time that the CPS is to be administered.

Master Formulation and Compounding Records

Some pharmacy labeling programs provide sterile compounding instructions directly on the label. However, when the labels do not provide compounding instructions or when CSPs are prepared *in a batch for multiple patients,* USP <797> requires that a **Master Formulation Record** be followed. Generally, a Master Formulation Record for each type of ordered medication can be found in the hospital software, the *USP-NF,* in an approved peer reviewed pharmacy-medical article, or at the website of the Professional Compounding Centers of America (PCCA). The Master Formulation Record lists the ingredients, specific procedures, equipment to be used, and testing required for each specific kind of CSP. (See Table 6.4.)

For every compounded product using a Master Formulation Record, a **Compounding Record**, with its specific medical order or batch lot number, must be established by the technician on the computer for each patient, as is done with nonsterile compounding. This record documents the ingredients, calculations, and compounding processes that were actually used for a particular preparation, allowing for traceability. It is critical that the record also describes in detail any deviations from the label directions or Master Formulation Record, any compounding problems or errors experienced, and the identities of the staff involved in its preparation and verification.

TABLE 6.2 Sterile Compounded Labeling Requirements

Each compounded product must have affixed upon it a label that encompasses most or all of the following information:

- Medication order number or batch lot number
- Name and identification (ID) number (barcode) of the patient for whom the medication is prescribed
- Name, concentration, and amount of base solution (such as *D₅W 500 mL*)
- Brand or generic name and amount (or concentration) of each drug or additive in the compound (such as *potassium chloride 20 mEq*)
- Infusion rate (such as *100 mL/hr* or *infuse over 20 min*), dosing interval, and/or administration time
- Form and route of administration (such as *for intravenous administration*)
- Beyond-use date (or manufacturer's expiration date)
- Storage requirements (such as *keep refrigerated or protect from light*)
- Auxiliary labels or special instructions (e.g., *Shake well before administering; Warm to room temperature before administering*; or *For wound irrigation only*)
- Any device-specific instructions (such as *MINI-BAG Plus must be activated and mixed prior to administering*)
- Preparer's and pharmacist's initials
- Address and contact information of the infusion pharmacy or compounder if the CSP is to be sent outside of the facility in which it was compounded

Note: Consult the hospital pharmacy's P&P manual for an institution's specific labeling requirements.

TABLE 6.3 Products used in Sterile Compounding

Small volume parenterals	25 mL, 50 mL, 100 mL, 150 mL, 250 mL with medications in normal saline or dextrose 5%
Large volume parenterals	250 mL, 500 mL, 1,000 mL with medications in saline or dextrose solutions, or with Lactated Ringer's solutions
Total parenteral nutrition solutions	Amino acid solutions, dextrose solutions, fat emulsions
Total parenteral nutrition additives	Electrolytes, trace elements, vitamins
Diluents	Sterile water for injection, lidocaine, sodium chloride, bacteriostatic water for injection
Pharmaceuticals	Antibiotics, chemotherapy, proton pump inhibitor, H2 blockers, etc.

TABLE 6.4 Sterile Master Formulation Record Components

A Master Formulation Record for sterile compounding should include the following information:

- Name, strength, and dosage form of the CSP
- Physical description of the final preparation
- Identities and amounts of all ingredients and appropriate container-closure systems
- Complete instructions for preparing the CSP, including equipment, supplies, and a description of the compounding steps
- BUD and storage requirements
- Quality control procedures (e.g., pH, filter integrity, and visual inspection)
- Sterilization method, if applicable (e.g., filter, steam, or dry heat)
- Any other information needed to describe the operation and ensure its repeatability (e.g., adjusting pH and tonicity and temperature)

Each Compounding Record must be reviewed and approved with the pharmacist's signature or initials and the date before the CSP is released. For sterile products that are assembled according to manufacturer's directions, such as in the standard reconstitution of powders for injectable medications, no Compounding Record is required.

Cleanroom and Air Quality Engineering Equipment

The standard sterile compounding area required by USP <797> is separated into two rooms: a preparatory **anteroom** (or transition area) and a **buffer room** (also known as the **cleanroom**) that provides space for the sterile compounding workstations or benches. (Some refer to the cleanroom as the two rooms together.) The workstations are called **primary engineering controls (PECs)** because they have **high-efficiency particulate airflow (HEPA)** filtered ventilation systems to protect the CSPs from contamination. Within the PECs, the direct compounding areas (DCAs) *must have an air quality rating that is ISO Class 5*, based on an international rating scale. (Less sterile air has higher particulate ratings; for example, an ISO Class 9 is general room air quality.) For sterile compounding, the air moves *horizontally* from the HEPA filter behind the grill over the CSP toward the compounder. The airflow must be unidirectional (going one way away from the CSP) with *positive pressure*, from filtered air pumped into the DCA toward the buffer room and outward to ever lessening air quality.

The buffer room and anteroom have HEPA ventilation systems called **secondary engineering controls**. The *buffer room must have at least ISO Class 7 air, and the anteroom must have at least ISO Class 8 air.* The common PEC for standard sterile compounding is called the **horizontal laminar airflow workbench (H-LAFW)**, known as the "hood." The ventilated airstream produced by the PEC and its hood create ISO Class 5 air quality for the DCA in the middle of the stainless steel workbench. Sterile compounding can also be done in a PEC called a **compounding aseptic isolator (CAI)**, which has an enclosed DCA inside a glove box. It offers even more protection for the compounding process.

The H-LAFW must be cleaned and sanitized according to USP standards at the beginning of each compounding shift and before preparing each batch. See Figure 6.2 for the order and process. The DCA must be cleaned after every 30 minutes of continuous compounding and after any spill or surface contamination. The PEC prefilters must be replaced every 30 days. The HEPA filters must be recertified every six months or any time the PEC is moved.

FIGURE 6.2
Hood Cleaning Order for the H-LAFW

Using a wipe with 70% isopropyl alcohol, the bar and hooks should be wiped, followed by ceiling, both sides of the hood, and finally the work surface.

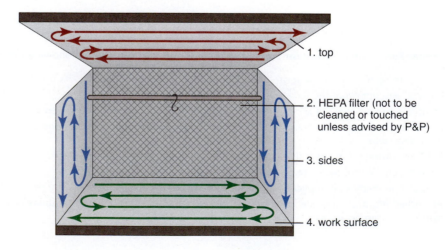

1. top
2. HEPA filter (not to be cleaned or touched unless advised by P&P)
3. sides
4. work surface

Also according to USP <797>, the counters, work surfaces, and floors of the buffer room and anteroom are required to be cleaned daily. The buffer area and ante area ceilings, walls, and shelving must be cleaned monthly. At specified intervals, the supervisor of the sterile compounding pharmacy will visually observe and document the cleaning and disinfecting techniques used by pharmacy staff.

In addition, routine environmental monitoring is required for quality assurance. Nonviable and viable airborne particle testing must be conducted at least every six months. Regular surface sampling is done to ensure cleaning and disinfecting procedures meet the required standards. If any area is out of compliance, corrective action has to be taken and documented.

Aseptic Technique and Protective Garb

For aseptic technique, technicians must put away outerwear, jewelry, and electronic devices before entering anteroom. In the anteroom, they must finish calculations, gather and wipe down supplies, and put on protective garb, also known as personal protective equipment as previously noted. The PPE garbing process for sterile compounding personnel follows a strict sequence, as shown in Table 6.5: first shoe covers, hair cover, and face mask. Then comes hand washing and arm scrubbing. The sterile gowns (with sleeves) and gloves are put on last because they must be the cleanest items; the gown goes on in the anteroom, and the gloves are donned in the buffer room. The gown must be clean, disposable, and nonshedding, with arms that fit snugly around the wrist. Goggles, face shields, nonpermeable gown, and two levels of heavy duty chemotherapy gloves are recommended when making hazardous CSPs.

TABLE 6.5 CSP Garbing and Hand Washing

In the Anteroom

Remove all personal outer garments (i.e., sweaters, jackets).

Remove jewelry from hands, wrists, or other visible body parts.

No artificial nails, nail polish, cosmetics, or perfume are permitted.

Put on first layers of PPE, in the following order:

- Shoe covers
- Hair cover
- Face mask (beard cover, if applicable)

Perform aseptic hand washing procedures.
Put on a nonshedding gown.

In the Buffer Area

Apply foamed, sterile, 70% isopropyl alcohol antiseptic hand cleanser.

Don sterile, powder-free gloves.

Sterile Compounding Calculations

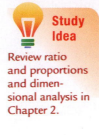

Study Idea

Review ratio and proportions and dimensional analysis in Chapter 2.

In the anteroom, before preparing the CSPs with aseptic technique, technicians need to do or double-check the calculations required by the medical order and/or the Master Formulation Record to fill in the Compounding Record. It is essential to memorize the equivalents and metric conversions provided in Chapter 2 to be confident in these calculations. You will also need to know conversions from standard time (clock time) to military time to interpret the labels for drug administration times. Knowing how to translate temperatures in Fahrenheit to Celsius and back is essential for checking the refrigerator and freezer storage conditions for IVs.

Some of the important calculations needed for sterile compounding include dosage concentrations, alligations, dilutions, specific gravity, millequivalents, base solution overfill, flow rates, and 24-hour supply for IVs. Some of these calculations are too complex and advanced for the certification exam, such as specific gravity, so it will not be covered in this text. Others are based on the knowledge already reviewed in Chapter 2 on calculations:

Safety Alert

Never rely solely on the directions on the CSP label or pharmacist's calculations, or on your own! The IV technician must *always* double-check the medication order, labels, and calculations, documenting them all in the Compounding Record.

- When doing conversions and a measurement is missing, the *ratio and proportion calculation method* is best (as reviewed on pages 65-66).

- For calculating dosages based on body weight or surface area, see pages 73-75.

- For multi-step dosage questions using conversions and concentration calculations, *dimensional analysis* is favored (as reviewed on pages 66-67, 70, 72).

- For calculating dilutions, use the formula: $is \times iv = fs \times fv$ to determine the final volume; then use the equation: $fv - iv = volume$ of diluent (as reviewed on pages 75-77).

- When combining two different concentrations of products for a midrange concentration, do an alligation calculation. One warning about alligation questions on the exam: it is common to see an incorrect answer choice that switches the concentrations. You can usually explore your answers to eliminate many of the distracter answer by logic, as demonstrated in Example 6.1.

Study Idea

Review alligation in Chapter 5 because it could be used in a problem like Example 6.1 to calculate the answer.

Example 6.1

How much D_5W and $D_{50}W$ should be mixed to prepare 1,000 mL of $D_{40}W$?

a. 700 mL of 5% and 300 mL of 50%

b. 777 mL of 5% and 222 mL of 50%

c. 222 mL of 5% and 777 mL of 50%

d. 222 mL of 40% and 777 mL of 50%

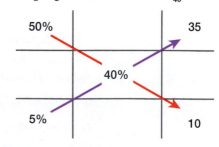

By process of elimination, it can be determined that:

- answer *a* is incorrect because an equal split in volume would provide a concentration that is too low; there should be more of the 50% to offset the low 5%.

- answer *b* has the correct numbers applied to the wrong solutions.

- answer *d* uses 40% as part of the answer. The *prescribed concentration cannot be part of a correct answer choice* because it does not even exist until it is mixed. Any answer choice that contains the final-strength solution or mixture must be incorrect.

- answer *c* must be correct.

If this were an actual test question, you could have arrived at the correct answer merely by inspecting your answer choices after setting up the alligation box (explained in depth in Chapter 5 on pages 146-148). Alligation problems take practice. Use the sample questions at the end-of-chapter test to sharpen your skills.

Overfill of Base Solutions

Study Idea

The 10% rule for overfill requires that if the added volume will be greater than 10% of the final volume, you should remove from the IV bag the amount equivalent to the volume of active ingredient(s) you will add.

Although manufactured base IV solutions are labeled to contain a set number of milliliters (e.g., 25, 50, 100, 250, 500, or 1,000 mL), the actual volume is greater because the containers include overfill. **Overfill** is the amount of solution manufacturers add to make up for the loss of water due to evaporation through plastic over time. This loss is somewhat dependent on conditions during transport and storage, the ratio of fluid volume to the surface area, and the time between manufacturing and use. The larger the IV bag base solution, the greater the potential loss, so the more overfill the manufacturers add to compensate.

Manufacturers are not the same or consistent in their addition of overfill amounts, and they do not always label the overfill percentages they use. (See Table 6.6 for an example of overfill amounts.) Some overwrap their non-PVC (a type of plastic) IV solutions to reduce evaporation. These wraps should stay on until right before compounding or administration.

TABLE 6.6 Examples of Overfill in IV Bags

- 100 mL bags contain 7 mL overfill
- 250 mL bags contain 25 mL overfill
- 500 mL bags contain 30 mL overfill
- 1,000 mL bags contain 50 mL overfill

  The amount of overfill varies with the manufacturer.

Overfill Policies

Each hospital and home infusion pharmacy will have written protocols for dealing with overfill calculations for base solutions. Small and large volume parenteral solutions compose the majority of sterile compounded solutions, and normally the overfill amount for these IVs does not appreciably affect the amount of fluids or drug dosages administered. However, in the case of IV premixed neonatal drugs or cancer chemotherapy drugs that must be reconstituted with a diluent before being transferred into a small or large volume parenteral solution, the combination of the overfill in the IV bag plus the diluent can cause an over-dilution of the prescribed dose, especially if the entire contents of the IV solution are not administered. A diluted dose of a critical drug may adversely affect the disease outcome.

Many pharmacies implement the 10% rule for overfill that states that *if the manufacturer's overfill plus any required additives equals 10% or more over the stock label amount for the base IV solution, then the overfill volume should be removed before adding the drug volume.*

Example 6.2

Mitomycin 40 mg in a 0.5 mg/1 mL sterile water dilution must be added to 1,000 mL NS to be infused over 6 hours. Will this CSP result in an overfill that needs an adjustment of the base solution?

Step 1 Mitomycin 40 mg is available as a dry powder that recommends a concentration of 0.5 mg/mL. The amount of sterile water diluent to be added must be determined.

Calculations are easier if you first convert 0.5 mg/1 mL from a decimal to a whole number ratio before doing the proportion equation:

$$\frac{10}{10} \times \frac{0.5 \text{ mg}}{1 \text{ mL}} = \frac{5 \text{ mg}}{10 \text{ mL}}$$

$$\frac{5 \text{ mg}}{10 \text{ mL}} = \frac{40 \text{ mg}}{y \text{ mL}}; \quad 5y = 400 \text{ mL}; \quad y = \frac{400 \text{ mL}}{5} = 80 \text{ mL}$$

Step 2 One liter (1,000 mL) of NS will contain approximately 50 mL NS of overfill if the manufacturer's proportion of overfill is similar to listed that listed in Table 6.6. Estimate the amount of overfill plus diluent.

1,000 mL + 50 mL (overfill) + 80 mL (diluent) = 1,130 mL

The final volume of the IV solution is equal to 1,130 mL, which is more than 10% of a liter (or 1,100 mL). Therefore, the volume of the base solution (NS) *must be adjusted.*

Step 3 The hospital protocol states the amount of the overfill plus diluent (130 mL) should be withdrawn from the normal saline before injecting the medicated solution into the 1,000 mL IV bag.

General Medication Addition to an LVP Base Solution With a typical LVP continuously administered, the problem of overfill diluting a medication does occur, but the measurements do not need to be precise because another IV with the same drug will be following it.

Precise SVP Compounding For medications that need to be the most precise, as in SVP chemotherapy, sterile compounding technicians need to work with accurate medication amounts, so all ingredients including the base solution and any diluent must be precisely measured and injected into a new sterile container. This can be done manually or in an automated compounding machine. Using a new container means that there will be no overfill to calculate or estimate.

An epidural pain medication must always be exact, with no overfill, so the base solution and the medication must be drawn into new syringes and then injected into a sterile medication reservoir cassette.

Study Idea

Return to Chapter 2 to study and apply the conversion, dosage, and dilution calculation skills explained there to parenteral solutions. Also, review and apply the compounding calculation skills in Chapter 5.

Calculating Sterile Compounding Doses and Dilutions

Injectable drugs and IV solutions use the same conversion, dosage, and dilution calculations explained in Chapter 2. Sterile compounding is particularly focused on working with liquids for IV solutions or sterile injections.

Calculating Weight-in-Volume Percents

Many IV solutions are ordered as a percentage of active ingredient weight based to solution volume. Premade preservative-free lidocaine, for instance, is available in 1% and 2% concentrations for parenteral use. To calculate dilution levels, you need to convert from percentages to fractions and sometimes from grams to milligrams of actual ingredient in a concentration. For instance, see Example 6.3.

Example 6.3

You are to prepare a 0.02% Nimotop solution administered in 1 liter of normal saline. How many mg of Nimotop are needed?

Step 1 Convert 0.02% Nimotop to a weight-in-volume.

0.02% = 0.02 g per 100 mL; converting the grams to milligrams would be

$$0.02 \text{ g} \times 1{,}000 = 20 \text{ mg}; \quad \text{so } 20 \text{ mg per } 100 \text{ mL}$$

Step 2 Set up a dimensional analysis to calculate what is needed for a 1 liter IV of Nimotop, as 1 L = 1,000 mL.

$$y \text{ mg} = 1{,}000 \text{ mL} \times \frac{20 \text{ mg}}{100 \text{ mL}}; \quad y = 200 \text{ mg}.$$

The tech must add 200 mg of Nimotop to a 1 liter bag of normal saline.

Study Idea

Remember: weight-in-volume percents are usually expressed as percentage of grams of the active ingredient per 100 milliliters of solution, as expressed in 1% = 1 g/100 mL.

Calculating Dry Powder Volume and Dilutions

At times, you will need to do calculations with dry powdered forms of active ingredients. For example, parenteral products are often reconstituted by adding a diluent to a lyophilized or freeze-dried powder to prepare an IV solution. The product is commercially manufactured in powder form because of the instability of the drug in a solution over a long period. The active ingredient (the powder) is expressed in terms of weight, but it also occupies a certain amount of space, or volume. This space is referred to as **powder volume (pv)**. It is equal to the difference between the **total volume (tv)** of the final product and the volume of the diluting ingredient, or the **diluent volume (dv)**, as expressed in the following equations:

total volume − diluent volume = powder volume [tv − dv = pv]; or

total volume = powder volume + diluent volume [tv = pv + dv]

For instance, a dry powder antibiotic must be reconstituted for use. The label states that the dry powder occupies 0.8 mL. In calculating amounts of powder and diluent, it helps to make a table of the information you know and don't know as seen in Figure 6.3 on the next page. Using the correct formula, determine the diluent volume for a total volume of 5 mL:

tv − pv = dv

FIGURE 6.3
Sample
Reconstitution
Table

Active Drug Weight	Concentration	Powder Volume	Diluent Volume	Total Volume of Final Drug Solution	How much to administer?
		0.8 mL	4.2 mL	5 mL	
		0.8 mL	5.5 mL	6.3 mL	

Total Volume		Powder Volume		Diluent Volume
5 mL	−	0.8 mL	=	4.2 mL

What is the total volume if you add 5.5 mL of diluent to 9.8 mL of powder volume?

Powder Volume		Diluent Volume		Total Volume
0.8 mL	+	5.5 mL	=	6.3 mL

Example 6.4

You are to reconstitute 1 g of dry powder. The label states that you are to add 8.3 mL of diluent to make a final solution of 100 mg/mL. What is the powder volume? Then if the patient's medical order is for 60 mg of the drug, how much must be drawn from the vial into the syringe?

Active Drug Weight	Concentration	Powder Volume	Diluent Volume	Total Volume of Final Drug Solution	How much to administer?
1 g (1,000 mg)	100 mg / 1 mL		8.3 mL		60 mg

Step 1 Calculate the total volume needed by using the equal ratio-proportion conversion method. The strength of the final solution must be 100 mg/mL, so you need to convert the grams of active ingredient into milligrams. Since you start with 1 g = 1,000 mg of powder, for a total volume y of the solution, it will have a strength of 1,000 mg/y mL.

$$\frac{100 \text{ mg}}{1 \text{ mL}} = \frac{1\text{g}}{y \text{ mL}}; \quad 100 \text{ mg} \times y \text{ mL} = 1 \text{ mL} \times 1{,}000 \text{ mg}$$

$$y \text{ mL} = \frac{1{,}000 \text{ mg} \times 1 \text{ mL}}{100 \text{ mg}}; \quad y \text{ mL} = 10 \text{ mL}$$

Using the desired solution concentration, you have determined you need to have a total volume of 10 mL.

Step 2 Using the calculated total volume of the final product and the given diluent volume, calculate the powder volume you must add to the diluent.

$$tv - dv = pv$$
$$10 \text{ mL} - 8.3 \text{ mL} = 1.7 \text{ mL}$$

Step 3 Now you have the final drug solution of 100 mg/1 mL, which means 1 mL contains 100 mg of the drug. You must have only 60 mg in the syringe. So how much drug volume should be put into the syringe?

$$60 \text{ mg} \times \frac{1}{100 \text{ mg}} = \frac{6 \text{ mL}}{10} \quad \text{which is 0.6 mL.}$$

You can finish filling in the chart and load the syringe with 0.6 mL of the drug solution.

Measuring Electrolytes

Study Idea

Review the abbeviations for commonly ordered electrolytes like potassium chloride (KCl) and sodium chloride (NaCl).

Many IV fluids used in hospital pharmacy practice contain dissolved mineral salts; such a fluid is known as an **electrolyte solution**, which provides needed electrical chemistry interactions for the body to rejuvenate.

Milliequivalents (mEq) are used to measure electrolytes in the bloodstream and/or in an IV preparation. The **equivalent (Eq)** weight is the number of grams of the substance that is able to fully dissolve in 1 mL of solution to react with another substance. The chemistry equation to determine the equivalent weight is based on each element's atomic structure. It is too complicated for this review and not needed for the certification exam. The Eq calculations are done by the pharmacy software. However, you do need to know that the milliequivalents in a drug solution are measured by the number of mEq per 1 mL. Then you can use a ratio and proportion equation to figure out the number of milliequivalents that should be dissolved in the IV solution to reach the prescribed concentration of electrolytes or other ingredients.

Example 6.5

You are requested to make a sterile preparation in the IV room by adding 88 mEq of sodium chloride (NaCl) to an IV bag. Sodium chloride is available as a 4 mEq/mL solution. How many milliliters (mL) will you need to add to the IV bag?

Step 1 Set up the equation, comparing the ordered solution to the available base solution.

$$\frac{4 \text{ mEq}}{1 \text{ mL}} = \frac{88 \text{ mEq}}{y \text{ mL}}; \quad y \text{ mL} \times 4 = 88 \times 1 \text{ mL}$$

Step 2 Solve for the unknown y.

$$4 \, y \text{ mL} = 88 \text{ mL} \quad y \text{ mL} = 22 \text{ mL}$$

Calculating IV Administration Flow Rates and Volumes

The **infusion rate** (or dosing rate) is the prescribed rate at which an amount of fluid is infused into a patient over a given period of time. The actual **flow rate** (how fast a fluid is traveling) is determined by the size and nature of the tubing.

Calculating Volume Delivered with Ordered Flow Rate

By knowing the flow rate and the amount of time that an infusion has to run, it is possible to calculate the exact amount of fluid that will be delivered. Example 6.6 uses a ratio and proportion equation to calculate a simple IV flow rate problem where you need to know how much fluid will be administered during a set amount of time based on its speed ratio of milliliters per hour.

Example 6.6

A patient has an intravenous normal saline infusion running in at a rate of 125 mL/hr. How much fluid will the patient receive during an infusion that lasts 8 hours?

Step 1 Set up a ratio and proportion by comparing the speed of mL/hr to the amount of hours the IV will run.

$$\frac{125\ \text{mL}}{1\ \text{hr}} = \frac{y\ \text{mL}}{8\ \text{hr}}; \quad 1y = 125 \times 8; \quad y = 1{,}000$$

Based on the original information, the units are milliliters. The patient will receive 1,000 mL or 1 L of fluid. On the exam, the answer may be written in either milliliters or liters, requiring you to think about the conversion between units.

Calculating Flow Rate Based on Volume Delivered

Now, one must apply a method for determining the IV flow rate. The equation is

Volume/Time = Rate.

The volume may be expressed in milliliters, liters, or drops. (Drop rates will be discussed later.) The time component of an IV flow rate may be expressed in terms of hours or minutes. Examples 6.7 and 6.8 give examples of these calculations.

Example 6.7

A patient receives 2.5 L of IV total parenteral nutrition over the course of 12 hours. What is the flow rate in milliliters per hour if the flow rate is consistent for the whole time period?

On the left side of your proportion equation, enter the amount of fluid infused and the amount of time it took. On the right side, determine the rate of flow based on the number of milliliters delivered in 1 hour.

Step 1 When you set up the ratio and proportion equation, make the units equivalent on both sides, converting liters to mL:

$$\frac{2.5 \text{ L}}{12 \text{ hr}} = \frac{y \text{ mL}}{1 \text{ hr}}; \quad \frac{2{,}500 \text{ mL}}{12 \text{ hr}} = \frac{y \text{ mL}}{1 \text{ hr}}$$

Step 2 Cross multiply to solve for the unknown y.

$$2{,}500 \times 1 = 12\,y; \quad y = \frac{2500}{12}$$

$y = 208.333$ mL. Round off, and the rate of flow is 208 mL/hr.

Example 6.8

A patient receives 2,640 mL of IV Lactated Ringer's solution over 24 hours. What is the flow rate in milliliters per minute?

Step 1 In this calculation, because you are both calculating the flow rate and converting it to minutes per hour, you can use a dimensional analysis equation.

$$y \text{ mL} = \frac{2{,}640 \text{ mL}}{24 \text{ hr}} \times \frac{1 \text{ hr}}{60 \text{ min}}$$

Step 2 Solve for y.

$$y = 264; \quad \frac{264 \text{ mL}}{144 \text{ min}}; \quad y = 1.83 \text{ mL/min; this is the flow rate.}$$

Be careful in your exam, because in a question like this, one of the distractor answers would probably be 110 ml/hr, which would be the right amount but the wrong unit of measure.

Calculating Time Duration for Infusion Based on Flow Rate and 24-Hour Supply

To answer the question, *"How long will this IV bag last (or take to administer)?"* you divide the total mL by the infusion rate at mL/min or mL/hr to find out how long it will take to empty. As you work it out the formula by adding a time conversion at then end, it is a dimensional analysis equation, as seen below. If you add a time conversion rate to the end, it turns into the same equation you would have used if calculating the problem with a dimensional analysis equation from the beginning (as in Example 6.9).

$$Time \text{ (hrs or min)} = \frac{Volume \text{ (mL)}}{Rate \text{ (mL/hr)}} \text{ ; can work into: } Time \text{ (min)} = volume \times \frac{hr}{mL} \times \frac{min}{hr}$$

Study Idea

When you work out the *Volume/Rate = Time* equation, you will note that, in order to divide the volume by a rate fraction, you have to flip the rate and multiply it by the volume. You end up with a dimensional analysis equation that can have the conversion rate of minutes/hour added to it, if needed.

Example 6.9

A 1,000-mL bag of solution containing 30 mEq of KCl is piggybacked into a continuous $D_{10}W$ solution. It is infusing into a patient at a rate of 3 mL/ min. How many hours will it take to complete the infusion of this one bag? And how many bags would you need to supply for 24 hours?

Step 1 Set up the dimensional analysis equation based on the formula, adding the conversion rate of minutes/hour. The tricky part is always setting it up so you are solving for the correct unit of measure. Arrange the conversion ratio so the desired unit of measure is in the numerator, and the

Safety Alert

When preparing IVs, remember tubing and bags made of PVC plastic can cause health problems because of PVC drug absorption or PVC leaching. Avoid using PVC IV sets for nitro-glycerin, amiodarone, most biotechnology drugs, fat emulsions. as well as for any drugs for pregnant women, neonates, children, and adolescent males.

undesired units are canceled out equally by having one similar unit in the numerator and one in the denominator, as seen in the equation below:

$$y \text{ hr} = 100\cancel{0} \cancel{\text{mL}} \times \frac{1 \cancel{\text{min}}}{3 \cancel{\text{mL}}} \times \frac{1 \text{ hr}}{6\cancel{0} \cancel{\text{min}}}; \quad y \text{ hr} = \frac{100}{18}; \quad y = 5.555 \text{ hr}$$

This IV bag will take more than 5 ½ hours, rounded off to 6 hours.

Step 2 Knowing how long each IV bag takes to be fully infused, how many bags would you need to supply? You can do a proportion equation:

$$\frac{6 \text{ hr}}{1 \text{ bag}} = \frac{24 \text{ hr}}{z \text{ bags}}; \quad 6z = 24; \quad z \text{ bags} = \frac{24}{6}$$

$$z = 4 \text{ bags}; \quad \text{you would need 4 LVP bags.}$$

The original proportion is based on hours, so the answer is rounded off to 4 bags for 24 hours. On the certification exam, be sure to provide your answer in the correct unit of measure.

Calculating Flow Rate in Drops

For extremely concentrated solutions, as in chemotherapy, a pharmacy technician may be asked to calculate the IV flow rates in terms of per milliliter instead of minutes or hours. Each IV infusion set has a particular drop factor based on the size of the tubing—the number of drops that will equal a volume of 1 mL, with **macrodrip tubing**, or **microdrip tubing** (often used for pediatric patients or chemotherapy)—as shown in Table 6.7. The infusion pumps can be set to regulate the infusion rate per drops (gtt).

TABLE 6.7 Common Drop Factors per Tubing Size	
Macrodrip tubing	10 gtt/1 mL
	15 gtt/1 mL
	20 gtt/1 mL
Microdrip tubing	60 gtt/1 mL

The larger the drop factor, the smaller each individual drop is, so more drops are needed to make up a milliliter. A 10-drop set requires 10 gtt to add up to 1 mL volume. Example 6.10 calculates an IV infusion rate in drops using dimensional analysis.

Example 6.10

A patient is to receive 200 mL of IV 20% fat emulsion over 10 hours, using a 15-drop infusion set. What should the flow rate be set to in the infusion pump in drops per minute?

The approach to this problem is the same as in earlier problems. You can use a rate proportion equation: 200 mL/10 hr = y mL/hr, cross multiply to solve for y, and then convert the answer into gtt/min. Or you can use a dimensional analysis equation to do it all in one equation, as shown below.

Step 1 Set up the equation: $y = \dfrac{200\text{ mL}}{10\text{ hr}} \times \dfrac{15\text{ gtt}}{\text{mL}} \times \dfrac{1\text{ hr}}{60\text{ min}};\quad y = \dfrac{30\text{ gtt}}{6\text{ min}};$

Then cancel out the same elements on the numerator and denominator (mL) and appropriate zeros:

$$y = \dfrac{5\text{ gtt}}{1\text{ min}}; \text{ so you have 6 gtt/min.}$$

Calculating Time For the New Supply Based on Infusion Rate

If you have been given or have calculated the infusion rate per hour and you know what time the first bag will be administered, you can figure out when the new IV bag will be needed.

Example 6.11

The prescriber orders

> ℞ **20 mEq of medication in 2,000 mL of D$_5$W to be administered at 125 mL/hr**

If the first bag of 1,000 mL (1 L) was hung at 9:00 a.m., when will the next bag for the full 2,000 mL order be needed by your watch?

Step 1 You can use the formula and turn it into a dimensional analysis equation with the conversion rate:

$$\frac{Volume}{Rate} = Time$$

$$\frac{1,000\text{ mL}}{125\text{ mL/hr}} = Time;\quad \text{or } 1,000\text{ mL} \times \frac{1\text{ hr}}{125\text{ mL}} = \frac{1,000\text{ hr}}{125} = 8\text{ hr}$$

One 1,000 mL bag will last 8 hours.

Step 2 Add the 8 hours to the last administration time of 10 a.m. to find the 24-hour clock time.

$$\left\{ \begin{array}{r} 0900 \\ +800 \\ \hline 1700 \end{array} \right.$$

So 0900 plus 8 hours equals 1700, or 5:00 p.m. by your watch.

The Sterile Compounding Process

After donning the gloves and cleaning the hood, compounding is ready to begin. (See Table 6.8 for an overview of the steps involved in the process.) It involves handling needles and syringes, and adding ingredients from vials and ampules to base solutions, often in IV bags in the protected space of the DCA.

TABLE 6.8   Overview of Steps in Sterile Compounding

This is a general outline of the process steps for sterile compounding in a two-room cleanroom area. Each facility is slightly different based on its layout and standard operating procedures. It is essential to take a sterile compounding course with practice labs to get a real sense of the detailed steps involved. USP Chapter <797> is the ultimate source for all sterile compounding guidelines.

1. In the main hospital pharmacy, receive medication orders and labels, and run drug utilization review. The pharmacist will do the initial calculations from the Master Formulation Record.
2. Receive the pharmacist's verifications, do any remaining calculations, and initiate a Compounding Record (may be done in pharmacy or anteroom, depending on area procedures).
3. After removing outerwear and entering anteroom, wipe down supplies and follow aseptic techniques for garbing and hand washing.
4. Transport compounding supplies, ingredients, and PEC-cleaning materials into the buffer room on a sanitized cart.
5. In the buffer room, sterilize hands and don sterile gloves.
6. Clean the primary engineering control (PEC) per manufacturing directions and USP <797>.
7. Compound the CSPs in the PEC according to USP <797>; processes often include withdrawing medications from vials or ampules and then injecting them into IV base solutions or containers.
8. Complete a quality check of each CSP by comparing label and medication order and doing a visual check.
9. Pharmacist will verify final CSP, label, and ingredients in buffer room or anteroom before applying the label and any auxiliary labels.
10. CSP will be delivered to nursing unit for administration.

Study Idea

You must work six inches from the outside edge of the H-LAFW.

The DCA is in the middle of the workbench six inches from the edge of the counter. The clean air flows over the DCA, so the compounder technician's hands, tools, and ingredients must never be placed between the grill and the CSP.

Wherever the air is blocked or interrupted from having unidirectional airflow, a **turbulence** of air is created. Turbulence occurs where the PEC airflow meets the buffer room air, behind the supplies, and wherever the body of the person compounding is moving or blocking the air. A **zone of turbulence** is created between the DCA and the compounding technician in the act of compounding. That is why technicians have to be very careful not to let their hands or supplies be closer to the air vent than the CSP or they will **shadow**, or block, the CSP from the cleansing airflow.

In preparation for compounding, to avoid shadowing, ingredients and instruments to be used must be arranged in a logical order to the sides of the DCA on the workbench.

Study Idea

Needlesticks during compounding may introduce contaminants into the CSP. Discard the product that may be contaminated.

Manipulating Needles and Syringes

Some of the main compounding instruments are needles and syringes. Needles come in gauge (or bore) sizes. Needles with the highest number have the smallest bore (opening), and needles with the lowest number have the largest bore. Pharmacy technicians need to be proficient in choosing the correct needle sizes and manipulating the syringe and needle properly. *You must never touch the critical sites of the needle, syringe tip, or syringe plunger*, because you may transmit pathogens, such as bacteria, viruses, or fungi from fingers, hands, and work surfaces. (See Figure 6.4 for the critical sites to avoid.)

During the compounding, universal precautions specify that needles used in patient care should not be recapped but should be placed uncapped into a puncture-proof sharps container. However, sterile compounding personnel are often required to

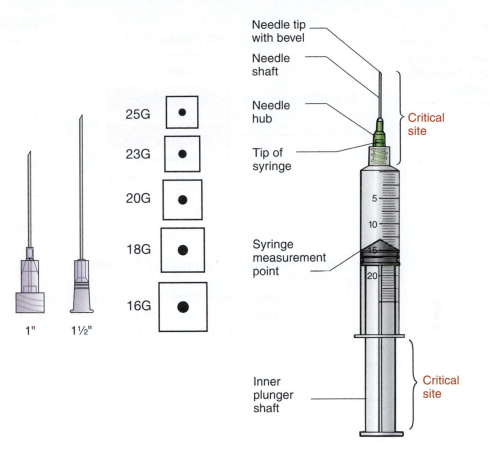

FIGURE 6.4
Common Needle Lengths and Gauges in Sterile Compounding and Critical Areas of a Needle and Syringe

Needle tip with bevel
Needle shaft
Needle hub
Tip of syringe
Critical site
Syringe measurement point
Inner plunger shaft
Critical site

25G
23G
20G
18G
16G

1"   1½"

perform compounding functions that require them to recap needles temporarily. So they use the "scoop" method with the needle to snag and scoop up the sterile cap without touching other surfaces.

Although there is no risk of exposure to patient blood or fluids during compounding, a needlestick could contaminate the final product with the healthcare worker's blood. If a needlestick occurs during compounding, the parenteral should be discarded and the whole aseptic garbing and compounding processes must be started again once the wound is treated and covered. When multiple vials of pharmaceuticals are compounded for medium- to high-risk parenterals, a different needle and syringe should be used for each vial.

Adding Ingredients from a Vial

A **vial** is a sealed glass or plastic sterile container with a rubber seal and hard plastic cap. Vials contain sterile diluents or medications in either a liquid or powdered form and are available in sizes ranging from 1 mL to 100 mL (for batch CSPs). Vials come as **single-dose vials (SDVs)**, which *do not contain preservatives*, and **multiple-dose vials (MDVs)**, which do contain preservatives. (Insulin often comes in MDVs.)

Information on the vial label includes the stock drug's concentration and the manufacturer's directions for reconstitution or use. (See Figure 6.5.)

The contents of the MDV are considered stable (with its preservatives) from its initial opening up to the manufacturer recommended BUD. (It is not generally longer than 28 days.) Once an MDV is opened, it must be marked with the beyond-use date and stored under appropriate conditions (usually refrigeration) to alert other

FIGURE 6.5
Identifying the Components of a Medication Label

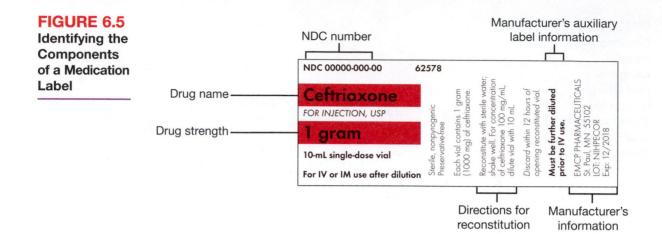

NDC number

Manufacturer's auxiliary label information

Drug name

Drug strength

NDC 00000-000-00   62578

Ceftriaxone

FOR INJECTION, USP

1 gram

10-mL single-dose vial

For IV or IM use after dilution

Sterile, nonpyrogenic Preservative-free

Each vial contains 1 gram (1000 mg) of ceftriaxone.

Reconstitute with sterile water; shake well. For concentration of ceftriaxone 100 mg/mL, dilute vial with 10 mL.

Discard within 12 hours of opening reconstituted vial.

Must be further diluted prior to IV use.

EMCP PHARMACEUTICALS
St. Paul, MN 55102
LOT: NIHPECOR
Exp: 12/2018

Directions for reconstitution

Manufacturer's information

Practice Tip

Because so much nitroglycerin is absorbed by PVC containers and IV sets, nitroglycerin is best compounded into a glass IV bottle and infused through a nonabsorbing IV line. The same is true for vitamin A acetate, warfarin, methohexital, terbutaline, lorazepam, and insulin.

pharmacy personnel of the opening and the medication's change from an expiration date to a BUD.

When removing contents from the vial, the plastic flip top must be removed, the rubber stopper wiped with 70% isopropyl alcohol (IPA), and the syringe needle inserted at a 45 degree angle to prevent **coring** (or the inadvertent introduction of a microscopic piece of rubber into the solution). Remove the solution by using the **milking technique**. This is done by inserting a little air and removing some solution and doing that a number of times if you are not using a **vented needle**. Using a vented needle, which has an opening in it, prevents air pressure buildup and makes it easier to remove the prescribed volume.

Adding Ingredients from an Ampule

An **ampule** is a small, hermetically sealed sterile glass container. An ampule stores a single dose of sterile medication in either a liquid (most common) or a powder. Ampules contain no preservatives, and some drugs are available only in an ampule because they are incompatible with the rubber top or any plastic sealing components of the vials.

Because an ampule is a completely whole glass container without an opening, it is designed with a **break ring**, or scoring on its neck. Before breaking, the neck must be wiped with a sterile 70% IPA swab to remove any microorganisms. Some technicians wrap a sterile 70% IPA swab around the neck of the ampule before breaking it *but gauze may not be used, per USP <797>*. Grasp the ampule body in your nondominant hand with thumb and fingers below the ampule neck away from the HEPA filter, exert a gentle but firm pressure, and snap the ampule's neck cleanly towards the side wall of the hood.

Because you have broken glass to access the medication, a blunt, **filter needle** or a **filter straw** must be used to withdraw the medication, according to USP <797> to catch any microscopic glass shards and impurities to prevent them from entering the CSP. The needle or straw must have a 5-micron (or finer) filter within its core and should be attached to the syringe just like a regular needle.

Filter needles are for one-directional use only, meaning that the needle may be used only to withdraw fluid from an ampule or inject fluid into an IV or IVPB. The same needle may not be used to do both. Before injecting the syringe contents into an IV, change to a regular needle in front of the DCA grill to prevent introducing glass or particles into the IV admixture. When delivering the final IV, *an inline filter should accompany the IV tubing* to screen out any microscopic glass shards that might still be in the admixture. This is particularly necessary for neonatal and pediatric patients.

Study Idea

A filter needle or straw should only be used to remove drug from the ampule and then be removed to attach a sterile needle to the syringe.

Using Automated Compounding Devices

In large hospitals and in many infusion compounding pharmacies for home care, an **automated compounding device (ACD)** is generally used. The ACD generally comes with 12 to 24 sterile fluid ports, and each dispenses a commonly needed nutritional additive for the total parenteral nutrition bags. The ACD uses a pumping system calibrated with metric measurements of volume or gravity to fill the bags with the correct elements. The technician who oversees the ACD must measure each compounded bag to check that it is of the desired volume or weight. The ACD must also be checked for accuracy and correct calibration each day, both of which must be documented.

Preparing Premade IV Solutions

Study Idea

Docked vial and bag drugs may be returned to the pharmacy if they are not activated to be relabeled and used on another patient with a similar order.

Other IV products come premixed but need sterile activation.

Vial-and-Bag IVs A **vial-and-bag system** provides a vial of powdered medication that will be attached with an adaptor to a specified IV bag solution. Though the technician does not compound the vial-and-bag product, it must be assembled, or **docked** (linking the vial and the bag with the connector device) in a DCA with aseptic technique. These products do not require sterile mixing, so they are not considered CSPs. Labels must be generated for the vial-and-bags with similar information as the CSPs, but they will come with manufacturer expiration dates rather than BUDs.

After scanning the product's labeled barcode, the nurse will use aseptic technique to break the seal of the attached powder vial, releasing the medication into the IVPB bag. This action "activates" the medication, which, once fully dissolved, is administered in short order to the patient via the secondary line tubing.

Premixed Frozen Solutions Manufactured frozen IV solutions, such as particular antibiotic solutions, are premixed products that are also not considered CSPs. When a frozen IV is ordered, it is thawed at room temperature or in the refrigerator (if there is sufficient time). After thawing, the technician prepares a patient-specific label. Once thawed, these frozen preparations cannot be refrozen.

Practice Tip

Manufacturers' recommendations for thawing frozen IVs vary among products, so be sure to check each product's label or package insert. The use of a warming bath or microwave to expedite the thawing process ("forced thaw") is not recommended.

Determining CSP Stability and Beyond Use Date

After the various types of CSPs and other IVs are prepared and labeled, they must be inspected once more by the technician and pharmacist and assigned a BUD or the manufacturer's expiration date on the label (if not preprinted), with a sign-off from both the preparer and pharmacist. As noted, the USP Chapter <797> guidelines specify the procedures for the dating, labeling, storage, handling, packaging, and transporting of CSPs in the hospital or infusion pharmacy. Improper procedures could adversely impact the sterility or stability of the products.

The BUD guidelines are based on the contamination risk or specific sterility testing provided by the hospital or manufacturer, as well as storage conditions and stability ratings (see Table 6.9). USP <797> provides the guidelines for risk levels depending on the number and sterility of ingredients, the presence or absence of preservatives, the number of transfers from vials or ampules, and the use of automated dispensing devices. (See Table 6.9.) Since CSPs may be compounded in anticipation of use, *the longer a compound is stored, the greater the risk of microbial and pyrogen formation*. Information about the chemical stability of a CSP is found in the Master Formulation Record, the manufacturer's literature, or specific product testing.

TABLE 6.9 Beyond-Use Dates for Compounded Sterile Drugs

Risk Category	Room Temperature	Refrigerator	Frozen (<+10°)
Immediate use	1 hour	1 hour	n/a
Low risk	12 hours	1 day	45 days
Lower risk	48 hours	14 days	n/a
Medium risk	30 hours	9 days	45 days
Medium high risk	24 hours	3 days	45 days

Note: Adapted from USP Chapter <797>

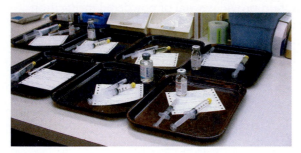

Medications compounded by the technician must await approval by the pharmacist.

Safety Alert

Total parenteral nutrition solutions have more compatibly and precipitate concerns because they contain so many additives.

Final Checks by Technician and Pharmacist

The technician checks to make sure there are no leaks in any of the IVs, precipitates, or incompatibilities, then lays out all the CSPs and all the components used in the compounding for the pharmacist's approval. The pharmacist's final CSP inspection will include checking the appearance and the accuracy in the proper selection and quantities of ingredients, technique for aseptic mixing and sterilization, packaging, and labeling that includes the BUD or expiration date. The pharmacist's inspection often includes rechecking the syringes used.

There should never be visible particles floating in the final parenteral solution. *CSPs with precipitates must be discarded, not filtered.* A precipitate is a nonsoluble particle or salt. A precipitate may clog an IV site or vein. A common cause of TPN precipitation is calcium gluconate and potassium phosphate added in too high of concentrations, in the wrong order, or without adequate mixing. Add the phosphate, then additives, and finally calcium. A colored multivitamin comes last. To verify ingredient compatibility, use a compatibilities handbook, such as *Trissel's Stability of Compounded Formulations*.

Hazardous Compounding

Any drug that is known to have a risk of at least one of the following six criteria is considered a **hazardous drug (HD)**:

- carcinogenicity (causes cancer)
- teratogenicity (causes developmental damage/problems)
- reproductive toxicity (causes reproductive damage/problems)
- organ toxicity (causes organ damage/problems)
- genotoxicity (causes genetic damage)
- drugs that mimic hazardous drugs in structure or toxicity

Because of the special dangers involved in hazardous compounding, the CDC and OSHA have teamed up in a special center for hazardous substances: the **National Institute for Occupational Safety and Health (NIOSH)**, which has published the "NIOSH Alert: Preventing Occupational Exposures to Antineoplastic and Other Hazardous Drugs in Health Care Settings." **Safety data sheets (SDS)**, also known as material safety data sheets (MSDSs), for each hazardous agent or investigational drug must be readily accessible so that employees can see what they are handling and know what should be done in the case of an accidental exposure or spill. The ASHP has also established new HD guidelines.

In addition, updated and expanded guidelines for hazardous compounding have been established in the new **USP Chapter <800>**, which must be fully implemented by July 1, 2018. USP <800> outlines requirements for receiving, storing, mixing, preparing, compounding, dispensing, and administering hazardous drugs to protect the patient, healthcare personnel, and environment. For more information about USP <800>, go to http://CertExam4e.ParadigmCollege.net/USP800PPT.

According to USP <800>, personnel in a hospital or compounding facility who come into *any level of contact* with HDs require specialized equipment, training, protective clothing, and procedures for handling, preparing, and disposing of these substances. Hospitals are required to develop written policies and procedures for each aspect of HD use to be in compliance with the USP and The Joint Commission, as well as state and federal regulations. Hospitals and compounding facilities must have intensive personnel training, protective primary and secondary engineering controls, personal protective clothing and gear, and specific techniques and supplemental engineering equipment. Routes of potential exposure are outlined on Table 6.10.

TABLE 6.10 Routes of Exposure to Hazardous Agents

- Receiving and unpacking HD orders
- Counting individual oral doses and tablets from bulk containers
- Crushing tablets or opening capsules to make oral solutions, suspensions, or syrups
- Pouring oral or topical liquids from one container to another
- Mixing topical dosage forms
- Weighing or mixing components
- Constituting or reconstituting powdered or lyophilized (freeze-dried) HDs
- Withdrawing or diluting injectable HDs from parenteral containers
- Expelling air from syringes filled with HDs
- Expelling HDs from a syringe
- Coming into contact with HD residue present on drug container exteriors, work surfaces, floors, and final drug preparations (e.g., bottles, bags, cassettes, and syringes)
- Inhaling HD residue or vapors
- Handling contaminated waste generated at any step of the preparation or dispensing
- Deactivating, decontaminating, cleaning, and disinfecting areas contaminated or suspected of being contaminated with HDs
- Undergoing maintenance activities for contaminated equipment and devices
- Spilling substances, cleaning up a spill, and disposing of cleanup materials

Medical Surveillance

With exposure to HDs, workers can suffer acute, chronic, and long-term health consequences if proper precautions, procedures, and training are not followed. To prevent any health issues, USP Chapter <800> requires a medical surveillance program by the hospital or compounding facility to collect and interpret data on HD workers to detect any changes in their health status due to potential exposure.

Any woman of reproductive age who routinely works with hazardous agents must confirm in writing an understanding of the risks and the importance of taking additional precautions to prevent pregnancy. A pharmacy technician who is pregnant, breast-feeding, or trying to conceive must notify her supervisor so that she can be reassigned to a different department position, take extra precautions, or have different work responsibilities to minimize contact with any hazardous substances.

Hazardous Compounding Engineering Controls

Hazardous substances and sterile hazardous substances must be compounded away from sterile products in a **containment secondary engineering control (C-SEC)** area with an exterior venting system. With this air-flow control, the trace hazardous substances do not flow into other CSP compounding areas, the hospital, or the rest of the compounding facility. The C-SEC rooms come in two kinds: one for the nonsterile and lower-risk nonsterile HDs, and one that has a buffer area with ISO Class 7 air for preparing sterile toxic HDs. Both C-SECs have to follow the appropriate USP <800> standards.

Hazardous compounding airflow goes in the reverse pattern of that in the sterile compounding cleanroom. C-SEC areas must provide **negative pressure**, with the ventilation system causing an unidirectional airflow that is suctioned out of the buffer room and away from the compounding technicians and outer rooms. A sink must also be available for hand washing and for emergency access to water. An eyewash station within the contained HD compounding area is necessary for removal of hazardous substances from the eyes and skin.

Containment Primary Engineering Controls

Per USP <800> standards, all HD compounding must be done in **containment primary engineering controls (C-PECs)**, which provide some level of shielding or isolation of the DCA, to contain the HD substances and protect the compounding personnel. These C-PECs should be a Class II-B biological safety cabinet (BSC) or compounding aseptic containment isolator (CACI)—see Table 6.11 for the various types and levels of protection. These C-PECs still provide ISO Class 5 air quality in the DCA but have **vertical airflow**, or downward moving air that is suctioned away from the compounding technician to prevent exposure.

Supplemental Protections

As mentioned when discussing aseptic garbing, extra personal protective equipment must be worn to do hazardous compounding: *goggles, a face shield with a respirator, a gown made of impervious material, and double heavy-duty chemotherapy gloves.* Upon completion of compounding activities, garb must be disposed of in a special hazardous waste container.

TABLE 6.11 General Types of Containment Primary Engineering Controls for Sterile Hazardous Compounding

Each C-PEC unit has vertical HEPA-filtered airflow, air exchanges, and some level of HEPA-exhausted air according to USP Chapter <800> standards.

Containment Primary Engineering Controls
Class II Biological Safety Cabinets
• **Class II-A Biological Safety Cabinets** (including the vertical laminar airflow workbench[V-LAF].)—partially shielded units with downward filtered airflow onto the DCA, with high amounts of recirculated air. (As of July 2018, Class II-A1 V-LAWs are not recommended for compounding HD products.) • **Class II-B Biological Safety Cabinets:** similar units to Class II-A (with barriers and vertical airflow) though with exterior filtered venting and little to no recirculated air
Aseptic Isolators
• **Compounding Aseptic Containment Isolator (CACI):** a unit with enclosed DCA in glovebox with external venting for sterile, hazardous compounding (for Class I or II hazardous substances)
Sealed Sterile Compounding Isolators
• **Class III Biological Safety Cabinet:** sealed unit for high-risk hazardous compounding; vented and filtered to outdoors with no recirculated air • **Radiopharmacy Isolator:** a lead-shielded, sealed unit designed specifically for compounding nuclear diagnostic and therapeutic agents

Study Idea

To ensure staff know how to properly clean a HD spill, mock HD spill drills are held for safety and quality assurance.

Supplemental Engineering Controls In addition, a few additional protective supplies are needed: a **chemotherapy compounding mat**, **closed-system transfer devices**, and **chemotherapy dispensing pins**. The devices and pins supply additional containment when transferring HD ingredients. These three types of protective supplies are called **supplementary engineering controls**.

Labeling All CSPs containing hazardous agents must be properly labeled. These CSP labels must contain the patient's name and room number, the solution name and volume, the drug name(s) and dosage, CSP administration information, and storage requirements. Hazardous agents also require additional labeling that clearly identifies the CSP as a hazardous agent, with a colored caution label.

HD Cleaning and Spill Kit A **spill kit** must be readily accessible in any area where HDs are handled, compounded, or administered. A spill kit is a container of supplies, warning signage, and related materials used to contain an HD spill. Table 6.12 lists the contents of a typical spill kit.

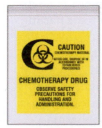

In general, the standard HD personal protective equipment, including eye and face protection and chemotherapy gloves, should always be worn for cleaning, disinfecting, decontaminating the C-PECs and CACIs, and deactivating HDs in the compounding area, using appropriate products. Chemical **deactivation** of a nonnuclear HD should be done with 2% sodium hypochlorite (chlorine bleach). Alcohol is not an effective deactivating or HD cleaning agent.

HD spills, however, must be contained and cleaned immediately. Only trained workers with appropriate PPE should manage an HD spill, and they must post warning signs to restrict access to the spill area. The goal is to ensure that the staff, patients, and visitors are not exposed and that the healthcare environment (both inside and outside the medical facility) is not contaminated.

TABLE 6.12 Typical Contents of a Spill Kit

A commercially available spill kit may be purchased, or one may be assembled with the following contents:

- absorbent chemotherapy pads and towels
- 2 disposable chemotherapy-resistant gowns (with back closure)
- 2 pairs of chemotherapy-resistant shoe covers
- 4 pairs of chemotherapy gloves
- 2 pairs of chemical splash goggles
- 2 respirator masks approved by the National Institute for Occupational Safety and Health
- 1 disposable dustpan
- 1 plastic scraper
- 1 puncture-proof container for glass
- 2 large, heavy-duty, sealable waste disposal bags
- 1 hazardous waste label (if bags are unlabeled)

Source: American Society of Health-System Pharmacists

Nuclear Compounding

A specific kind of hazardous compounding occurs in a **nuclear pharmacy**, which prepares radioactive materials to diagnose and treat specific diseases. Nuclear medicine scans records radiation that is emitting from elements injected into the body, rather than from external elements like x-rays. **Radiopharmaceuticals** are an irradiated form of HDs.

Unlike hazardous CSPs, these preparations are not prepared in a hospital pharmacy. They are most commonly prepared off-site in a nuclear pharmacy by specially trained and certified nuclear pharmacists and pharmacy technicians. The federal Nuclear Regulatory Commission (NRC) regulates the medical use of radioactive materials to minimize radiation exposure to patients and medical staff. **USP Chapter <823>** provides nuclear compounding guidelines.

A **nuclear pharmacy technician (NPT)** prepares the radioactive pharmaceuticals. Working knowledge of these nuclear drugs and their risks and benefits is essential, as these technicians often advise medical providers regarding their toxic nature and their dangers. A nuclear pharmacy technician works under the direct supervision of a nuclear pharmacist and receives special training and education on radiation safety. They must wear protective garments to reduce radiation exposure, and follow strict guidelines with regard to the receipt, handling, disposition, disposal, and transfer of radioactive materials. The radiopharmacy compounders must use leaded glass or tungsten syringe shields, transfer devices, and containers in the radiopharmacy isolator.

Worker protection and medical surveillance programs for the nuclear pharmacy workers are even more strict than those for chemical hazardous drugs. Pharmacists, technicians, and others working in a nuclear pharmacy wear badges to monitor their exposure on a weekly, monthly, quarterly, annual, and lifetime basis. In addition, nuclear hazardous wastes are handled differently from other hazardous wastes or pharmaceuticals, as regulated by the NRC.

Although USP Chapter <823> has outlined rules for radioactive compounding, in 2015, the USP decided to begin revising and updating these guidelines. There are in development two new USP Chapters: <1821> Radioactivity: Theory and Practice and <1823> Positron Emission Tomography: Information. As with the revision of compounding standards and the creation of Chapter <800>, the USP has been soliciting public comments before proceeding. So these chapters will take time before becoming accepted standards.

Waste Handling and Disposal

Sterile and hazardous compounding produces waste that must be properly disposed of. Traces of hazardous wastes and residual pharmaceuticals have been found in the surface water, groundwater, and drinking water in the United States, which has raised concern about the environmental consequences of inappropriate disposal of waste from sterile and hazardous compounding as well as from general pharmaceuticals.

Hazardous Waste Disposal

During the admixture and administration of chemotherapy, any unadministered medication left in the IV bags and tubing, bottles, and vials must be disposed of in a hazardous waste container with a yellow label identifying it as hazardous waste. The US Environmental Protection Agency (EPA) defines **hazardous waste** as waste that causes or contributes to an increase in mortality or an increase in irreversible or incapacitating reversible illness. The definition also includes waste that poses a threat to human health when improperly treated, stored, transported, disposed of, or otherwise mismanaged. Table 6.13 lists examples of hazardous pharmaceutical waste based on the EPA's waste determinations. Further information about hazardous waste is available on the EPA's website at www.epa.gov and from state environmental protection agencies.

Nuclear hazardous wastes are handled differently from other hazardous wastes or pharmaceuticals, and are regulated by the NRC.

TABLE 6.13 Hazardous Pharmaceutical Waste

Waste Determination	Example
Ignitable	Flammable liquid or gas/aerosol or oxidizer, ethanol, ethyl chloride spray, silver nitrate swabs
Reactive	Nitroglycerin
Heavy metals	Products with thimerosal preservatives, burn ointments with silver compounds; m-cresol preservatives; selenium, mercury, silver sulfadiazine, and barium
Corrosivity	Acids and bases; acetic acid
Specifically listed drugs	Highly hazardous unused pharmaceuticals and chemicals; nicotine, physostigmine, chlorambucil, and warfarin

Sterile Compounding and General Pharmaceutical Wastes

Even small concentrations of certain drugs or a multitude of drugs can have detrimental effects on aquatic and terrestrial wildlife species and on human health and development. A pharmacy technician must be aware of disposal requirements for sterile compounding and individual pharmaceuticals based on the employer's policy and procedures. The EPA and state governments monitor pharmaceutical waste disposal. There are significant fines for the inappropriate disposal of any waste. Black waste containers are used for pharmaceutical waste, which must be labeled as to its contents. Storage and removal of filled containers must be handled in accordance with the federal hazardous waste regulations.

Unused medications at healthcare facilities, pharmacies, and patient homes should not be flushed down the toilet or sink, because for they flow into the wastewater system and work their way in to rivers, groundwater, reservoirs, and the oceans. This results in unintentionally "medicating" any person or animal drinking the water with trace elements. These substances often accumulate in bodily tissues and fat and in aquatic plants, having unintended and often damaging effects. That is why the EPA is now more concerned about pharmaceutical wastes and asks for careful disposal.

Certain wastes are even more dangerous than others, such as used fentanyl transdermal patches and other controlled substances. Because of their danger to children and pets, these patches should be folded in half and put into a sealed container with unappealing food waste like coffee grounds or kitty litter and then put into a sealed trash container, away from child access. The FDA still recommends flushing down them down the toilet, but this causes the other problems mentioned.

For patients with pharmaceutical remainders, many pharmacies have established their own safe medication return containers. The National Community Pharmacists Association (NCPA) offers the Dispose My Meds program that allows patients to use their zip codes to find a disposal site at the closest community pharmacy of the NCPA's for over 1,600 participating independent pharmacy members. The National Association of Boards of Pharmacy (NABP) Foundation has worked with police departments and sheriff offices to set up permanent medication disposal drop-boxes through its AWARxE program.

For pharmacies, outdated stock that can be returned to the manufacturer for credit is exempt from waste disposal regulations. If credit is not available, the pharmacy must dispose of outdated pharmaceuticals in accordance with hazardous waste regulations.

STUDY SUMMARY

The certification exam will require you to have a basic knowledge of the guidelines set up by the USP, OSHA, NIOSH, and NRC for safe compounding. Each hospital will also have its own P&P manual that includes these and additional guidelines. Personal protective equipment, hand washing, and aseptic technique should be reviewed.

Many different types of parenteral products are compounded. Be aware of the procedures for compounding, calculations you will need to be able to compute, beyond-use dating based on level of risk of contamination of the sterile product, documentation of the compounding process, and maintenance of equipment. You should be versed in the appropriate procedures for the disposal of waste from sterile and hazardous compounding and drug dispensing.

ADDITIONAL RESOURCES

For more in-depth explanations, check out *Sterile Compounding and Aseptic Technique* from Paradigm Education Solutions. To master and extend the material presented in this chapter, take advantage of the resources available through the eBook resources links. These include digital supplements, study resources, and a practice exam generator with 1,000+ exam-style questions. End-of-chapter tests are accessible through the eBook for individuals using the self-study course and through Navigator+ for individuals enrolled in the instructor-guided course.

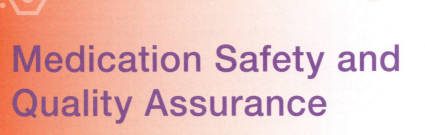

7

Medication Safety and Quality Assurance

Learning Objectives

1   Identify the various agencies involved with medication safety, including the FDA, ISMP, and CPSC.

2   Differentiate between generic, trade, and chemical drug names.

3   Understand the steps required to develop and manufacture a new drug or generic equivalent.

4   Identify FDA-mandated sources of information on medications for healthcare professionals and patients.

5   Explain FDA categories for use of drugs in pregnancy.

6   Identify high-risk/high-alert medications.

7   Know the restrictions on the use of clozapine, isotretinoin, and thalidomide.

8   Define the pharmacy technician's role in the Drug Quality and Security Act.

9   Understand the provisions of the Poison Prevention Packaging Act of 1970.

10 List innovations and techniques to reduce medication errors.

11 Recognize look-alike/sound-alike medications and techniques to prevent errors.

12 Identify strategies to prevent data entry errors.

13 Define the components of the NDC number and its significance in medication error prevention.

14 Recognize when pharmacist intervention should occur.

15 Identify quality assurance and improvement techniques.

16 Explain how PSQI will improve medication error reporting.

Access eBook links for resources and an exam generator, with 1,000+ questions.

According to the Centers for Disease Control and Prevention, 48.7% of patients have used at least one prescription drug in the last 30 days, 21.8% have used three or more in the last 30 days, and 10.7% have used five or more in last 30 days. With each drug added, the risk for errors, drug-drug interactions, and adverse drug reactions multiplies. Pharmacy technicians have very hands-on ways to provide safe medications to patients by following pharmacy procedures, rules, and standards. That is why domain 4 of the PTCE (12.5%) is dedicated to medication error prevention and safety questions, and these types of questions are woven throughout all of the topic areas of the ExCPT, especially 3.

Medication safety is a subset of the larger push in the pharmacy industry for quality control and improvement, which use systematic approaches to analyze and reduce errors, prevent and control infection outbreaks, and improve overall safety, productivity, profitability, and patient satisfaction. Quality assurance questions are addressed in domain 5 of the PTCE and throughout the ExCPT.

Medication Safety Systems

One of the first challenges about medication safety is to make sure that drugs themselves are safe for human use. The federal and state governments have created laws to address drug manufacturing and safety issues that have already arisen to prevent them from happening in the future. The FDA, DEA, CDC, OSHA, the Consumer Product Safety Commission (CPSC), and the Federal Trade Commission (FTC) are agencies set up by the federal government to enforce the laws but also to do research and establish prevention processes. The state boards of pharmacy also advocate for safety laws on the state level.

The major nongovernmental agencies involved in safety efforts are the US Pharmacopeial Convention (USP), the National Coordinating Council for Medication Error Reporting and Prevention (NCC MERP), the Institute for Safe Medication Practices (ISMP), Centers for Medicare & Medicaid Services (CMS), and The Joint Commission (TJC), which oversees healthcare institution accreditation. Within each pharmacy and compounding facility, the policy and procedures (P&P) manual lays out the safe procedures for pharmacy filling, dispensing, and compounding based on the laws, regulations, standards, and counsel from all of these organizations.

FDA New Drug Oversight

> **Study Idea**
>
> Brand names may only be on the prescription label if the proprietary product is dispensed. If the less expensive alternative is used, you must put the generic name on the label.

The FDA is responsible for the review and approval of all prescription and over-the-counter (OTC) medications, including generic drugs. Although the manufacture of vitamins and herbal and diet supplements is not under FDA control, the FDA does monitor adverse reactions and marketing claims.

It is important to understand that every new drug approved by the FDA has a chemical name, a generic or nonproprietary name, and the manufacturer's recommended brand or trade name. Table 7.1 lists the different types of names used for a commonly used pain medication. A chemical name describes the chemical structure of the drug molecule. The brand name is owned by the company that develops the drug, gets FDA approval (which will be explained later), and first markets it. The generic or nonproprietary name (USNA) is developed to provide an identifier that is not protected by a patent. Once the original patent of the brand drug expires (usually 17+ years after the patent is filed), any manufacturer can apply to the FDA with an **Abbreviated New Drug Application (ANDA)** to market a generic version, which usually sells for a reduced price.

TABLE 7.1 Drug Names

Name Category	Drug Name
Chemical	2-(4-isobutylphenyl)propionic acid
Generic	ibuprofen
Brand	Advil, Motrin, Motrin IB

Investigational Drugs and New Brand Drug Approvals

For all new brand drugs, manufacturers must file an **Investigational New Drug Application (IND)** with in-depth animal studies before the new drug can be tested with human subjects. In its application, the developer must offer a compelling case for the human need for the drug, the results of the animal studies, an explanation of how the drug would be manufactured, and a detailed description of the proposed clinical studies on humans. The research study must then be submitted and approved by the **Institutional Review Board (IRB)** of the university or hospital where the research will be conducted before the human clinical studies are allowed to begin. This IRB, also known as the Human Use Committee, is comprised of scientists and practitioners from various disciplines, plus consumers. The committee must review, approve, and monitor all medical research involving humans. Each study participant must sign an **informed consent form**—a document that states the purpose and risks of the research in easily understandable terms.

After the IND is approved by the FDA and the IRB, non-FDA scientists conduct three phases of human clinical studies as part of the drug approval process. Phase 1 is the initial study or trial of the new drug, usually completed on a small number of healthy volunteers. The Phase 2 study aims to evaluate the effectiveness as well as the safety of a drug for a specific indication or disease state on another slightly larger number of patients. If the results of Phase 1 and Phase 2 studies are promising, Phase 3 studies are conducted in larger clinical trials (larger groups) to better assess the overall benefits and risks of the investigational drug on patients (see Figure 7.1).

FIGURE 7.1
The Three Phases of the Drug Approval Process

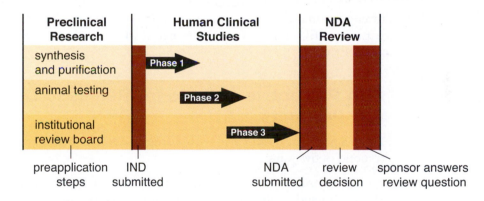

Technicians often work on the dispensing, documentation, and inventory management of the investigational drug in the studies, following all the special FDA regulations for safety and tracking. All investigational drugs must be documented and stored separately from the regular pharmacy drug inventory. The informed consent forms and the documentation of each dispensing and administration must also be filed.

If the investigational drug shows promise after Phase 3 studies are completed, the pharmaceutical manufacturer can submit a **New Drug Application (NDA)** to the FDA. The results of the scientific studies are evaluated by an independent advisory panel of experts, and recommendations are forwarded to the FDA. If the benefit of the drug outweighs the risk, the drug is generally approved. The FDA, however, may request additional studies be completed. The drug approval process takes a year or longer in most cases.

FDA Drug Reaction Tracking

Once drugs are released, dangers can still arise as the large population using the drugs increases the statistical chances of problems showing up, so the FDA tracks adverse drug reactions through different feedback processes. The FDA **Adverse Event Reporting system (AERS)** is a centralized database that stores information from two separate federally sponsored reporting programs: MedWatch and VAERS.

MedWatch Run by the FDA in collaboration with the ISMP, **MedWatch** is a voluntary program that offers healthcare professionals *and consumers* an avenue to anonymously report a serious adverse event associated with any specific drug, biological device, or dietary supplement.

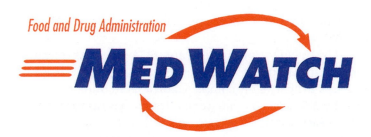

Food and Drug Administration

Vaccine Adverse Event Reporting System Cosponsored by the CDC, the **Vaccine Adverse Event Reporting System (VAERS)** is a safety surveillance program, collecting information from those who provide vaccinations and from the public about adverse events (possible side effects) that occur after the vaccine has been released in the United States.

Healthcare personnel are mandated by the National Childhood Vaccine Injury Act of 1986 to report serious adverse reactions from vaccines. Technicians may contribute to this safety effort, as they are often the ones who patients confide in and report reactions to recent vaccinations. The technician should document the information on the patient profile and notify the pharmacist who can discuss the reaction with the patient further.

FDA Protective Actions for Released Drugs and Products

When a problem is identified with a drug or durable medical equipment, the FDA may respond in five ways:

1. Issue safety alerts to healthcare professionals or consumers on the drugs (including drug recalls), biologicals, dietary supplements, and counterfeit drugs;

2. Request medication labeling changes to the product package insert, including contraindications, warnings, black box warnings, precautions, and adverse reactions.

3. List the drug as a high-risk medication and require that it be dispensed with a MedGuide for provider and patient education. (This action may also be required before market release because of the results of the clinical studies.)

4. Require Risk Evaluation and Mitigation Strategies (REMS). These, too, may be required before market release.

5. Remove the product from the market in a drug recall, as described in Chapter 3.

Product Labeling Warnings

The FDA requires manufacturers to include safety information in the **product package insert (PPI)** attached to each stock bottle. Technicians often use these PPIs for information on precautions, contraindications, warnings (including black box warnings), and adverse reactions. This information is also published in the *Physicians' Desk Reference (PDR)*.

Avandia, Paxil, Adderall, Accutane, and Coumadin are examples of drugs that require additional alerts in the PPI—called **black box warnings**—and communications to pharmacists and prescribers. Black box warnings are significant warnings assigned to products approved and regulated by the FDA. *These warnings must be observed and followed when dispensing these products.*

Study Idea

Look at the drug package insert for the pregnancy, lactation, and reproductive warnings.

Pregancy Labeling The FDA can also require specialized patient container labeling. A good example is the case of new labeling for pregnant and nursing women. Until 2015, the FDA categorized the risks of taking a drug or biological product during pregnancy under a five-letter system (A, B, C, D, and X) based on what was known about that product. However, for easier-to-understand patient education, the FDA now requires the product labeling to include explanatory sentences and/or paragraphs that address the categories and subcategories listed in Table 7.2. Technicians need to learn to look for these warning descriptions on the labels and recommend counseling with the pharmacist when patients seem to fall into these categories. OTC drugs are not yet required to have this information.

TABLE 7.2 New Labeling for Drugs that Affect Pregnant and Lactating Mothers

Pregnancy (includes mothers in labor and delivery)	Pregnancy exposure registry Risk summary Clinical considerations, Data
Lactation (includes nursing mothers)	Risk summary Clinical considerations Data
Females and Males of Reproductive Potential	Pregnancy testing Contraception Infertility

Study Idea

MedGuides are required for commonly prescribed medications like antidepressants, NSAIDs, and stimulants for ADHD.

MedGuides for High-Risk Medications

For select high-risk drugs used by the general population or vulnerable populations, such as those listed in Table 7.3 on the next page, the FDA requires by law the pharmacy to provide additional written information in the form of the MedGuides. These patient guides include black box warnings and guidelines on the safe and effective use of a high-risk drug and to minimize the risk of serious adverse reactions.

TABLE 7.3   Examples of Drugs Requiring a MedGuide

Drug	Risk Factor
Accutane	Causes birth defects in women of childbearing age; women must be on some form of birth control or be advised not to get pregnant while on this medication
ADHD drugs (e.g., Adderall XR, Concerta, methylphenidate, Ritalin, Strattera)	May cause insomnia, loss of appetite, and changes in pulse and blood pressure; may interfere with growth and weight in children; monitor vital signs
Antidepressants (SSRIs, such as fluoxetine, sertraline, paroxetine, citalopram, escitalopram, venlafaxine)	May be associated with an increase in suicide risk, especially in adolescent patients; watch for changes in behavior
Ciprofloxacin	May cause tendon rupture
Cordarone	May cause lung/liver damage, abnormal heartbeats and thyroid dysfunction; limited to life-threatening conditions due to its side effects; monitor vital signs and symptoms
Coumadin	Reduces blood clotting, so the patient must be careful when working with sharp objects, shaving, and participating in contact sports while taking this drug; interacts with many drugs
Fentanyl transmucosal drug products (various forms)	Indicated only for breakthrough pain in cancer patients tolerant of and maintained on around-the-clock opioid therapy; risk of respiratory depression and even death
NSAIDs (e.g., hydromorphone, morphine, naproxen)	May cause increased risk of stomach ulcers; take with food, no longer than necessary
Xarelto	May cause bleeding; avoid other drugs that can cause bleeding, such as aspirin, and NSAIDs, such as ibuprofen; monitor uncontrolled bleeding of nose, gums, etc., and discoloration of urine/stools
Zolpidem	May cause confusion, sleepwalking, next-day sleepiness and driving issues, especially in higher doses in women and the elderly; do not combine with alcohol; use lower doses in high-risk groups

Risk Evaluation and Mitigation Stategies Medications

For some high-risk drugs, MedGuides are insufficient. For drugs that are both particularly and uniquely needed but also pose great health risks, the FDA requires manufacturers develop **Risk Evaluation and Mitigation Strategies (REMS)** for providers and patients to follow. Community and institutional pharmacies (and prescribers) must register with the drug manufacturer or federal REMS program for each drug they will be dispensing (or official wholesaler) and receive drug-specific REMS training. The pharmacist must pledge to go over the MedGuide with patients and do other required counseling and monitoring activities.

REMS programs are individually designed to closely track patients on these high-risk drugs and make periodic assessment reports to the FDA on their status. You can become familiar with these drugs at http://CertExam4e.ParadigmEducation .com/REMS. Some of the more common REMS drugs technicians must know are described below.

Web

Thalidomide   Though at first rejected for FDA drug approval, thalidomide (Thalomid) was eventually approved for treatment of leprosy or severe nerve inflammation and pain. However, because of its known harm to children in the womb, or **teratogenicity**, the FDA requires the REMS program called **STEPS (System for Thalidomide Education and Prescribing Safety)**. It is intended to mitigate the risks for both women and men.

Isotretinoin and the iPLEDGE Program Isotretinoin (a synthetic analog of vitamin A) is a common generic drug for intense acne and other skin problems that has a very high incidence of teratogenicity. Common brands of this drug are Accutane and Claravis (see Table 7.4 for others). The **iPLEDGE Program** is a REMS that was designed for isotretinoin and related drugs to prevent fetal exposure and the resulting birth defects, and to educate all patients (both female and male) on the drugs' risks and proper uses. All patients must be registered and agree to meet all conditions required during treatment. Pharmacies may receive the drug only from a certified wholesaler and can only dispense written prescriptions authorized by a certified prescriber. An assigned Risk Management Authorization (RMA) number must be placed on each prescription, and prescribers must agree to provide contraception counseling to patients prior to and during treatment with this drug. The prescription quantity *is limited to a 30-day supply with no refills, and all pregnancies must be reported*. Patients must agree not to share their medication or donate blood while on the medication and for one month after discontinuing use.

If patients are sexually active, prescribers must document the forms of contraception the patients are currently using. Women of childbearing potential must agree to monthly pregnancy tests and have a negative result prior to prescribers issuing a new or refill prescription. If sexually active, they must commit to two forms of contraception while on the drug and for one month after drug discontinuation. In addition, they must agree to pick up the prescription within a specified period (usually within seven days) or the prescription is void.

Study Idea

A patient has 7 days from the last pregnancy test to fill the prescription for isotretinoin.

TABLE 7.4 Isotretinoin and Isotroin Drugs in the iPLEDGE Program

The generic drugs isotretinoin and isotroin come in the following brand names:

- Absorica
- Accutane (generic only)
- Amnesteem
- Claravis
- Epuris (Canada only)
- Isotroin (Canada only)
- Myorisan
- Sotret
- Zenatane

Pharmacists who dispense these drugs and patients who use them must agree to the terms of the iPLEDGE Program as part of these drugs' REMS.

Transmucosal Fentanyl The REMS for fentanyl seek to limit the medication access to only the appropriate opioid-dependent cancer patients or those in palliative care and to promote patient education and safe storage to avoid accidental exposure to children. Prescribers must agree to initiate therapy with the lowest dose, follow up on efficacy of dose titration, and document any signs of misuse or abuse. Pharmacies are also responsible for training all staff, including pharmacy technicians; hospital pharmacies can dispense transmucosal fentanyl to inpatients only. Patients must review and study the MedGuide, sign an agreement with the prescriber, and follow prescribed instructions exactly.

Buprenorphine Transmucosal Products for Opioid Dependence These medications, including Subutex and Suboxone, are prescribed by doctors certified to treat opioid dependence. Certified physicians have DEA numbers that all start with an "X," indicating their ability to prescribe these medications. Subutex (buprenorphine HCL) is a sublingual tablet formulation commonly prescribed to pregnant females and patients who cannot tolerate Suboxone. Suboxone is available as a film and sublingual tablet used to control relapse with opioid addiction. Other products available are Bunavil and Zubzolv. The REMS goals are to prevent accidental overdose, misuse, and abuse, and to inform patients of serious risks.

Clozapine and Olanzapine An atypical antipsychotic drug, clozapine (Clozaril, Fazacio ODT, Versacloz, FazaClo, and generics) has been found to cause a life-threatening decrease in white blood cells. Technicians, again, participate in the documentation, facilitating patient access to the pharmacist, and any monitoring. Clozapine registry requirements state that the patient must be registered with the dispensing pharmacy and the prescribing physician. There must be appropriate laboratory monitoring of the patient's blood.

Before the long-acting injectable formulation of the antipsychotic medication olanzapine (only available as Zyprexa Relprevv) can be administered to a patient, the prescriber, healthcare facility, patient, and pharmacy must be enrolled in the Zyprexa Relprevv Patient Care Program. Postinjection delirium/sedation syndrome (PDSS) may occur in patients after administration. Patients must be monitored for at least three hours after every monthly injection. Everyone in the pharmacy involved with the process must be aware of the high risk associated with olanzapine injection.

Addyi The adverse reactions for Addyi (flibanserin)—the new sexual drive enhancing drug for women—include extreme hypotension and loss of consciousness (syncope) due to a drop in blood pressure when taken with alcohol. The drug poses other dangers as well. Prescribers and pharmacies, as with the other REMS drugs, must complete training and enroll to be authorized to handle this drug. Patients need to be directly counseled by pharmacists on how to use the drug properly and to avoid alcohol when taking this medication.

Drug Supply Chain Security Tracking

In 2012, the New England Compounding Center prepared a solution for injection of methylprednisolone that was provided to healthcare clinics and institutions throughout many states. Because the drug was contaminated, it caused the deaths of at least 64 patients and the serious injury of at least 750 more. In 2013, Congress passed the Drug Quality and Security Act, also known as the Drug Supply Chain Security Act and the "Compounding Act." It aimed to increase compounding safety guidelines and establish a national database to "track and trace" drug products through the supply chain from the manufacturer to the pharmacy. As of 2016, it requires the following:

- verification that all trading partners and practitioners are properly licensed
- drug-tracking documentation to be completed by the compounder/manufacturer, wholesalers and distributers, pharmacies, and administering clinicians and kept on file for a minimum of six years

Study Idea

Special DEA licenses are issued to prescribers of buprenorphine products for treating opioid dependence. Their DEA numbers begin with "X".

Study Idea

When dispensing clozapine, if the patient has not had their absolute neutrophil count (ANC) done, you cannot dispense the drug.

Study Idea

Signs a drug package may be counterfeit include: packaging looks different from previous ordered product, missing product insert, product shipped from foreign entity, or package label containing foreign language, misspelled words, or missing information.

- inspection of all drugs upon receipt to remove any suspicious products for further investigation

The key points of drug checks and documentation occur at delivery by the compounder/manufacturer to the wholesaler, by the wholesaler to the pharmacy, from the pharmacy to the medication administrator, and of course, at the point of administration (for which documentation was already required by the healthcare facility). Technicians take part in the documentation at the points of drug inventory delivery and dispensing. It is important to file invoices from all wholesale purchases and only purchase from FDA-approved wholesalers and manufacturers. During the receiving process, technicians must be able to recognize signs of drug tampering and counterfeiting and know how to report to the FDA all suspicious products.

Consumer Product Safety Commission

The Poison Prevention Packaging Act of 1970 is enforced not by the FDA but by the US Consumer Product Safety Commission. The incidence of childhood deaths, emergency room visits, and calls to poison control centers has been considerably reduced since the law was enacted. Toxic substances that require this packaging include prescription and OTC drugs and common household products.

A child-resistant container is defined as one that cannot be opened by 80% of children but can be opened by 90% of adults. Exceptions include:

- prescriptions sent from a community pharmacy to a nursing home or hospital because the medication will be administered by a nurse and stored in a locked area,
- certain emergency medications, such as sublingual nitroglycerin for chest pain, that need quick access,
- specific drugs with packaging that already limits child access, such as metered-dose inhalers (MDIs), birth control medications, and Medrol Dosepaks.

As noted in other chapters, elderly patients or patients with certain disabilities can opt out of special packaging requirements. Then the technician may dispense the medications using a non-safety lid. A signed opt-out document should be on file.

Reuse of plastic prescription vials and lids on refills is also prohibited by the Poison Prevention Act to prevent potential contamination and defect due to previous use.

Preventing Medication Errors

The pharmacy technician, as a member of the healthcare team, works to deliver the right drug, at the right strength, in the right route of administration and form, with the right frequency and time of administration, with the right documentation, and the right education material to the right patient with 100% accuracy. (See Figure 7.2.)

Yet in 2012, 700 pharmacists from various settings responded to a survey by the ISMP and American Pharmacists Association (APhA), and 44% admitted making errors. Of these, 37% admitted that they *did not report the errors they made*. That shows how underreported prescription errors are and how necessary it is for effective checks and balances systems.

FIGURE 7.2 Patient "Rights" in Prescription Drug Dispensing

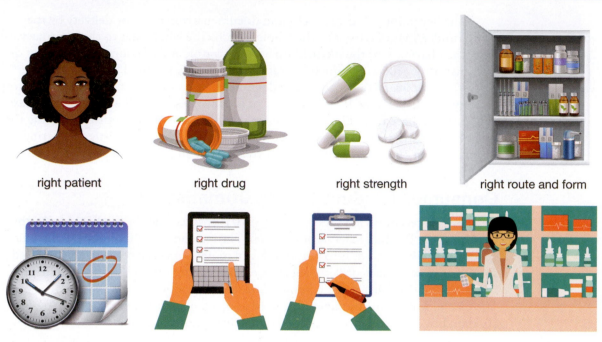

| right patient | right drug | right strength | right route and form |

| right time | right documentation | right education |

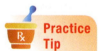

Study Idea

Know the rights of medication safety.

The National Coordinating Council for Medication Error Reporting and Prevention defines a **medication error** as "any preventable event that may cause or lead to inappropriate medication use or patient harm while the medication is in the control of the healthcare professional, patient, or consumer." A medication error often results in an **adverse drug reaction (ADR)**, which is an appreciably harmful or negative consequence to a patient from taking a particular drug. It may be a short-term acute reaction, long-term injury, or even death.

Practice Tip

Technicians need to watch out for medications that look alike (e.g. bupropion/buspirone), or sound alike (e.g., Xanax / Zantac) or both (e.g., guanfacine / guaifenesin).

Failure Modes and Effects Analysis

To try to discover the root causes of medication errors to proactively prevent them, many independent pharmacies, chain and mail-order pharmacies, hospital and other healthcare pharmacies, and compounding facilities are using **failure modes and effects analysis (FMEA)**. Failure modes means the ways in which something can fail, and effects analysis looks at the results or consequences and analyzes prevention techniques. Getting to root causes often entails asking the question, "Why did this happen?" and when an answer is given, asking, "Why did that happen?" to each succeeding answer at least five times. In pharmacy, causes fall into four levels, as seen in Table 7.5.

TABLE 7.5 Categories of Cause Levels and Human Errors

Category	Definition	Examples
Root Causes		
Manufacturing	The drug, administration method, packaging, or educational materials provided.	The packaging for one product looks nearly alike in coloring and branding to another.
Organizational	The rules, policies, or procedures are inadequate or training in them is insufficient. Excessive workload and a culture of fear of not being productive enough or saying something when something seems wrong.	An outdated policy on sterile compounding leads to compromised sterility of an admixture. Technicians and pharmacists too rushed to double-check calculations or selections.
Technical	Equipment is not calibrated or working properly.	The pharmacy's automatic dispensing machine is malfunctioning. A computer glitch mixes a prescription for one patient with another patient's.
Human	An error is caused by an individual not following procedures, missing or ignoring a step, or lacking training.	A technician pulls a bottle of medication from the shelf to fill a prescription from memory and does not read the label. Stores frequently relocate medications.
Prescriber Errors		
Illegible handwriting or misspelled e-script	Questionable information on prescription due to writing or spelling.	Look-alike drug names are highly susceptible to misspellings, especially since prescriptions commonly do not have rationales to guide selection.
Insufficient knowledge of drug for problematic prescription	Prescriber is not aware of special prescribing requirements of a drug.	REMS requirement for drug prior to dispensing.
Use of high-risk abbreviations and measurement notations	Abbreviations that can be misinterpreted.	Writing "u" for units can lead to a tenfold increase in dose.
Dispensing Errors		
Wrong drug error	A drug that was different from the prescribed drug was selected and dispensed.	A look-alike medication or one with a similar name was selected from the shelves or placed into wrong slots in the robotic dispensing machine or automated dispensing cabinet.
Adverse drug error	A DUR warning alert is missed or ignored.	Patient on warfarin is prescribed Bactrim, interaction warning overridden.
Wrong amount/dosage error	The dose given is 5% greater or less than the dose prescribed.	Synthroid 0.025 mg dispensed as Synthtroid 0.25 mg.
Wrong label/mislabeling error	Incorrect data is entered on the label.	Wrong patient profile selected to enter prescription data onto.
Wrong formulation error	Different dosage forms or salt are not interchangeable without a prescriber authorization.	The patient has an order for Ondansetron oral disintegrating tablets but is dispensed oral swallowing tablets.
Documentation error	Essential information is missing or wrong.	Med list in computer is not updated with recent med changes.
Medication education error	Proper education material is not passed on to patient.	Medguide is not dispensed with drug.
Contaminated product error	Medication that is supposed to be removed from stock is still on shelves for dispensing.	Drug recall is not addressed timely.

Causes of Dispensing Errors		
Incomplete information	Policy is not followed on completing the patients medication profile.	Allergies are missing from profile.
Incorrect assumption not checked	Wrong assumptions are made on missing or questionable information.	Wrong drug is selected based on assuming you can read the doctor's questionable writing.
Selection error	On a pull-down menu or shelf, drugs with similar names or labeling are present, and you select the wrong one.	A look-alike or sound-alike drug is selected.
Capture/habit error	Error or inattention and habit cause a wrong selection or calculation.	Used to dispensing the usual adult dosage for a medication, the technician fills the adult dose for a child, and the pharmacist approves without noticing.
Rushed error	Pressures to meet deadlines or quotas cause an error and the double checking is skipped.	You cut corners to decrease time it takes to fill prescription.
Distraction error	Interruptions during critical filling phases cause missed steps or wrong actions.	The phone's ringing, customers are demanding your attention, and you miss a step.
Fear error	Fear of speaking up and bothering the pharmacist or other technician allows medications with suspected errors to be dispensed without double-checking them.	Pharmacist has been angry with you in the past for asking too many questions, so you stop asking for help.
Administration Errors		
Omission error	The prescribed dose is not given/taken.	A patient forgets to take the medication or nurse neglects to administer.
Extra dose(s) error	The patient receives more doses than prescribed.	A nurse gives two tablets but the order is for one; or a patient thinks more is better of another medication and takes an extra dose to get well more quickly.
Wrong dose	The calculations done are incorrect, or the weighing instruments were not calibrated properly.	The dose given is 5% greater or less than the dose prescribed.
Wrong time	The medication is given too early or too long after the intended time of administration.	A patient in the hospital is to receive an intravenous antibiotic at 8 a.m. but does not receive the medication until noon.
Wrong mixture with other drugs and supplements	Patient or nurse do not attend to the accompanying educational warnings.	A patient takes a few drinks of alcohol while on the medication or drinks grapefruit juice while taking statins.

Pharm Facts

FMEA encourages finding problems with the system instead of blaming individuals. Do not point fingers, but help identify why the error happened and how it can be prevented from happening again.

Resources to Fight Medication Errors

In addition to the FDA's MedWatch and VAERS, a number of nonprofit and professional agencies track and/or work to minimize medication errors, including:

- The ISMP tracks, collects, and disseminates information to healthcare personnel regarding safe medication practices using the following tools (among others):

  ~ **Medication Errors Reporting Program (MERP)** is a voluntary medication error reporting program administered by the ISMP. It allows healthcare providers who have made a medication error to self-report anonymously. The confidential information submitted to MERP may be used as part of future case studies and for the education and training of healthcare professionals. It helps ISMP seek out trends and address causes with innovations and guidance. In a study of 26,604 reports, 60% occurred in the dispensing

Web

process—*and pharmacy technicians were involved in nearly 40% of these errors.* Major contributing factors included inexperience, distraction in the workplace, and excessive workload.

~ The ISMP distributes lists of high-alert medications to dispense with great care in different settings: acute care, community and ambulatory healthcare, and long-term care (found here: http://CertExam4e.ParadigmEducation.com/HighAlertMeds). To accompany these lists, the High-Alert Medication Modeling and Error-Reduction Scorecards (HAMMERS) tool was developed to help pharmacies track and improve their policies to reduce errors.

~ ISMP also has assembled a List of Error-Prone Abbreviations, Symbols, and Dose Designations (found here: http://CertExam4e.ParadigmEducation.com/Error-ProneAbbrev). Both are important to study.

~ The ISMP with the FDA has also been fighting against look-alike drug names and labeling. They have established a warning list of drug names that are too close for safety and have recommended **TALL MAN LETTERING**. This style of capped bold lettering calls out the differences between two or more names that are too close, as with bu**PROP**ion and bus**PIR**one., or aceta**ZOLAMIDE** and aceto**HEXAMIDE**. (For the full list, go to: http://CertExam4e.ParadigmEducation.com/TallManLetters.)

• The USP provides safety recommendations throughout the chapters of the *US Pharmacopeia-National Formulary (USP–NF)*. It also makes recommendations to have manufacturers change formulations and packaging, such as revising the labels on Heparin Lock Flush Solution and Heparin Sodium Solution to be bright red with with the warning "HIGH ALERT" on them.

TABLE 7.6 The Joint Commission's Official "Do Not Use" Abbreviation List

Do Not Use	Potential Problem	Use Instead
U, u (unit)	Mistaken for "0" (zero), the number "4" (four), or "cc"	Write "unit"
IU (International Unit)	Mistaken for IV (intravenous) or the number 10 (ten)	Write "International Unit"
Q.D., QD, q.d., qd (daily)	Mistaken for each other	Write "daily"
Q.O.D., QOD, q.o.d, qod (every other day)	Period after the Q mistaken for "I" and the "O" mistaken for "I"	Write "every other day"
Trailing zero (X.0 mg)*	Decimal point missed	Write X mg
Lack of leading zero (.X mg)	Decimal point missed	Write 0.X mg
MS	Can mean morphine sulfate or magnesium sulfate	Write "morphine sulfate"
MSO_4 and $MgSO_4$	Confused for one another	Write "magnesium sulfate"

NOTE: This information applies to all orders and all medication-related documentation that is handwritten (including free-text computer entry) or on preprinted forms.

*Exception: A "trailing zero" may be used only where required to demonstrate the level of precision of the value being reported, such as for laboratory results, imaging studies that report size of lesions, or catheter/tube sizes. It may not be used in medication orders or other medication-related documentation.

- The Joint Commission also publishes a "Do Not Use" list of abbreviations (see Table 7.6) for prescribers in the healthcare facilities that seek to gain or maintain accreditation, and this influences all prescribers (go to http://CertExam4e.ParadigmEducation.com/JointCommission).

Web

- The American Society of Health-System Pharmacists (ASHP) publishes comprehensive guidelines on the prevention of medication errors in hospitals.

ALWAYS TRACE IV LINE
Heparin   Heparin
Heparin   Heparin
⚠ *HIGH ALERT!* ⚠
✓ DOUBLE CHECK ✓

Technology, Automation, and Manufacturing Innovations

As some of the other chapters have noted, some of the biggest innovations in medication safety have arisen from technology and innovation: e-prescriptions (e-script), electronic health records (EHRs) and profiles, drug utilization reviews (DURs) and insurance adjudication, robotic and automated filling and compounding, barcode scanning, barcoded patient wristbands, computerized prescriber order entry (CPOE), and electronic medication administration records (eMARs), to mention the most common. Automated compounding is being used to prepare commonly used, complex IV products such as total parenteral nutrition (TPN).

Studies have shown that these automated systems decrease medication errors; however, healthcare workers need to be aware that technology may create new errors. So technicians must be double-checking the accuracy as they work, doing computer software updating and data storage back up, and maintaining the automation and technology.

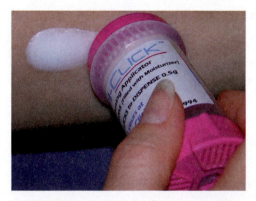

Topi-CLICK is a patented delivery system to accurately dose hormone creams and gels.

Manufacturing Improvements

Besides implementing the recommended tall-man lettering on their labels, manufacturers are often offering improvements in packaging. Unit packaging for hospitals has helped patients get just the right dose per day. The Target brand ClearRx packaging provides different colored container neck rings for different members of a family. The PillPack pharmacy offers all of a nonhospital patient's pills for one day. They come in a roll like a cash register receipt paper roll, and you merely tear off the pillpak for the day. The Topi-CLICK is a patented delivery system to dose compounded hormone creams and gels accurately. These are just examples.

Technician Techniques to Reduce Errors

The pharmacist is ultimately responsible for the accuracy and dispensing of prescriptions, but the pharmacy technician plays an important role in ensuring safety. *The pharmacy technician has a moral and ethical obligation to raise questions to protect patient safety.* It is better to err on the side of caution than make a hasty decision and risk harming or killing a patient.

The work area should be uncluttered and well-lit, and drug stock bottles should be returned to inventory after dispensing. When dealing with look-alike/sound-alike names, the pharmacy should *separate the stock containers in the inventory so that similar-sounding and similar-looking products are not next to each other on the shelf.* Actions must be focused—even while multitasking—to prevent errors. Personal calls or cell phones distract attention and compromise safety. Technicians need to know and follow the policies and procedures manual and state and federal laws and apply them.

Using NDC Numbers and Barcodes for Safety

Technicians should verify all their drug selections with the NDC number and barcode scanning of the stock label. The NDC number plays a crucial role in the prevention of medication errors. For example, if the prescription is for the antibiotic clarithromycin 500 mg but the technician inadvertently selects clarithromycin 500 mg XL and scans the label, the computer will indicate the error. See Figure 7.3 and Table 7.7 for how to find the NDC numbers on the labels and scan the barcodes.

FIGURE 7.3 NDC Numbers and Barcodes

All stock medication labels include a unique, product-specific National Drug Code (NDC) in both numeric and barcode form. The first number set (4–5 digits) identies the manufacturer, the second set (3–4 digits) indicates the product code, and the last set (2 digits) shows the packaging size and type.

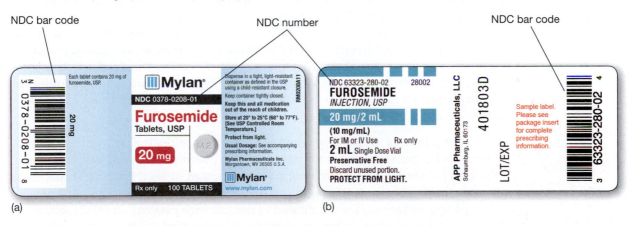

(a)   (b)

TABLE 7.7   Reading NDC Numbers

Manufacturer		Product Code		Packing Size and Type	
NDC	Name	NDC	Product	NDC	Size
(a) 0378	Mylan Pharmaceuticals, Inc	0208	furosemide 20 mg tablet	01	100 tablets
(b) 63323	APP Pharmaceuticals, LLC	280	furosemide injection 20 mg/2mL	02	2 mL vial

NOTE: (a) and (b) refer to labels in Figure 7.3.

Times for Pharmacist Intervention

At what point should a technician filling a prescription or medication order consult the pharmacist? Any time that the technician is unsure, it is better to ask than make a mistake. There are also key points in the processes for verification: after entering the profile and prescription, during the DUR and online adjudication if there are any alerts, after the prescription is filled but before applying the label, as well as any time there is a question.

Drug Utilization Review Issues When alerts arise during the DUR, the technician should consult a pharmacist before proceeding. *A patient's allergy list should be updated every time he or she presents a new prescription because new allergies may have occurred since the last update.* Common allergies to medications include penicillin, sulfa, codeine, and allergies to foods include eggs and nuts. Some pharmaceuticals, including vaccines, are grown in egg cultures and should not be dispensed to patients with egg allergies. The pharmacist will use his or her professional judgment to decide whether to contact the prescriber or fill the prescription.

Adjudication and Prior Authorization Issues Adjudication alerts on similar therapeutic medications and other alerts need to be addressed by the pharmacist. Insurance companies may refuse reimbursement for some high-cost or brand-name medications and recommend therapeutic substitutions. Commonly, this occurs for such medications as proton pump inhibitors, antihyperlipidemic-like statins, antidepressants, and nonsteroidal anti-inflammatory drugs (like naproxen). When prior authorization is required, it is up to the prescribing physician to justify the use of the more expensive drug. The technician or pharmacist will need to contact the prescriber for review and action; the pharmacist may be able to expedite the clarification process by telephone, particularly if a delay would harm the patient (waiting for an antibiotic needed to treat an infection, for example). Often, the prescriber will change to a comparable medication that is covered.

Study Idea

Know the crucial points in the filling and compounding processes when a pharmacist needs to be consulted.

Counseling Issues At the dispensing of each prescription, the technician is bound by law to offer counseling from the pharmacist. A pharmacist should always be consulted if a patient requests counseling on a prescription or OTC product. If specifically asked, the technician may point out the location of an OTC product. In some states, pharmacy technicians are allowed to consult with patients on OTC medications. In other states, technicians are permitted only to read the medication label to the patient and then refer the patient to the pharmacist for more information. Pharmacists are allowed to recommend an OTC product for a self-limited condition. Pharmacists do not diagnose, however, so if the patient is unsure what is wrong, the pharmacist must advise the patient to see a physician.

Patients often have questions at the time they pick up medications or after beginning a medication. The pharmacy technician is permitted to answer questions about the price or what a tablet looks like but should not advise about issues such as missed doses or improper use of a medication. If a patient requests a therapeutic substitution, mentions a use of the medication that is incorrect, or says that a dose has been missed, the pharmacist must be alerted to talk to the patient.

Adverse Drug Reactions If a patient ever reports an adverse drug reaction or event, *the pharmacist must be immediately notified.* Adverse reactions will be assessed by the pharmacist who will determine if the reaction should be added to the patient's profile as an allergy and/or be reported to the MedWatch program.

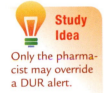
Safety Processes at Every Step

The average prescription may take only 15 minutes to fill. Even so, experienced technicians have built in habits of safety into every step. Simple things are important, such as always doing the barcode scanning or using the leading 0 when inputting into the computer decimals below the value of 1, and not using a zero after whole numbers (also known as "eliminating the trailing zero"). For example, .5 mg is wrong, whereas 0.5 is right; 5.0 is wrong, whereas 5 mg is right. Here is an overview of the types of special attention that needs to be built into every step.

Step 1: Reviewing Profile and Prescription Each element of the profile must be checked (especially allergies), and prescription checked against it. Double-check the patient name (first, middle, and last and spellings), date of birth, and address to make sure the correct patient's profile is being accessed and updated. Are all the ID and contact information present for the prescriber (including DEA number)? Is the prescription complete with the date, the inscription, signa, and prescriber's signature?

Step 2: Inputting and Checking the Drug Information This is where the technician must check the prescription against the computer's drug choices and spellings, available routes of administration and formulations, and the decimals and measurement units. Make sure that you avoid inputting any of the dangerous measurement notations and abbreviations listed by the ISMP or The Joint Commission. Have the pharmacist check the transmitted prescription or what you input with the hard copy and/or profile.

Step 3: Drug Utilization Reviews and Adjudication This is where the screening for allergies, drug-to-drug and/or drug-to-supplement interactions, and formulary issues occurs, and the computer raises red flags. But the technician and pharmacist are also responsible to be on the lookout for any issues having to do with the physical condition of the patient, such as with children, elders, and pregnant or nursing women. See Table 7.8 and the end-of-chapter supplements linked in the eBook.

Step 4: Generating the Prescription Label Recheck the label with the original prescription to make sure everything matches up correctly.

Step 5: Retrieving the Proper Medication Now it is necessary to scan the stock label and verify correct brand/generic, manufacturer, strength, formulation, and route of administration. If automatic dispensing is done, the technician needs to double-check the drug dispensed by the robot or dispensing cabinet.

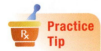
Step 6: Filling or Compounding the Medication Calculations are crucial for verifying at this stage to get the right dosage or compounding measurements and days supply, or compounding calculations. Counting cannot be done with tools or automated equipment that has been used for drugs known to induce allergic reactions, because there is a risk of residue cross-contaminating other drug products.

Step 7: Preparing for Pharmacist Review The medication, prescription, label, notes for calculations and conversions, the computer screen profile, and other pertinent elements must be presented in an organized fashion to facilitate clear review. The proper patient education materials (including MedGuides and potential auxiliary labels) must also be included.

Step 8: Storing Medication Properly The medication must be placed in proper conditions in terms of temperature, lighting, and humidity. It needs to be sufficiently separate from other patients' medications and well organized for easy retrieval.

TABLE 7.8 Drug Utilization Reviews and Special Populations

Information to Check	Resources to Verify Information	Potential Errors Resulting from Failure to Check/Verify Information
Drug Screening: Does the prescribed medication interact with other conditions or medications listed on the profile?	Patient, physician, family member, patient profile, interaction screening program, insurance provider electronic messages, drug information resources (e.g., books, call centers, package inserts, patient information handouts)	Contraindicated drug dispensed; drug–drug or drug–disease interaction occurs
Pediatric Patient Dosing: Are the prescribed dose and frequency of dosing in a pediatric patient consistent with manufacturer recommendations and pharmacy references?	Original prescription, physician, package inserts, electronic database, reference texts, pharmacist experience	Serious overdose (or underdose) leading to side effects, adverse reactions, or treatment failure
Geriatric Patient Dosing: Are the prescribed dose and frequency of dosing in a geriatric patient consistent with manufacturer recommendations and pharmacy references?	Original prescription, physician, package inserts, electronic database, reference texts, pharmacist experience	Serious overdose leading to side effects or adverse reactions
Pregnant (or Potentially Pregnant) and Lactating Patient Dosing: Is the prescribed drug indicated in pregnant women or women of childbearing age? Does the drug pass into the breast milk?	Physician, package inserts, electronic database, reference texts, questions to patient, pharmacist experience	Congenital birth defects, side effects in breast-feeding infants

Study Idea

Identify the times in the filling process that require pharmacist intervention or review.

Step 9: Delivering Medication to Nurse, Patient, or Caregiver Before delivering or filling a unit dose cart, the technician must double-check the patient information to ensure the right patient will receive it. A barcode scan will verify this too. The medications in dispensing cabinets and machines *must be scanned as they are filled into the proper shelves and when they are removed* for administration or dispensing. The patient must be offered counseling and the educational materials. If the patient asks if the medication is right, double-check the prescription. Also, if the look of the medication has changed since the last refill, explain this. If there are more in-depth questions, again, refer them to the pharmacist. The information the patient must know about the medication is listed on Table 7.9.

TABLE 7.9 Information Patients Must Know About Their Medications

1. Brand and generic name
2. The medication's proper appearance
3. The purpose of the medication and the duration of treatment
4. The correct dosage and frequency and the best time or circumstances to take a dose
5. How to proceed if a dose is missed
6. Medications or foods that interact with the prescribed medication
7. Whether the prescription is in addition to or replaces a current medication
8. Common side effects and how to handle them
9. Special precautions necessary for each particular drug therapy
10. Proper storage for the medication

Quality Control and Assurance

Within pharmacies and healthcare facilities medication errors are difficult to track because *there are no national laws requiring the reporting of pharmacy personnel errors.* To encourage more medical and medication error tracking and analysis by pharmacies and healthcare institutions, the federal government passed the 2005 **Patient Safety and Quality Improvement Act (PSQI)**. It encouraged the creation of **Patient Safety Organizations (PSOs)** that can collect confidential information on medical errors to develop systematic changes for safety. Those who report errors are legally protected from being sued or being punished in the workplace by loss of responsibilities, pay, or promotions.

Quality assessments include product integrity and safety (patient and staff members), as well as customer service, productivity, efficiency, and profitability. In addition to safety processes being outlined in a pharmacy's policies and procedures manual, each pharmacy can set up systems to track and rate their success based on these different criteria, and seek ways to improve.

Continuous Quality and Performance Improvement

Continuous quality improvement (CQI) is a process used to evaluate systems and errors. It includes these basic steps:

- Describe the process and the sources of variation from the intended outcome.
- Conduct a team analysis to clarify the source of variation and the extent of problem.
- Discuss alternatives and make decisions on how to reduce variations.
- Implement a plan and measure its effectiveness.

A full discussion of CQI is beyond the scope of this chapter, but it is important to note that it is a team process. The process does not stop with the initial implementation of a plan; it is a continuous process that cycles and is updated as new data becomes available or healthcare rules change. Cooperation is needed at all levels to effectively manage errors and prevent future errors. The failure of a hospital or employer to change work practices in the P&P manual that may cause errors and harm to patients is called organizational failure.

Staff Quality and Safety

The quality of the workforce is an essential component of any high-quality business. To ensure that pharmacies and institutions employ the best qualified people, the human resource department investigates all potential employees' credentials and employment histories. Credentials are the education and licensing requirements to practice your job. As a pharmacy technician, certification will be one of your best credentials.

Advanced Technicians for Safety

Technicians who gain experience and responsibilities are also improving safety. The **tech-check-tech** system, where advanced technicians check the work of less experienced technicians before the pharmacist verifies a medication, has been found to greatly reduce medication errors. Technicians who serve as medication profile specialists or medication reconciliation specialists in hospitals have also reduced many of the errors and omissions that admitting nurses do not have the knowledge base to catch or query.

Employee Safety and Satisfaction

Study Idea

Review the proper technique for hand washing and hand hygiene.

Practice Tip

Safety needles, where the needles retract into the syringe or have attached sheaths, can really help to prevent needle-sticks in staff. All needles and other sharps need to be properly disposed of in a sharps container.

Pharmacies and healthcare institutions must protect the safety of their workers as well as their patients. That is why they follow OSHA regulations and the recommendations of the USP, The Joint Commission, and the CDC. They require hand-washing standards and personal protective gear, sharps disposal containers, medication disposal processes, and hazardous spill kits, They encourage or require annual flu vaccinations, and they implement the CDC's Universal Precautions against the transmission of bloodborne pathogens. (See Table 7.10.)

Besides safety on the job, personal satisfaction is also an important aspect of a career as a pharmacy technician. Job satisfaction is more than about earning a paycheck. Satisfaction comes from doing the best job possible every day. This includes showing commitment to the profession by continuing to improve your skills and knowledge through training and continuing education. Employers often provide avenues of advancement in training, responsibility, position, and compensation to retain their experienced and qualified staff members, putting their skills and expertise to greater use. They also often send out employee satisfaction surveys to better understand the needs of employees that will improve the worksite and hopefully lead to better care of patients and improve their satisfaction.

TABLE 7.10   Universal Precautions for Prevention of Bloodborne Infection Transmission

- Universal Precautions apply to all individuals within the hospital.
- Universal Precautions apply to all contact or potential contact with blood, other bodily fluids, or body substances.
- Disposable gloves must be worn when contact with blood or other bodily fluids is anticipated or possible.
- Hands must be washed thoroughly after removing gloves.
- Blood-soaked or contaminated materials (such as gloves, towels, or bandages) must be disposed of in a wastebasket lined with a plastic bag.
- Properly trained custodial personnel must be called if cleanup or removal of contaminated waste is necessary.
- Contaminated materials (such as needles, syringes, swabs, and catheters) must be placed in red plastic containers labeled for disposal of biohazardous materials. Proper institutional procedures generally involve incineration.
- A first aid kit must be kept on hand in any area in which contact with blood or other bodily fluids is possible. The kit should contain, at minimum, the following items:
    - ~ adhesive bandages for covering small wounds
    - ~ alcohol
    - ~ antiseptic or disinfectant
    - ~ bottle of bleach, which is diluted at the time of use to create a solution containing 1 part bleach to 10 parts water, for use in cleaning up blood spills
    - ~ box of disposable gloves
    - ~ disposable towels
    - ~ medical adhesive tape
    - ~ plastic bag or container for contaminated waste disposal
    - ~ sterile gauze for covering large wounds

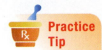

Practice Tip

Healthcare Associated Infections (HAI), also known as nosocomial infections,

Hospital Quality and Patient Satisfaction

Hospital accreditation is a sign of quality healthcare for patients. The Joint Commission places a strong emphasis on patient and personnel safety and in quality healthcare service and products. It sets standards, evaluates facilities against the standards, and monitors progress toward facility and national healthcare goals. It also initiates and supports medication safety efforts, as with the "Do Not Use" pharmacy abbreviation list.

Within the hospital, there are committees working on safety and quality control and assurance. They track medical and medication errors to ensure that root causes are found and processes improve. The Infection Control Committee (ICC) specifically works on preventing inadvertent passing on of infection and disease. It tracks and works to stop patients and staff from acquiring any healthcare associated infections. The hospital staff are trained in standard hygiene, infection controlling protocols, and universal precautions.

How can a healthcare provider or institution know if the patient is happy with the care provided? Many hospital and healthcare institutions use surveys (e.g., Press Ganey) to measure patient satisfaction. Also, hospital pharmacies can survey their "customers," the physicians, surgeons, and nurses who order or administer the drugs. Survey results can identify trends, areas that work well, and areas that need improvement. Institutions can also use survey results to compare their own performance over time, and compare their institution's performance against others. Such analysis can lead to improvements.

In community pharmacies, satisfaction is less likely to be measured by a formal survey. Repeat business is one measure of satisfaction. Patients who return again and again are usually content with the level of service. Magazines and newspapers in many areas can offer another means of assessing consumer satisfaction through annual "Best of" contests and surveys. These offer positive reinforcement that the institution is satisfying its clientele.

Quality assurance is an ongoing activity, and one in which the pharmacy technician has an important role to play. Only by identifying areas of weakness can pharmacy professionals and the institutions they serve become better at serving patients safely and protecting workers.

STUDY SUMMARY

Medication safety and the quality assurance programs established in healthcare are integral to containing costs and protecting patients. Pharmacy technicians need to be aware of the work being done by the FDA, ISMP, and various other organizations to protect the safety of both patients and employees.

As a technician studying for certification, you need to be always watchful for potential errors and how to prevent them. Understand the importance of the NDC, barcodes, sound-alike/look-alike lists, high-risk/high-alert medications, and policies and procedures used to correctly select medications and fill prescriptions. Know strategies you can employ to prevent filling errors. Be aware of the importance of having your work double-checked by a pharmacist and knowing when you should ask for help. Understand the importance of quality assurance and performance improvement strategies to ensure patient safety and satisfaction.

ADDITIONAL RESOURCES

For more in-depth explanations, check out *Pharmacy Practice for Technicians*, 6e from Paradigm Education Solutions. To master and extend the material presented in this chapter, take advantage of the resources available through the eBook resources links. These include digital supplements, study resources, and a practice exam generator with 1,000+ exam-style questions. End-of-chapter tests are accessible through the eBook for individuals using the self-study course and through Navigator+ for individuals enrolled in the instructor-guided course.

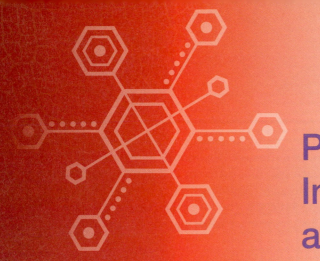

8

Pharmacy Information Systems and Automation

Learning Objectives

1. Understand the use of database management systems in both community and institutional pharmacies as they relate to prescription or medication order processing.

2. Know the importance of interoperability of pharmacy systems as they relate to online adjudication, DURs, and e-prescribing.

3. Identify the various components used in informatics, including input devices, output devices, hardware, and software.

4. Understand how the various software programs with software technologies help decrease errors, maintain patient health records, process claims, and provide reports of safety and productivity.

5. Know the importance of maintaining and updating patient profiles.

6. Discuss the advantages of information technologies, such as e-prescribing, medication dispensing robots and cabinets, telepharmacy, kiosks, automated compounding devices, and online adjudication.

7. Understand the many uses of barcode technology in medication dispensing and administration.

8. Understand the functionality and maintenance of the POS cash register.

9. Describe the uses of automation for sterile and hazardous compounding.

Access eBook links for resources and an exam generator, with 1,000+ questions.

Safe, effective, and efficient pharmacy practice depends upon electronic information technologies and their interconnected communication highways. That is why 10% of the PTCE, categorized as domain 9, is related to the technological applications in pharmacy, including electronic medical and health records, data storage and manipulation of records, software documentation for drug diversion, error tracking, inventory reports, and medication therapy resources and monitoring, and more. The ExCPT has information systems and automation questions woven throughout its topical areas.

Pharmacy Computer Basics

The pharmacy technician needs to gain a working knowledge of how to use pharmacy-specific software programs and automation through labs, simulations, externships, and on-the-job training. Exact use of each system is different and part of your orientation at a new pharmacy technician job. Because technology is key to every aspect of the technician's responsibilities, some technicians who love pharmacy practice and information technology are specializing in pharmacy **informatics**, or pharmacy software application, storage, and retrieval.

Pharmacy Software Interoperability

To process prescriptions and accomplish the other pharmacy functions, almost all community and institutional pharmacies are now equipped with specially designed pharmacy **database management systems (DBMSs)**. These are pharmacy-oriented computerized information systems with software that integrates and interfaces (communicates) with the many different software programs and databases needed for various pharmacy operations and online transmissions and networking. Some examples of pharmacy software management systems include Rx-1, Rx30 Pharmacy System, SRS Pharmacy Systems, Pioneer Rx, ScriptPro Central Pharmacy Management System, and Prodigy's PROscript 2000.

The ability to exchange and process information between various internal and external databases, software, and technology is called **interoperability**. It enables different pharmacy functions and out-of-pharmacy stakeholders (like the prescriber and insurance representatives) to work together for the best care of the patient. Interoperability also provides the most economical and time efficient pharmacy practices in both community pharmacies and institutions.

Usually the DBMS software is menu-driven or Windows-based, allowing the technician to choose fields or functions easily from a menu of options on the screen by typing a single keystroke or function key on the keyboard. The fields of information can be sorted or queried using the patient's name, address, phone number, and date of birth; the prescription's number, drug name, National Drug Code (NDC) number, dosage and quantity of the drug, and number of refills; and the prescriber's name, address, phone number, and DEA number. Having these different fields of input information allows the software to sort and retrieve many different types of information for reports, audits, and work lists. *Errors in data entry will affect all processing connected through the database interfaces.*

Having the patient's history of medication, allergies, drug interactions, and pertinent elements of medical history allows the software to run comparisons with the external medical science database called the **clinical decision support system (CDSS)** for the drug utilization review (DUR). With this informational cross-checking, the DUR provides automatic warnings about possible drug interactions with other drugs (drug-drug), potential allergic reactions to the drug (drug-allergy), drug interference with illnesses or medical conditions based on patient diagnosis (drug-disease), and drug reactions due to food or alcohol consumption (drug-food). **Therapeutic drug duplications** are also identified during the DUR and insurance adjudication to prevent a patient being dispensed multiple drugs for the same diagnosis (**polypharmacy**). Most software applications even provide a picture or description of the prescribed medication to prevent errors. The pharmacy software for hospitals and other institutions must provide the DUR in addition to **intravenous compatibility data** for compounding sterile products.

Up-to-date pharmacy software programs and DBMSs interface with e-prescribing, barcode scanning technology, laboratory data reporting, computerized physician orders, and electronic record systems. The DBMS also interfaces with medical databases for medical and pharmacy literature searches, pharmacy benefits management databases and government insurance programs for claims adjudication, and the DEA databases for compliance with drug enforcement regulations.

Prescribers depend upon this interoperability within their clinics and hospital networks for medical information and to transmit e-prescriptions. (See Figure 8.1 for an example of DBMS interoperability in e-prescribing.) Most of the pharmacy database systems also are capable of tracking expenses; generating profit and loss statements, productivity and inventory reports; controlled substance and restricted drug sales logs; and performing special dosing calculations, among many other functions.

FIGURE 8.1 Interoperability and E-Prescription Flow

This diagram shows the direct pathway of information from and back to the patient (1, 2, 3), as well as the supportive resources and systems supplying and exchanging information.

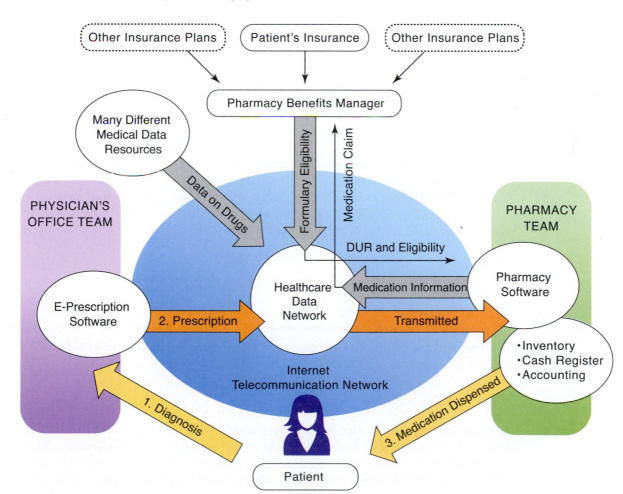

These interoperability functions are growing with the push for universal **electronic health records (EHRs)**. An EHR is a record that encompasses all of a patient's care information in one data file that can be shared among appropriate healthcare professionals and facilities.

Besides being familiar with the pharmacy software or operating system, the technician should be knowledgeable of the hardware used in the pharmacy. Hardware is the actual equipment that the software application is used on. The **processor** is the "brain" of the workstation. Computer input devices include the keyboard, mouse, trackball, microphone for voice recognition, touch screen, and light pen. Computer output devices are the display or monitor, speakers, and printer.

Because of computer integration, computer availability for technicians affects workload and efficiency. Some computers are **smart terminals** that are microcomputers or personal computers (PCs) with their own storage and processing capabilities. Others are **dumb terminals**, which are computer devices with a monitor and keyboard that do not contain storage and processing capabilities.

Some chain pharmacies have a terminal dedicated for each pharmacist and pharmacy technician. In independent pharmacies, both pharmacists and technicians may be working at one or more computers throughout the pharmacy during a shift. Technicians sign on with their usernames and passwords for each computer they will be working on; pharmacists do likewise. After completing a shift or leaving the terminal, each technician must log out. The log in and out function provides a means for confidentiality and securing the sensitive patient data contained on the pharmacy computer. Confidentiality and security are required by the Health Insurance Portability and Accountability Act (HIPAA). This function also provides accountability for the user, allowing for all the data entered and computer access during a shift to be tracked and attributed to a person or device.

The dumb terminal is connected via a **local area network (LAN)** to a remote computer that stores and processes the data. Remote computers are often **mainframe computers** at the main pharmacy or company headquarters, or **minicomputers** (smaller scale mainframes). This computer communication involves the transmission of data signals through modems and cables or the air via wireless transmitters, receivers, and satellites. *The DBMS needs regular and nightly storage backups, on-site or at a remote site or Internet cloud location. There should always be a monthly or regular backup that provides an extra off-site location for data storage in case of a natural disaster.*

Community Practice Information Technology and Automation

Electronic information software programs and interconnected automation systems have been designed uniquely for community pharmacy practice.

E-Prescribing

An **e-prescription**, or e-script, allows a prescriber to transmit a patient's prescription directly to the pharmacy computer. It is important for pharmacy technicians to know the state and federal laws and regulations that pertain to electronic prescribing. In addition, the federal Drug Enforcement Administration regulates e-prescriptions for controlled substances (discussed in Chapter 3), and individual states may have additional rules. **SCRIPT standards**, established by **National Council for Prescription Drug Programs (NCPDP)**, are followed for electronic transmission of medical prescriptions. SCRIPT standardizes the formatting protocols of the electronic transfer of prescription and medical history data between pharmacies, prescribers, and other entities. The NCPDP and the pharmacy industry are responsible for developing real-time claims adjustment, eligibility and benefit verification, e-prescribing, and medical history sharing.

Physicians generally submit e-prescriptions to the pharmacy while documenting the information in the **electronic medical record (EMR)**, which is the digital version of the traditional paper chart at a single facility. This is a time-saver for physicians. E-prescriptions also reduce prescription forgery and medication errors stemming from a physician's hard-to-read handwriting. The e-prescription capability saves time within the pharmacy by reducing time spent talking on the phone and entering information from written prescriptions, and it reduces wait time for patients. In many cases, a prescription can be ready before the patient arrives at the pharmacy.

For hard copy prescriptions, the technician or pharmacist must enter the information into the proper fields in the pharmacy computer and then scan the prescription into the patient profile database for a visual record.

Prescription Processing

Within the pharmacy, the DBMS supports many different software programs and functions during the prescription filling and dispensing processes. The pharmacy technician should be knowledgeable about how to manipulate the necessary components of the patient profile, handle overrides for DUR, deal with claims handling, select drugs, and track restricted drugs.

Patient Profile

The patient profile database includes fields for patient demographics, insurance, medications, supplements, and allergy information. Changes can be easily made to any of these fields, new prescriptions entered, and medication labels printed. It reminds technicians about HIPAA forms that need updating and store the forms so technicians can quickly find out who they are legally able to have pick up prescriptions and share prescription information for each patient.

Medication Therapy Management Tracking

The pharmacy software also assists in tracking medication use, compliance, complications, and prescription modifications for medication therapy management (MTM). The technician can use the software to assemble patient reports to provide the pharmacist with the information needed for proper patient MTM recommendations and follow-up instructions.

Drug Utilization Review

As noted, the drug utilization review (DUR) draws from a database of drug manufacturer, medical, and pharmaceutical information sources to automatically alert pharmacy staff of duplicate therapeutic prescriptions and any potential adverse drug reactions due to drug-drug, drug-allergy, drug-diagnosis, and drug-food interactions. For example, if a patient has an existing prescription for nitroglycerin 0.4 mg

FIGURE 8.2 E-Prescription

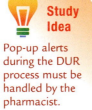

sublingual and brings in a new prescription for Viagra 25 mg oral tablets, the computerized DUR will alert the technician to a potential drug interaction, as seen in Figure 8.2. It also shows the patient's allergies for codeine and sulfa drugs.

Pharmacy technicians receiving any DUR warning *should not continue further with filling the prescription but instead alert the pharmacist*. The pharmacist will decide upon the course of action and may contact the physician. The pharmacy technician will notify the patient that the prescription is taking longer to fill than anticipated, and the pharmacist will be out to talk to them.

Study Idea

Pop-up alerts during the DUR process must be handled by the pharmacist.

Online Third-Party Claims Adjudication

Study Idea

Online real-time adjudication is important to the financial bottom line of a pharmacy.

The pharmacy software connects with the databases of the pharmacy benefits managers (PBMs) for the patient's insurance company. It allows the pharmacy's computer to submit a prescription claim directly to the insurer's PBM and receive a rapid response—real-time **claims adjudication**—often in less than 30 seconds. The response includes the amount the pharmacy should charge the patient for a medication and the amount the pharmacy will be reimbursed. It alerts the pharmacy if the medication is not covered by the insurer or if the patient needs to meet a deductible before payment is available. The PBM can also notify the pharmacy if the patient has filled the prescription at another pharmacy or has a prescription at another pharmacy that may cause an adverse drug interaction. Chapter 10 on billing and claims covers the information a technician must correctly enter into the system, issues resolutions, chargebacks, and audits.

For patients who have more than one type of prescription coverage, online adjudication also makes it possible for the pharmacy to bill the primary insurer first and then bill the unpaid balance to the secondary insurer. This is referred to as **coordination of benefits**, which will be explained more in Chapter 10.

Study Idea

Durable medical equipment billing requires ICD-10 diagnostic codes.

Medical Coding and Terminology For proper PBM adjudication for some medical devices, Medicare B and some insurance companies require medical diagnosis coding, or ICD-10, which went in to effect October 1, 2015. **ICD-10** stands for International Classification of Diseases, Tenth Edition. It is a system used by the healthcare industry to classify and code all diagnoses, symptoms, and procedures recorded in connection with healthcare. Technicians do not need to know how to code but need to know how to get the common codes for adjudication of durable medical equipment (DME), which also requires a certificate of medical necessity from the medical provider.

The Pharmacist Services Technical Advisory Coalition was established to improve the coding infrastructure necessary to support pharmacy billing. Coalition activities include updating electronic data interchange standards, modifying coding structures, and supporting provider identifiers.

Drug Selection and Filling

Computer software allows pharmacy technicians to prepare prescriptions, freeing up time for the pharmacist who needs only to perform a final check. Most of the information the pharmacist needs for final verification of a prescription is available on the computer, including an image of the tablet or capsule, the national drug code, an image of the prescription, and drug utilization review information. This leaves the pharmacist more time for patient counseling, MTM, vaccinations, and other patient care services.

Study Idea

Barcode scanning prevents selection errors when retrieving the drug to fill a prescription.

As explained, technicians use the NDC barcode scanning programs to select and verify the correct medication from stock. The system can automatically deduct the amount of medication taken from the stock in the inventory management system to keep it up-to-date in real time. Reports on prescription drug usage are a valuable asset to pharmacy management for ordering and inventory requirements.

Restricted Drug Documentation

Study Idea

Study what is required to sell pseudoephedrine to a customer.

Pharmacy software alerts remind technicians to do the proper legal documentation on controlled substances and restricted products like pseudoephedrine/ephedrine. It provides the sales logging software and electronic storage needed to meet the legal documentation outlined in Chapter 3. Pharmacy inventory management software works with the DBMS during ordering, receiving, posting, tracking, theft/loss and disposal reporting, and auditing for prescription medications, controlled substances, OTC medications and supplements, and other inventory stock. Controlled substance fill reports should be run by the technician at the end of business day for the pharmacist to review and sign.

Pharmacy Robotics and Automated Filling in the Community Pharmacy

Study Idea

Remember never to use automated pill counting machines for any drug substance known to be a common allergen, such as a penicillin-based antibiotic.

Medication dispensing machines are often used to count and fill prescriptions in busy pharmacies. The robot uses barcode scanning to identify and select drug products. The pharmacy technician is responsible for making sure all pharmaceuticals have barcodes and are loaded in the correct location in the robot. Attention to detail is important to ensure accuracy. Reports can be run on the amounts and types of medications dispensed automatically and the time each dispensing task took.

Pill counting machines count tablets or capsules as they are propelled through a beam of light. The technician should make sure the machine is cleaned regularly. Automated pill counting machines *should never be used to count penicillin, sulfonamide, or codeine products because cross-contamination with other products could be life threatening for a patient who has medication allergies.*

As healthcare needs increase, other forms of technology are being used in pharmacy to bring the pharmacist to the patient. **Telepharmacy** technology brings pharmacy care to the patient via videoconferencing for real-time counseling. **New drug dispensing kiosks**, such as Walgreens' MedAvail MedCenter, allow patients to step up to an automated prescription kiosk with their prescription, connect with a pharmacist and, in ten minutes, walk away with a filled prescription. Kiosks are changing pharmacy for underserved areas just as ATMs have done for banking, providing service at easy-to-reach locations and at the time the patient needs the prescription. Pharmacy technicians may find themselves sent out to fill and service the kiosks.

Point-of-Sale Cash Register, Sales, and Inventory Reports

Study Idea

Maintenance of the cash register includes replacing the receipt paper, replacing the ink cartridge, and running end-of day-reports.

Pharmacy database management systems can also be aligned or interactive with the pharmacy's cash registers and credit processing. The point-of-sale (POS) cash registers have buttons denoting Rx (nontaxable prescription items) and other retail sales (taxable). Keeping sales in the correct categories is essential to the accounting tasks of the pharmacy and technicians. By using barcode scanning at the register, a new prescription fill can be flagged to alert the technician to stop the sale and call the pharmacist over to counsel the patient.

Technicians often run end-of-shift or end-of-day reports. The cash remaining in the register along with the credit, debit, gift, and flex card receipts must be totaled and **reconciled**, or matched, with the reports to find any discrepancies and resolve them. Then these totals must be added to those of other registers to find the full amount of business for the day. The complete total will be checked against the total of the purchase prices of the prescriptions filled and merchandise sold according to the barcode scanners, minus the insurance reimbursements expected.

Sales and reimbursement reconciliation is complicated, but automation does a great deal of the work. The barcode scanning technology works in concert with the POS cash register. A POS cash register provides the advantage of automatically reordering inventory at the end of each day. The retail software systems can process average wholesale price, sales markups, discounts, and profit margins. Ordering and inventory software is also connected to the other software systems so they can communicate together.

In larger pharmacies with multiple technicians, it is not uncommon for each technician to have a sign-on and password code to enter when starting the shift on a certain register, just as with the computer terminals. This allows a tracking of sales transactions and reconciling the receipts at the end of the day or shift. A technician can then be held accountable for all customer receipts at his or her register during the shift. It is common to be off a few cents or dollars once in a while, but frequent or large discrepancies are brought to the attention of the pharmacist. Major cash discrepancies during a technician's shift, especially if there is a pattern of such discrepancies, will require explanation and should be discussed privately. Surveillance cameras protect the pharmacy from money loss or drug diversion by staff or customers.

Study
Idea

In the community pharmacy, productivity and profit must be balanced with safety and accuracy, with the emphasis on the latter two.

Safety and Productivity Reports

DBMS and pharmacy informatics can also generate a pharmacy's safety and productivity reports. The safety reports, however, can only be generated if the pharmacy has put in place an electronic system for logging errors. Reports can then be run on the type of errors, timing, or situation, and DUR alert overrides, depending on what information fields are input into the tracking system.

Productivity reports are generated by the software totaling the prescription filling and sales done by each staff member working that shift. The productivity reports compare staff time to prescriptions filled and other income-generating activities. The pharmacy can also use these reports to determine the amount of staff needed for which shifts and duties to optimize staff to patient/consumer ratios. These reports can be formatted in different ways, such as by individual or group staff hours versus prescriptions generated, or by individual or group hours versus sales income and reimbursements.

The productivity reports then need to be compared to safety reports for the same time periods. Do safety errors go up as productivity or swiftness of prescription filling goes up? Does customer satisfaction go up as productivity goes up (and perhaps waiting times decrease), or does it go down because fewer people are expected to do more, and waiting times actually increase along with less personal attention to each customer? For a community pharmacy to do well, it must have safety first and customer satisfaction emphasized while being productive to make income. Experienced technicians can help establish and run needed reports, and also design customer satisfaction surveys and safety tracking mechanisms.

Institutional Pharmacy Information Technology and Automation

Hospital pharmacy also have DBMSs, and they align the medication orders with the patients, electronic health records, and hospital billing, automated inventory counts and pharmacy ordering, and documentation. Within hospitals and other healthcare institutions, the software coordinates the centralized functions (within the pharmacy) and decentralized pharmacy-related activities (outside the pharmacy), including in the nursing units, in billing and accounts receivable, in inventory management and purchasing, and in quality control.

Study
Idea

Barcode scanning during medication administration requires all medications to have a barcode, either from the manufacturer or assigned by the pharmacy technician and attached to the packaging.

Electronic Records, Orders, and Administration Tracking

Hospitals are moving to be fully computerized systems from admission to discharge. At admission, an electronic medical record is initiated (or accessed from a former visit) for each patient, and aligned with it, the patient is given a barcode ID wrist band with a unique patient identifier—a personal number code.

Hospital prescribers transmit medication orders to the pharmacy through computerized physician order entries (CPOEs) from computer terminals, laptops, or from the room or cart computers. Pharmacists and technicians check the orders and run the DURs. Technicians then use the orders to print work lists to fill the medication carts and automatic dispensing cabinets, or compound the products.

Nurses who administer the medications scan both the medication and the patient's wrist band, and these must align with information on the medication order to fill in the electronic medication administration record (eMAR).

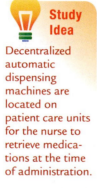

Study Idea

Centralized automated dispensing systems help manage the inventory in the pharmacy.

Study Idea

Decentralized automatic dispensing machines are located on patient care units for the nurse to retrieve medications at the time of administration.

Study Idea

Review the sterile compounding chapter for guidelines on safe compounding of sterile products, with and without an ACD.

Hospital Dispensing Robots and Automated Dispensing

Since most hospital medications are dispensed in unit-dose packaging, if the manufacturer does not supply the product in a single-dosage package, the technician must repackage the medication and label the dose with the drug name, strength, lot number, expiration date, beyond-use date, and barcode. (Technicians must also do this for home meds, brought in by the patient for continued use while in the hospital.) Software programs, such as the WaspLabeler, print sheets of the unit-dose labels with barcodes for the repackaging of medications.

In high-volume institutions, the repackaging is done by pharmacy robots, and the cart filling is also done by the robots. Technicians must oversee and check the work, filling the robotic stations with medications in the proper places using barcode scanning. Then the pharmacists verify their work. These types of automated dispensing machines are called **centralized automated dispensing systems**.

Nursing stations are equipped with automated dispensing cabinets, such as Omnicell and Pyxis. They are known as **decentralized automated dispensing systems**. Nurses can withdraw medications based on the eMAR if the dispensing system is connected to the medication order. These automated medication storage units provide a secure, accurate, and efficient means of dispensing and tracking patient medications. The dispensing cabinets need to be programmed with minimum stock levels for each drug triggering fill lists for refilling. As the technicians fill the units, they scan the barcodes of the dispensing drawers and the medications they place within them so they match up. Besides saving technician time, these medication storage units provide diversion prevention, improve inventory control, reduce costs, increase compliance protocols, monitor for violations, and help eliminate mistakes. Decentralized automated dispensing systems have replaced the filling of medication carts with individualized patient drawers in many hospitals and nursing homes.

Some larger hospitals also use a pneumatic system to deliver medications to the floor, usually for stat doses. Some companies are developing motorized robots to deliver medication to patient care units.

Sterile Compounding Automation and Administration

Technology is helping to prepare compounded products in the hospital pharmacy. The pharmacy software is able to track the ingredients, compounded products, and patients as necessitated by the Drug Quality and Security Act (DSQA).

Automated compound devices (ACDs) are used to compound injectable pharmaceuticals, especially in large medical centers that produce a high volume of total nutrition parenteral medications. ACDs improve efficiency and reduce labor costs. The machines are programmed to reliably add electrolytes or additives to many different batches, reducing the potential for medication errors and contamination. The automation interfaces with the pharmacy software to ensure that USP Chapter <797> guidelines are followed, so that ACD records are accurately maintained. Pharmacy technicians must know how to program and calibrate the ACDs for accuracy and the documentation required.

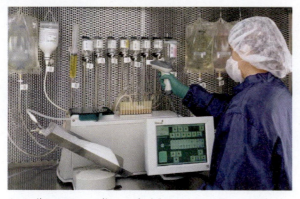

A sterile compounding technician uses an Exacta-Mix 2400 from Baxa, which is an automated compounding device that allows up to 24 ingredients to be inserted in total parenteral nutrition bags, producing a sterile 3 L bag in about four minutes.

Hazardous Infusion Compounding, Administration, and Disposal

As noted in Chapter 6, hazardous compounding adds additional responsibilities on the technician in terms of safety, protection, and documentation. Automated compounding of hazardous substances for chemotherapy helps protect the compounding technician and the patient from compounding errors. The Occupational Safety and Health Administration (OSHA) requires the documentation of worker health assessments and monitoring, worker training and protection, ingredient registration and safety data sheets, and disposal procedures and tracking. The hazardous compounding software has programs designed for these uses, data storage, and report generation. These programs interface with the other pharmacy functions.

Pharm Facts

When patients are allowed to control the rate of administration of analgesics, they tend to have lower narcotic usage during recovery.

Smart Pumps and Patient Controlled Analgesia Pumps

Once the IVs are delivered to the nursing unit, infusion pumps are used to guarantee that the correct volume of a parenteral is administered to the patient. The nurse attaches an in-line filter on the tubing and the pump, and then programs in the correct infusion flow rates and the medication is ready for administration.

A new approach to sterile drug delivery is through **patient-controlled analgesia (PCA) devices**—or patient controlled system (PCS)—which allow the patient to have greater power in managing the rate of drug administration, especially for pain medications. One example is intravenous admixtures of pain medications that come stored in medication reservoir cassettes, such as the CADD-Prizm PCS II. Experienced sterile compounding technicians may fill these cassettes with narcotic solutions, such as meperidine, morphine, fentanyl, or dihydromorphone. (Some drug manufacturers offer prefilled medication cassettes.) Technicians must remember to dispense the special IV tubing to the nurse to accompany the PCA device.

Another new sterile delivery device is a small, solution-filled sterile plastic ball attached to a sterile catheter line that is sewn into a surgery site. The ball, such as the ON-Q Fixed Flow Rate Pump, slowly deflates, administering the pain medication as the patient heals. Sterile compounding technicians are now filling these balls with the medications ordered for the patients' specific needs.

Technology and automation in the pharmacy allow the staff to work smarter with safer outcomes for patients. Pharmacy technicians must become the experts on the use, calibration, checking, maintenance, and repair of these tools and be willing to learn new skills as advances are made. That is why the certification exams test to see if pharmacy technicians are up-to-date and ready to utilize these tools effectively in practice.

STUDY SUMMARY

The pharmacy technician must be able to work with the technology used in today's pharmacies. For the exam, the pharmacy technician should:

- Be knowledgeable about computer basics.

- Be familiar with the terminology used to describe the various hardware and software and the importance of interoperability to the sharing of healthcare information.

- Understand how the drug utilization review works in terms of data information sharing and how software assists in medication therapy management.

- Be familiar with the various types of automation used in community and institutional pharmacies.

- Describe how technology improves patient care and decreases medication errors.

- Understand the necessity of the various reports that will be generated by the pharmacy software and how they are used in pharmacy to better care for the patient and save healthcare dollars.

- Be aware of the national organizations that have helped establish pharmacy coding infrastructure and standards for pharmacy electronic transmission of health-related information.

ADDITIONAL RESOURCES

For more in-depth explanations, check out *Pharmacy Labs for Technicians*, 3e from Paradigm Education Solutions. To master and extend the material presented in this chapter, take advantage of the resources available through the eBook resources links. These include digital supplements, study resources, and a practice exam generator with 1,000+ exam-style questions. End-of-chapter tests are accessible through the eBook for individuals using the self-study course and through Navigator+ for individuals enrolled in the instructor-guided course.

9

Pharmacy Inventory Management

Learning Objectives

1 Identify components in profitable inventory management, including the differences in AWP and acquisition costs, markup, and profit.

2 Understand the different systems of reordering: PAR versus maximum/minimum levels.

3 Discuss the advantages and disadvantages of a formulary.

4 Become familiar with purchasing concepts.

5 Understand the receiving process and the DQSA requirements in it.

6 Explain stock rotation using expiration dates.

7 Discuss storage requirements for refrigerated and frozen products, and look-alike packages.

8 Discuss beyond-use dates for insulin.

9 Identify product removal requirements related to overstock, outdated drugs, and medications returned by patients.

10 Understand the handling of controlled substances, including the special DEA forms for purchasing, recording diversions, and documenting destruction.

11 Calculate inventory turnover rates and how these calculations relate to good inventory management.

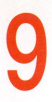 Access eBook links for resources and an exam generator, with 1,000+ questions.

One of the responsibilities of a pharmacy technician is inventory management. Drug inventory is one of the pharmacy's largest investments, and a busy retail pharmacy may have $400,000 or more in inventory on the shelves. Proper ordering, receiving, posting, pricing, documenting, rotating, and other ways of managing pharmaceutical and over-the-counter inventory are important to the pharmacy's bottom line. The pharmacy needs to keep sufficient drug stocks on hand to meet customer needs while minimizing costs, including the cost of stock sitting on the shelves and waste generated from expiring pharmaceuticals. At the same time, insufficient inventory can cost a community pharmacy individual and future sales if the pharmacy is not able to fill customers' prescriptions. In an institutional pharmacy, stock shortages may force the pharmacy to purchase products at higher prices.

The pharmacy technician is often responsible for ordering and receiving medications, durable medical equipment, and over-the-counter (OTC) products. Knowledge of inventory management, purchasing, and receiving is so important that it takes up domain 7 in the PTCE and is included in topic area 1 of the ExCPT.

Inventory Accounting

A community pharmacy operates under the same principles as any other business—it must make a **profit** to survive. In other words, it must have more income than expenses to continue to provide services.

A **profit and loss statement**, or report, is the financial statement that summarizes the revenues, costs, and expenses incurred for a specific period of time.

Study Idea

AWP is the highest price or upper limit of what a pharmacy would pay to buy a drug from a wholesaler. Acquisition cost is what the pharmacy actually pays for the drug.

Acquisition Costs versus Pharmacy Reimbursements

Like all businesses, pharmacies purchase their products from a wholesaler or supplier at a generally lower-than-retail price called the **acquisition cost**.

In contrast, the **average wholesale price (AWP)** of a drug is the benchmark price or "sticker price" that wholesalers list for each drug, dose, and package size. There is a difference between the AWP and the actual acquisition cost because the AWP does not include the discounts pharmacies receive for volume purchasing, prompt payment, or rebates from manufacturers for brand name drugs.

Estimating Third-Party Reimbursements

Usually, the insurance companies and other third parties reimburse pharmacies at a brand drug's AWP minus the third-party discount agreed upon in a negotiated contract, plus a pharmacy dispensing fee (in the range of $2.50 to $4.00 per prescription). The dispensing fee is for the services rendered with the drug, and it is supposed to cover the pharmacy's personnel costs.

Insurance companies and their pharmacy benefits managers (PBMs) calculate a prescription reimbursement price to the pharmacy with the following formula:

AWP × reimbursement percentage rate + dispensing fee = reimbursement amount

To maximize the pharmacy's income, it is essential to purchase a stock quantity from a wholesaler at less than AWP to make up for low reimbursement percentages. Consider Examples 9.1 and 9.2.

Example 9.1

You receive a prescription for 30 tablets of a cholesterol-lowering drug. The drug comes in a stock bottle that contains 90 tablets. The AWP for the bottle is $300. The insurance PBM has contracted with the pharmacy to pay the AWP less 4% (converted to 0.04) plus a $6.00 dispensing fee. What is the reimbursement fee the pharmacy will receive?

$$\frac{X\$}{30\,tab} = \frac{\$300}{90} = 100 - 4\% + \$6.00 = 102$$

Step 1 Begin by calculating the AWP for 30 tablets with dimensional analysis:

$$y = \frac{\$300}{90 \text{ tabs}} \times 30 \text{ tabs}; \quad y = \frac{\$900}{9}; \quad y = \$100$$

Step 2 Calculate the discount:

$$\$100 \times 0.04 = \$4.00$$

Step 3 Calculate the amount of reimbursement (AWP − 4% + $6.00):

$$\$100.00 - \$4.00 + \$6.00 = \$102.00$$

Example 9.2

Now it is important to be able to determine the potential gross profit when considering a product purchase. Calculate the pharmacy's gross profit if the pharmacy has contracted with the supplier to pay AWP minus 5%.

Step 1 Calculate the discount amount on the entire bottle (*AWP × discount % = discount*):

$$\$300.00 \times 0.05 = \$15.00$$

Step 2 Calculate the acquisition cost of the stock bottle of 90 tablets (AWP − discount amount = acquisition cost):

$$\$300.00 - \$15.00 = \$285.00$$

Step 3 Determine the cost of the prescribed quantity (30 tablets).

$$y = \frac{\$285}{90 \text{ tabs}} \times 30 \text{ tabs}; \quad y = \frac{\$855}{9}; \quad y = \$95.00$$

Step 4: Find the gross profit by subtracting the acquisition cost from the reimbursement (use the reimbursement of $102 from Example 9.1).

$$\$102.00 - \$95.00 = \$7.00$$

As you can see, the lower the pharmacy's acquisition cost, the more money there will be to cover operating costs and, hopefully, generate a profit.

Markup and Profits

Pharmacies also buy their nonprescription products from wholesalers and sell them at higher prices. The pricing of nonprescription items is primarily determined by competition in the marketplace and customer expectations.

The difference between the store acquisition cost and customer price is called the **markup**. It is determined by the pharmacy and used in the following formulas:

pharmacy acquisition cost + markup = retail selling price

retail selling price − acquisition cost = markup

The accumulation of profit from the retail sales, patient pharmaceutical sales, and third-party reimbursements add up to the business's **gross profit**. The gross profit must cover the **overhead**, or operating costs, including personnel and benefits, facility costs, technology, utilities, marketing, and other expenses. What is left after all the expenses are paid is the **net profit**. A **loss**, or negative profit, occurs when the total of the customer prices with claims reimbursement is lower than the total of the acquisition prices plus overhead. Having the right retail markup can help balance the bottom line toward profitability. Too high a markup drives customers away. Too low a markup means the pharmacy cannot meet its expenses and make enough profit to stay in business.

Each independent pharmacy or chain determines the percentage of each sale that must go toward the operation costs and profit. This percentage is called the **markup percentage**. To determine the exact **markup amount** to charge per item, whether prescription or retail, you start with the acquisition cost from the wholesaler (supplier price) and multiply it by the pharmacy's markup percentage. (Pharmacies may set different retail markup percentages than prescription drug markup percentages.)

To calculate this markup amount, turn the markup percentage into a decimal by dividing it by 100, which is your **markup rate**. Then multiply the acquisition cost of the item by that rate. Add that markup amount to the acquisition cost to get the customer price. The formula steps are as follows:

$$markup\ \% \div 100 = markup\ rate$$
$$markup\ rate \times acquisition\ cost = markup\ amount$$
$$acquisition\ cost + markup\ amount = cash\ price$$

You can see the formulas applied in Examples 9.3 and 9.4.

Example 9.3

One case (12 bottles) of ABC All Natural Fish Oil 1200 mg capsules are acquired for $180, and there needs to be a 34% markup to determine the customer price. What will be the cash price for one bottle of Fish Oil?

Step 1 Convert 34% to a decimal by dividing by 100 to find the markup rate:

$$34\% \div 100 = 0.34 \quad \left\{ or\ \frac{34\%}{100} = 0.34 \right\}$$

Step 2 Multiply the markup rate by the acquisition cost:

$$0.34 \times \$180 = \$61.20$$

Step 3 Add the acquisition cost plus markup price for the cash price:

$$\$180 + \$61.20 = \$241.20\ (for\ 12\ bottles)$$

Step 4 Divide the cash price for 12 bottles by 12: $\frac{\$241.20}{12} = \$20.10$

$20.10 is the retail cash price for one bottle of ABC All Natural Fish Oil.

$180 + 34\% = $241.20
$241.20 ÷ 12 = $20.10 one bottle

Pharm Facts

Markup for OTC items may seem high, but the profit on these front end items help make up for the small profit realized on the prescription drugs due to the insurance contract pricing agreements.

Example 9.4

One bottle of Senna with stool softener, 100 count, sells at the pharmacy at the cash price of $34.95 and costs the pharmacy $22.45. What is the markup amount, and what is the markup rate?

Step 1 Determine actual price markup from selling price by subtracting product expense from selling price:

cash price − *acquisition cost* = *markup amount*
$34.95 − $22.45 = $12.50 is the markup

[handwritten: $12.50 / $22.45 × 100 = 56?]

Step 2 The markup percentage is computed as follows:

markup ÷ *acquisition cost* = *markup rate*
$12.50 ÷ $22.45 = 0.555679 (round up to 0.56)

Step 3 Convert 0.56 rate to percentage by multiplying it by 100, which equals 56%.

The pharmacy's profit/operating expenses markup for this item is 56%.

Managing Inventory Value and Turnovers

Inventory value is defined as the total value, or costs to acquire, the entire stock. The inventory includes prescription and OTC drugs, dietary supplements, medical and home health supplies and equipment, front-end retail, and impulse merchandise. To determine inventory value, a careful count of each product must be kept. This can be done manually or through technology.

Maintaining a Perpetual Inventory

As each drug prescription is filled, the pharmacy operations software and the point-of-sale (POS) cash register (which is connected electronically to the product barcode scanner and pharmacy inventory software) automatically deduct the product unit from the inventory count. This provides a **perpetual inventory**, or a continually up-to-date inventory count.

Each item in stock must also be counted once a year, and the manual counts are compared to the software's perpetual inventory to reconcile them. For example, the software may indicate that there are 120 tablets of 300 mg ranitidine remaining in stock. If the minimum reorder level is 100 tablets, the drug will not be on the generated reorder list. However, if you retrieve the drug from the shelf and find only 25 tablets remaining, you will update the actual inventory count in the system so that the drug can be ordered for the next business day. You and the pharmacist will need to try to figure out where the extra stock went.

One of the responsibilities of the pharmacy technician is to help keep track of the inventory and ensure that the inventory turns over by making wise purchasing orders. To do this, it is important to know the inventory **turnover**—the number of times the whole inventory sells out per year—to make any necessary adjustments in stock ordering levels and ranges for more profitability. A high turnover rate without any shortage gaps is good. It means the pharmacy has closely estimated the individual stock movement needed to meet patient needs, but not so closely that the pharmacy runs out of the medications and loses sales or customers. A low turnover rate indicates the inventory has been sitting on the shelves too long. If the inventory turns over every other month, the turnover rate is 6 (or 6 turns in a year). If the inventory turns over

Pharm Facts

Whenever a pharmacy is in the process of being sold, an inventory count is required and the value of the drug stock is included in the purchase price.

every month the rate is 12. Pharmacies generally aim for a turnover rate of approximately 10 to 12 times a year, though most pharmacies do not usually exceed 10 turns. Most pharmacies average between 8 to 10 annual turnovers.

Practice Tip

A turnover ratio can be applied to an individual product as well as to the inventory as a whole to determine how many times a single product's stock turns over in a year.

Calculating Inventory Turnover Ratios and Rates

To calculate the annual inventory turnover, you must calculate the annual total of costs for inventory compared to its current value based on its acquisition costs (or average value). This is the **turnover ratio**. Divided out the turnover ratio gives you the number of turnovers in a year, or **turnover rate**, as seen in the formula below.

$$inventory\ turnover\ rate = \frac{annual\ acquisitions\ costs}{current\ inventory\ value}$$

You can see how to apply this formula in Example 9.5.

Example 9.5

The pharmacy purchases $60,000 in stock per month and has $140,000 invested in the inventory on hand. What is the inventory turnover rate?

Step 1 First multiply $60,00 by 12 months for the annual acquisition costs or investment into the inventory:

$$\$60,000 \times 12 = \$720,000$$

Step 2 Set up the turnover ratio to determine the amount of annual turnover:

$$y = \frac{\$720,000}{\$140,000} = 5.1$$

The annual turnover rate is rounded to 5; the inventory turns over about 5 times a year.

As this example shows, this pharmacy is not controlling its inventory well, because a turnover rate of 5 is low. Several important inventory questions must be asked:

1. Which products are the fastest moving, and which are the slowest?
2. Which are the products that require the most investment to maintain, and how much are they needed by your patient population? Do they have to be on the shelves, or could they be ordered as needed?
3. Which drug products are absolutely necessary for local patients, and how much of each drug should be maintained?
4. Where should they be shelved or stored?
5. Is there sufficient room for new products or should other items counts be adjusted to make room?

In addition to these questions (which will be addressed in-depth in this chapter), other factors that need to be considered for inventory management decisions include the amount and type of new products being released that will need to be added, floor space allocation, design and arrangement of shelves, and demands on available refrigerator or freezer space. Adjustments may include returning a portion of the current drug stock to a wholesaler, selling or transferring stock to another pharmacy, and lowering automatic restock levels.

Inventory Levels and Ordering Strategies

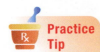
With the exception of Schedule II drugs, ordering and purchasing often are initiated by the pharmacy technician. In addition to pharmaceuticals, the pharmacy technician is also responsible for ordering pharmacy supplies, prescription vials, bottles, labels, information sheets, measuring devices, syringes, needles, and other items. In a hospital, the technician is responsible for ordering supplies (including personal protective equipment and intravenous base solutions for compounding) from the materials management department, which is in charge of ordering supplies for the entire institution.

In community pharmacies, medications are frequently ordered daily to minimize inventory costs and promote stock turnover. Most of the time, drugs are ordered from a wholesaler or corporate warehouse to be delivered to the pharmacy the following day. This is known as **just-in-time (JIT) ordering**—receiving medications just in time to sell. JIT purchasing can also refer to waiting to order an expensive, rarely prescribed drug until someone needs it to avoid the outlay in investment of carrying it on the shelf until it is needed.

Chain pharmacies generally receive warehouse deliveries only once a week, and they rely heavily on JIT ordering to cover potential shortages during the week.

Investigational Drugs

Institutional pharmacies that work with research institutions acquire investigational drugs directly from the lead investigator or manufacturer instead of the wholesaler. A **drug accountability record** must be maintained to account for the receiving and dispensing of the investigational drugs. This is generally done by a dedicated technician who also assists in the dispensing. The drugs in the investigational study must be labeled and stored separately from the rest of the institution's pharmacy stock.

Periodic Automatic Replenishment Levels and Reorder Ranges

In business, **economic order quantity** is the principle that you want to order the optimal number of units to minimize the total cost associated with purchase, delivery, and storage of the product. In pharmacy, that means ordering the highest amount of each drug possible that can move fast enough off the shelves to receive a quantity discount without wasting money and shelf space with too many units sitting on the shelves too long or having them expire.

On the one hand, you want to buy in volume to get a drug at the lowest cost possible, but it must be in a quantity that the pharmacy can use in a reasonable time. It may be cheaper per tablet to purchase 1,000 tablets, but if you only sell 50 tablets a month, it could take 20 months to use up the bottle. This is money sitting on the shelf.

Unlike some businesses, pharmacies often keep some slow-moving products on their shelves as a service to the few customers who will need them medically. If the pharmacy frequently runs out of needed supplies and medications, this causes great inconvenience to patients who will often just go to a different pharmacy, losing sales. So pharmacies set a **periodic automatic replenishment (PAR)** level in their software for each item, or the minimum level at which each stock item will generate automatic reordering. To accommodate fluctuations in demand, seasonal adjustments are made to the PAR levels of certain stock, such as stocking more allergy products in the spring, sunscreen products in the summer, flu vaccines in the fall, and antibiotics in the winter. If a new medication is increasingly prescribed in your geographical area, its PAR level will need to be increased.

Pharmacies that do not have an automated inventory ordering system must track drug stock by hand. These pharmacies usually have inventory ranges for each item—a minimum and maximum number of units to have on hand. The maximum number is the **safety point**, which allows a level of **safety stock** for more than average sales. Orders are calculated from these levels. The minimum level marks the point when the stock must be ordered, as with a PAR level. When inventory falls below the minimum level (or PAR level), an order is made. The order is for product that will take the inventory closest to the maximum level without going over the maximum level.

Stickers on the shelves list the minimum and maximum quantities for each drug. To calculate the amount to order use the following equation:

$$\textit{maximum inventory level} - \textit{present inventory} = \textit{order amount}$$

When quantities get low, the technician notes it on the inventory control sheet and calculates the quantity needed by using this formula, as shown in Examples 9.6 and 9.7.

Example 9.6

The pharmacy's maximum inventory of sertraline 100 mg tablets is 600 tablets and the minimum is 200 tablets. By the end of the day there are 100 tablets left on the shelf. How many bottles of sertraline 100 mg #100 per bottle should the pharmacy order?

600 tablets – 100 tablets = 500 tablets; $500 \text{ tablets} \times \dfrac{1 \text{ bottle}}{100 \text{ tablets}} = 5 \text{ bottles}$

The pharmacy needs to order 5 bottles of 100 tablets.

Example 9.7

The pharmacy buys sertraline in bottles of 30 tablets each that only need to be labeled before dispensing, saving the pharmacy the cost of a prescription vial. With the same maximum inventory level of 600 tablets, how many bottles of 30 tablets should be ordered?

$$\dfrac{500 \text{ tablets}}{30 \text{ tablets per bottle}} = 16.67 \text{ bottles.}$$

Round down to 16 bottles so the order does not exceed the maximum level.

Excessive inventory ties up capital in the inventory; hinders the ability to invest in other areas, like marketing and staffing; and incurs wastage due to product expirations. It also increases the likelihood of theft. Therefore, *inventory levels must be kept adequate but not excessive, with a rapid turnover of drug stock on the shelf.*

ABC Classification System for Stock Management

PAR levels and ordering ranges need to be set based on a thorough knowledge of pharmacy stock movement and costs. There is an 80/20 rule in business that can be applied to inventory analysis, where 80% of the costs are attributed to 20% of the products, and often 80% of the profit comes from abundant sales of the lower end items. By classifying products into categories of costs, the pharmacy can more easily monitor the most expensive and high-use products and use just-in-time ordering for these products to keep inventory costs down.

Inventory can also be sorted by product type, as in Table 9.1, where 80% fits a pharmacy's core mission: to sell prescription drugs. The other two product types (the 20%) will have the most mark-up to make a profit.

TABLE 9.1 ABC Classifications

Category	% of Resource $	Product Type
A	80%	Prescription drugs
B	15%	OTC and supplements
C	5%	Retail items

Poor management of a few products in category A is more detrimental to the bottom line than inadequate attention to a large number of items in category C. That is why it is particularly important to track the movement of these high-dollar drugs and order *only when necessary, without making patients wait for medications*. Many pharmacies dispense these drugs with auxiliary labels that read, "This item is special ordered for you; please call a few days prior to needing refills."

When ordering, it is important to know how soon the product will be available, which is the **lead time**—the time between ordering or compounding a product and its delivery or payment. A compounding pharmacy must also consider the time it takes to compound or mix as part of the lead time.

If the pharmacy runs out of a medication before more stock arrives and cannot fill prescriptions, the pharmacy experiences what is known as a **shortage cost**. Shortage cost is difficult to measure, because it is made up of differing elements. For instance, because of being out of stock, the pharmacy may need to deliver medications to the patients at home, incurring extra costs. Or if medications are unavailable too often, the pharmacy may lose customers. These are all part of shortage costs.

To ensure the pharmacy does not run out of a specific product, pharmacies often keep a safety net of supply on hand. The safety stock provides a cushion so that if orders exceed the daily average, the pharmacy can still fill every prescription for this product in a timely manner. To calculate safety stock, the technician must know the maximum potential daily usage, the average daily usage, and the lead time. You can then use the required amount of safety stock to calculate the level at which the pharmacy should reorder. This is called the **reorder point** for the PAR or ordering range. Example 9.8 shows how to calculate the amount of safety stock and the reorder point needed for atenolol (a beta blocker used to treat high blood pressure and overly rapid heartbeats), by using the following formulas:

$$safety\ stock = (highest\ usual\ level - average\ usage\ per\ unit) \times lead\ time$$
$$reorder\ point = (average\ usage\ per\ unit \times lead\ time) + safety\ stock$$

Example 9.8

A chain pharmacy dispenses an average of 400 atenolol 50 mg tablets daily, but it has sold as many as 550 tablets in one day. How many bottles of atenolol 50 mg 100 tablets should the pharmacy keep as safety stock if it takes 2 days of lead time to receive a new supply? What is the reorder point?

Step 1 Set up equation by inserting information, with 100 tablets per bottle:

$$y = (5.5 \text{ bottles} - 4 \text{ bottles}) \times 2 \text{ days lead time}; \quad y = 3 \text{ bottles}$$

The safety stock is 3 bottles of 100 tablets of atenolol 50 mg.

Step 2 Use the safety stock to calculate when the pharmacy should reorder.

$$z = \frac{4 \text{ bottles}}{1 \text{ day}} \times 2 \text{ day} + 3 \text{ bottles}; \quad z = 11 \text{ bottles}$$

The reorder point is 11 bottles of atenolol 50 mg.

The pharmacy should have at least 11 bottles of atenolol available at the beginning of the day to make sure it can fill every prescription.

Shelf Maintenance and Rotating Stock

> **Study Idea**
>
> Highly automated pharmacy computer systems generate the daily reorder list based on PAR levels. Some pharmacies still use the paper order book system in which, if an item is used, it is reordered.

As a purchasing agent, you have to consider shortage costs as well as counts of waste due to expired or almost expired medications. Once a month, or per store policy, technicians have to check and reposition the stock, placing the oldest items in front and the new stock behind—unless the new stock has an earlier expiration date than the packages on the shelf. This repositioning is known as **rotating the stock** to make sure that pharmaceuticals with the earliest expiration dates are used first. Products close to expiration dates need to be removed. Each pharmacy has a policy for an acceptable range of shelf dates. A typical requirement might be that products have expiration dates of at least twelve months from the date of wholesaler receipt, and products on the shelves must have a four- to six-month shelf life.

The goal is to have low wastage and shortage costs while taking advantage of volume discounts and other good deals negotiated through established purchasing relationships.

Purchasing Relationships and Contracts

Before any ordering or purchasing can happen, relationships with those who distribute, store, or manufacture specific drugs must be established. Purchasing contracts can be negotiated by an individual pharmacy or with other pharmacies as part of a group purchase contract. This can help independent pharmacies obtain greater discounts to better compete with chain stores that can buy in far larger quantities as a group.

Every month, a report is sent by each wholesaler to the pharmacy inventory manager called a **compliance report**. It lists all the purchases made that did not comply with the contract bid and notes cheaper alternatives. Reviewing these reports for strategic changes in purchasing can save the pharmacy money in the future and help them determine if they want to remain in their current wholesaler relationships or forge new ones.

Primary Wholesaler Purchasing

Independent pharmacies generally each secure a **primary wholesaler purchasing contract** with a local drug wholesaler to be its primary supplier so it can receive the fastest moving products from a single source for the best negotiated price to be delivered on a daily basis. (Chain pharmacies negotiate as a group or have their own wholesalers.) The advantages include scheduled deliveries and ordering, automatic online ordering, reduced turnaround time for orders, lower inventory and lower associated costs, discounts, and reduced commitment of time and staff. The turnaround time for receipt of drug orders is usually the next business day, with the exception of weekends and holidays. Disadvantages include higher purchase costs for individual stock items, occasional supply shortages (called *back orders*), and unavailability of some pharmaceuticals.

Prime Vendor Purchasing

In some situations, pharmacies need to work with more than one vendor, getting a large amount of stock from two or more suppliers. The pharmacy may be able to set up a **prime vendor purchasing contract** with one of these vendors to secure a discount for high-volume purchasing. This is an exclusive agreement to continually purchase a specified percentage or dollar amount toward different types of ordering and delivery methods. Prime vendor purchasing offers the advantages of lower acquisition costs, competitive service fees, electronic order entry, and emergency delivery services. Prime vendor purchasing is common in both retail and hospital pharmacies.

Closed or Open Formularies

Beside considering delivery times and drug costs, the selection of wholesalers for primary and prime vendor purchasing relationships may also be influenced by a drug formulary and which wholesaler can supply the drugs on the list most cost-effectively. A formulary is a list of medications approved for use or coverage. With a **closed formulary**, drugs not on the list are not allowed or covered by the insurer or institution. Hospitals try to control expenses by reducing the number of pharmaceuticals of the same drug class in its formulary according to best practices established by the medical community and what is available economically in purchasing groups. For example, the hospital may purchase one proton pump inhibitor (PPI) drug and make a therapeutic substitution for any other kind of PPI ordered. If omeprazole is the least expensive, then any medication orders for lansoprazole, esomeprazole, or pantoprazole would be changed to omeprazole. Typically, any nonformulary order has to be approved by the Pharmacy and Therapeutics (P&T) Committee, which includes members of the medical staff.

Community pharmacies have **open formularies**. They stock pharmaceuticals to serve all of the patients in their community. However, insurers sometimes have closed formularies, though most use a more open, multi-tiered formulary as will be explained in Chapter 10. If the pharmacy is owned by a health maintenance organization, private insurer, or the Veterans Health Administration, for example, the pharmacy may have a formulary based on the larger organization's accepted standard of care.

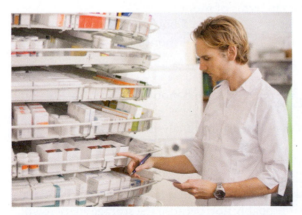

Technicians need to keep close track of the inventory, especially the most frequently purchased pharmaceuticals, to assist in deciding what needs to be purchased and how quickly.

Handling Purchasing Orders

The technician reviews and verifies each of the drugs listed on the end-of-the-day reorder list and purchase orders to process them, alerting the pharmacist to the Schedule II drugs needing attention. If the pharmacy is on a strict daily drug budget, you need to exercise good judgment and prioritize which drugs will be ordered for the next business day and which can wait. It is not uncommon for an independent pharmacy to wait to order an expensive drug rather than keep it in stock on the shelf.

When ordering next-day inventory, the technician assesses the predicted new prescriptions or refills for (1) **out-of-stock (OOS)** items, (2) partial fills, and (3) stock replenishment. Special orders for seldom stocked high-cost injectable products often require additional delivery time directly from the manufacturer if they are not in the wholesaler's on-site inventory.

For "fast movers," the purchase decision is often based on the most economical order quantity or best value (such as ordering capsules in a 1,000 count size rather than 100 count size, or buying a case of liquid antacid rather than one or two bottles). As noted, before purchasing a large quantity of a product on sale, the technician must estimate the additional time it will take to sell the larger quantity at a profit using the following formula implemented in Example 9.9:

$$time\ till\ all\ stock\ is\ sold = \frac{quantity\ to\ sell}{sales\ history\ (units\ sold/time\ unit)}$$

Example 9.9

The supplier offers a sale on calamine lotion: buy six cases, get the seventh case free. Each case sells for $6 and contains 12 bottles. All invoices must be paid in 30 days or the pharmacy will be charged interest. Last year, the pharmacy sold 60 bottles of calamine. If sales remain the same, how long will it take the pharmacy to sell all seven cases or turnover this stock?

Step 1 Find out the quantity to sell:

$$\frac{12\ bottles}{1\ case} \times 7\ cases = 84\ bottles$$

Step 2 Find out the sales history in terms of months:

$$\frac{60\ bottles}{12\ months}\ is\ reduced\ to\ \frac{5\ bottles}{1\ month}$$

Step 3 Divide the quantity by the time it takes to sell:

$$\frac{84\ bottles}{5\ bottles\ per\ month} = 16.8\ months$$

You could also do it in one dimensional analysis equation:

$$y = \frac{12\ bottles}{1\ case} \times 7\ cases \times \frac{12\ months}{60\ bottles} = \frac{1008\ months}{60} = 16.8\ months$$

If it takes more than 16 months for the pharmacy to realize its return, is it a good idea to buy the product even if it is on sale? Probably not, because the storage space it will take up will prevent a faster moving item from being shelved. The gross profit from the discounted price will be absorbed into the overhead costs, leaving little net profit. Calamine lotion is a low-dollar inventory item. What if this scenario involved an expensive pharmaceutical like Vytorin, which is used for treating hyperlipidemia? The pharmacy pays $100 or more for a bottle of Vytorin. In that case, the pharmacy would not want to wait almost 17 months to see a return on its investment.

Processing Order Deliveries

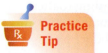

Practice Tip

When a delivery arrives without a medication because it has been discontinued or is no longer manufactured, you need to ask the pharmacist to discuss an alternative medication to order.

Once an order is delivered from a wholesaler, warehouse, or other pharmacy, the technician must go through a number of key processes that require documentation.

Receiving

When the wholesale delivery arrives, the process of **receiving** begins, which is a set of procedures to legally check in and accept the order. The pharmacist or technician first must sign an invoice from the wholesale representative, verifying the receipt of the correct number and type of totes or boxes. **Totes** are the plastic containers that contain specialized medications, including those for refrigerated items (in cold packs) and controlled substances, which all come sealed. (A separate invoice and receipt are required for controlled substances. The pharmacist should check for and document intact seals and the content of these totes, which will be explained in more depth later.)

To check a delivery, you must carefully match the pharmaceutical products received against the purchase invoice for the correct products—matching the names, NDCs, barcodes, manufacturers, quantities, product strengths, and package sizes. You must also check for their delivery condition. In the case of a missing item or an incorrect, damaged, or improperly shipped product (not stored properly), notify the wholesaler and pharmacist immediately. Return the defective shipment and replace the ordered items as soon as possible.

Occasionally, a pharmaceutical product is temporarily or permanently unavailable from a wholesaler. First determine the reason for the unavailability—for example, the drug is (1) on back order, (2) being recalled by the manufacturer, or (3) being discontinued. If the product is not expected to be received the next day, the pharmacist should then identify a therapeutically equivalent product with permission from the prescriber. Alternatively, the pharmacy could consider borrowing the drug from another local pharmacy or one in the corporate chain if the drug is available.

Posting

As the inventory order is checked and approved, it is important that the order is accurately posted. **Posting** is the process of updating inventory in the pharmacy software database and reconciling any differences between the new and current stock. This

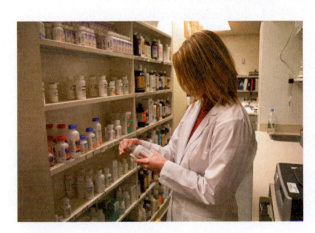

process includes checking the newly received drug inventory for NDC numbers, expiration dates, and drug cost updates.

Once the posting of the invoices is complete, a copy should go to accounts receivable for payment and the original should be filed in the pharmacy. (Controlled substance invoices should be filed separately for auditing convenience.)

The technician must also handle the Drug Quality and Security Act (DQSA) documentation. It includes noting the delivery transaction information and the full history or statements of the compounder/manufacturer on the lot number of the delivered medication. The DSQA documentation must be kept on file for six years. Many wholesalers do not send a written copy of these reports but have them available online.

Storage

After medications are received, they must be stocked or shelved according to their proper labeling and storage requirements. Instructions for special storage and handling requirements for the pharmaceuticals are included on their product package inserts. These requirements are in line with the *United States Pharmacopeia and National Formulary (USP-NF)* reference standards.

For instance, nitroglycerin has strict storage requirements. The sublingual tablets are unstable in the presence of air, moisture, and light, and must be stored in their original brown glass container from the manufacturer or a specially designed airtight container. Nitroglycerin should be kept at temperatures below 77°F, or 25°C. Even body temperature will decrease its potency. To ensure potency, patients should purchase a new bottle of 25 tablets every three months. Intravenous nitroglycerin must be protected from light by covering the solution during administration.

Refrigerated and frozen pharmaceuticals are delivered in specially marked storage totes packed with ice or dry ice. These drugs should be posted and stored as soon as possible. Do not touch the dry ice. Place it in a well-ventilated area until it completely dissolves.

Vaccines come in a tote with a color-coded tracking device that indicates whether the vaccine has been exposed to temperatures outside the proper storage range. If the temperature fluctuated out of the proper range in transport, the vaccine must be discarded, and the supplier should be contacted for credit or replacement. Zostavax and other vaccines and intravenous pharmaceuticals that need to be kept frozen should be stored at 5°F, or –15°C. Zostavax must be used within 30 minutes after it is reconstituted with a diluent.

Remember to check and log the freezer and refrigerator temperatures daily. Pharmacy refrigerator temperatures are kept in the range of 36°F to 46°F, or 2°C to 8°C. Refrigerated drugs include insulins, suppositories, some eyedrops and soft gels, many vials, and injectable drugs. Chemotherapy agents that require refrigeration should be stored either in a separate refrigerator or isolated to prevent contamination if a leak or spill occurs. Any open refrigerated drug must be dated with its beyond-use date to ensure it is discarded at the appropriate time.

Medications and items stored at room temperature should have a designated space and shelf label organized to minimize dispensing errors. Some pharmacies have stock alphabetized by brand name with the generic stock next to each item. Others have different systems or exceptions for look-alike or sound-alike drugs. For example, metformin 500 mg (a common diabetic drug) should not be placed on the shelf next to metformin ER 500 mg.

In the hospital pharmacy, the technician is often responsible for restocking the floor stock medications stored in automated dispensing units, such as the Pyxis and Omnicell. The automated units include a perpetual inventory system and electronically charge the appropriate patient account at the point of administration.

Patient Prescription Storage Patients should be informed about how to properly store medications at home. For example, a reconstituted antibiotic suspension is stable for a limited time, about 10 days, and should be discarded once the treatment is complete. Penicillin-based solutions need to be stored in the refrigerator after they have been reconstituted. Other antibiotics such as azithromycin, clarithromycin, and cefdinir are stored at room temperature, which is generally considered to be below 86°F, or 30°C. Some temperature variation may occur during a short-term power outage, but any long-term storage above room temperature can affect medications, and patients should contact the pharmacy or manufacturer of the product for more information.

Patients need to be made aware that if an insulin vial or syringe is frozen or left in the heat of a car or in light, the medication should not be used and should be discarded. In warm climates or in summer, patients may be advised to transport their insulin home from the pharmacy in a cooler, especially if they are not returning home immediately.

Once opened, most insulins have a beyond-use date of 28 days, though newer agents may be good for up to 60 days. Check the package insert for the manufacturer-recommended BUD. Patients need to be instructed that insulin should be stored in the refrigerator until first use, and then discarded after the BUD. Patients do not need to refrigerate a vial or insulin pen after first use.

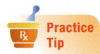

Practice Tip

It is good customer service for technicians to call customers when the remainder of an out-of-stock or partial-fill medication is available for pickup.

Study Idea

On a partial fill, if the patient does not pick up the medication balance, the insurance claim must be adjusted, or the pharmacy could be charged with fraud.

Handling Out-of-Stock and Partially-Filled Medications

After receiving, posting, and shelving/storing of the inventory is complete, it is important to initiate the prescription filling process for any OOS or partial-fill prescriptions from the day before. The OOS prescription orders are processed, verified, and filled first so they can be available for the patients to pick up later that same day, as promised. If possible, you should notify the patients that the prescriptions are now ready for pickup. The completion of partial-fill orders takes priority next. These patients have commonly received 3 to 5 days worth of medication to hold them over until the order is received.

Handling Controlled Substances

Controlled substances demand special purchasing, receiving, and recordkeeping of inventory, according to the Controlled Substances Act. Each pharmacy must register with the DEA to purchase and dispense controlled substances, and the FDA requires that all controlled-substance containers be clearly marked with their "schedule" on the product label.

Schedule III, IV, and V Drugs

In most pharmacies, the technician can order Schedule III–V medications. However, per store policy, the pharmacist may have to verify and sign for their receipt at delivery. After comparing the invoice with the ordered drug name, dosage, and quantity, the receipt can often be signed by the technician and verified by the pharmacist. These drugs can then be stored by the technician among the rest of the drug stock, usually alphabetically by generic drug name. All Schedule III, IV, and V prescriptions and records, including purchasing invoices, are commonly kept separate from other records and must also be kept in a readily retrievable form.

Schedule II Purchasing

Schedule II controlled substances follow stricter protocols per DEA law and regulations. Similar to other medications, PAR levels for most C-II drugs generate automated inventory alerts in the pharmacy software for reorders or special out-of-stock or partial-fill orders. However, purchase of Schedule II controlled substances must be specifically initiated and authorized by a pharmacist and executed on a DEA 222 form, either online or on paper (see Figure 3.1 and Table 3.8 DEA forms in Chapter 3).

Schedule II Receiving and Documentation When receiving the Schedule II tote, the technician should check that the seal is not broken, then break the seal and verify the contents with the invoice. After verification, the pharmacist must document the following information on the DEA 222 delivery receipt section: the date, the name and amount of Schedule II drugs received, and the corresponding NDC numbers. You, as the technician, can then post the Schedule II drug inventory to the database, including the NDC numbers, prices, and expiration dates.

Controlled Substance Disposal As Schedule II substances in the inventory expire or are defective (such as a case of broken tablets), they must be disposed of properly. Any controlled drug disposal must be itemized, recorded, witnessed, and signed by a second pharmacist on the DEA Form 41. In most cases, Schedule II drugs are delivered or sent to an authorized destruction depot after the proper documentation of DEA Form 41 has been completed with a copy to accompany the drugs, a copy mailed to the DEA, and a copy kept on file.

Schedule II Perpetual Inventory Record Community pharmacies use automated or manual perpetual inventory to maintain inventory counts and close control of all Schedule II drug stock. A perpetual inventory record for all Schedule II medications must be kept on a tablet-by-tablet (or other dosage form) basis that includes product, dosage, quantity, date received or dispensed, prescription number, remaining inventory, and signature or initials of the pharmacist.

Biennial Inventory Count In addition, according to DEA regulations, *a biennial (every two years) inventory of controlled substance drugs must be taken.* Some states (and pharmacies) have even more stringent requirements, such as a yearly inventory. These inventories should closely approximate the perpetual inventory record. For Schedules III, IV, and V substances, an estimated count and/or measure of units remaining in stock containers is permitted, unless a container holds more than 1,000 capsules or tablets. Then an exact count is required. For Schedule II drugs, each unit must be accounted for. The Schedule II inventory count should not vary by more than four days from the calendar month and date of the last biennial inventory. An original hard copy of the biennial inventory must be filed, another sent to the DEA, and one may also be sent online to the DEA. Major deviations in actual counts and numbers listed in the Schedule II drug inventory must be investigated and reported if not resolved.

Additional tracking mechanisms exist by state and federal authorities to monitor the distribution of Schedule II drugs. If there is evidence of overprescribing by a physician, overdispensing by a pharmacy, or overselling of Schedule II drugs by a wholesaler, the DEA—after a thorough investigation—has the authority to temporarily or permanently revoke the DEA license of that physician, pharmacy, or wholesaler. A wholesaler can limit the monthly amount of controlled substances distributed to a community pharmacy if it deems that there has been excessive use.

Drug Returns and Credits

Sometimes, drugs must be returned to the wholesaler for credit in their original stock bottles or unit-of-use packaging *and in their original condition*. These returns may be caused by pharmacy overstocks, patient declining medications at pickup or neglecting to pick them up, soon-to-be-expired drugs, manufacturer or FDA recalls, reformulated drugs, or drugs in out-of-date packaging. The different reasons for returns result in slightly different ways to handle them.

Study Idea

DEA Form 41 is for destruction of expired or damaged controlled substances. DEA Form 106 is to report theft of controlled substances. DEA Form 222 is used to order controlled substances.

Study Idea

When a new pharmacy opens or a new director of pharmacy starts, an initial inventory of all controlled substances must be done on the first day of business, whether it's a community or institutional pharmacy.

Study Idea

Once a drug has left the community pharmacy, it cannot be returned and resold, even if unopened. In an institutional pharmacy, if a patient declines a unit dose and it is unopened, it may be restocked and used on another patient.

Return of Recalled Drugs

When an official drug recall alert occurs, the wholesaler will typically email or mail the drug recall information: drug name, strength, dose, NDC, lot number, and expiration date as well as the date and type of recall (voluntary, mandatory). This form is then returned to the wholesaler with the stock pulled from the shelves.

Return of Declined Medications

At times, patients do not pick up their filled medication within seven days, even after reminder messages. Consequently, you must "reverse" or cancel the online insurance billing, store the prescription in the patient profile for possible future use, and return the stock to drug inventory or the wholesaler. For example, if a patient declines to pick up the expensive diabetic drug Tanzeum (albiglutide), you can store it in the refrigerator and then return it to the wholesaler for credit if the box is unopened and the prescription label (perhaps attached by rubber band) can be removed without altering the manufacturer's label.

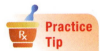
A return-for-credit form must be completed that lists the drug(s) and quantities to be returned. You and the wholesale driver must verify the contents of the return totes or boxes, and sign for the credit. Your signature guarantees under penalty of law that the product was purchased directly from the wholesaler and that the drugs have been stored and handled in accordance with manufacturers' guidelines and all federal, state, and local laws. The containers are then sealed and returned to the wholesaler for credit. The signed form is filed for future reference.

Expired Medications

As noted, pharmacy technicians must check the dating on stock and rotate the products (including OTC drugs and dietary supplements) on a monthly basis, or per store policy. Remove all expired or nearly expired (within three to six months) medications and return them to the wholesaler or manufacturer, but no credit may be issued. This process of returns and credits is time-consuming, involving a lot of paperwork. Many pharmacies now hire **reverse distributors** to handle outdated inventory. They come to your pharmacy, prepare the drugs for return, and provide the return documentation.

Wrongly Filled Prescriptions

At times, the wrong medication has been filled in a prescription, which occasionally happens despite safety checks. If the drug did not leave the pharmacy, the prescription can be corrected and the drug can be returned to stock. However, if the patient left the pharmacy, discovered the mix-up, and then came back to the pharmacy later with the medication unopened, the incorrect drug can be returned to the pharmacy and the correct medication dispensed, *but the incorrect drug must be discarded per law and pharmacy protocol*. The pharmacy cannot redispense or recover the cost of the incorrect prescription.

As you can see, inventory information takes time to get to know well. Technicians need knowledge and experience working with the various aspects of inventory management before they move into positions of such responsibility. That is why technicians taking a certification exam need to be well versed in the basic terms and concepts of inventory management.

STUDY SUMMARY

The task of inventory management in a pharmacy requires an in-depth knowledge of the amount and types of drugs being prescribed and the rate of purchases in each pharmacy. Sales reports and turnover rates are used to set up inventory PAR levels or establish maximum and minimum levels of each drug. Technicians must be aware of:

- the different wholesaler relationships and ordering procedures for prescription controlled and non-controlled drugs as well as OTC products.

- procedures for purchasing, receiving, and stocking of pharmaceuticals.

- inventory terminology.

- the importance of DQSA, FDA, and DEA rules and documentation on drug inventory.

- the proper forms to order and report issues of controlled substances. Be aware of the special storage requirements for select pharmaceuticals.

- the methods to return and be reimbursed for recalled products.

- the importance of monitoring, reversing claims, and returning to stock prescriptions that are filled or not picked up by patients.

ADDITIONAL RESOURCES

For more in-depth explanations, check out *Pharmacy Practice for Technicians*, 6e from Paradigm Education Solutions. To master and extend the material presented in this chapter, take advantage of the resources available through the eBook resources links. These include digital supplements, study resources, and a practice exam generator with 1,000+ exam-style questions. End-of-chapter tests are accessible through the eBook for individuals using the self-study course and through Navigator+ for individuals enrolled in the instructor-guided course.

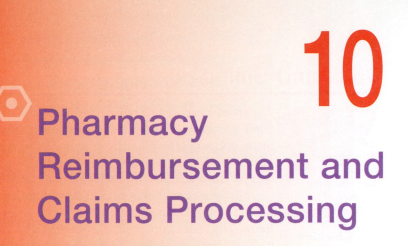

10

Pharmacy Reimbursement and Claims Processing

Learning Objectives

1 Understand the importance of correct cash register entry during sales.

2 Identify different sources of payment.

3 Understand the different insurance payment options and structures available, including coinsurance and copayments.

4 Be familiar with the tiered copayment system used by insurers.

5 Determine eligibility for third-party reimbursement by identifying key components of a patient's prescription insurance card.

6 Understand coordination of benefits for patients with more than one prescription drug plan.

7 Calculate days supply accurately for tablets, capsules, liquids, and otic or ophthalmic solutions or suspensions.

8 Identify rejected insurance claims and the process for notifying both patient and prescriber.

9 Determine the reason for a chargeback on a prescription claim and the documentation needed for an insurance audit.

10 Identify systems in place to help patients with medication assistance, including lower cost generics, manufacturer's coupons, discount cards, and low-fee and charity clinics.

Access eBook links for resources and an exam generator, with 1,000+ questions.

Since over 90% of patients have some form of private or government health insurance, pharmacy technicians provide a valuable service to patients by having the knowledge and skill to properly enter insurance information into the pharmacy computer and correctly interpret insurance regulations and requirements. Domain 8 of the new PTCB and topical area 3 of the ExCPT exam test knowledge of pharmacy billing and reimbursement processes and procedures.

Cash and Billing

Study Idea

Many items are exempt from state sales tax. Be aware of the category of items that are nontaxable items according the federal categories and the additional items listed in your specific state, as you may need to pass a state exam too to practice.

As part of working in a retail pharmacy, you are responsible for collecting payments from customers. The price of each prescription, medical supply, OTC drug, supplement, and retail item is either scanned with a barcoder to pull the price into the point-of-sale (POS) cash register, or it is hand entered into a less automated one. Cash register procedures differ with each pharmacy and its technology.

FDA-approved prescription drugs for humans (not animals) and certain medically necessary supplies are federally exempt from any state sales tax, so these are **nontaxable items**. The tax-exempt medical supplies include disposable or consumable medical items (such as glucose test strips and nutritional drinks for diabetic patients) and durable medical equipment (such as canes, walkers, crutches, orthopedic and diabetic shoes, but not hospital beds). Other nontaxable items include prescribed devices, such as neck collars, ankle braces, slings, and wrist and arm braces. Each state may add other items they deem as "necessary. Charges must be entered into the cash register in the correct tax category and product code to ensure the correct product is removed from the inventory count with the sale.

Customers often pay for their purchases using various cards (credit cards, debit cards, Flex cards, and gift cards), cash, or checks. Each payment option has a unique processing method; these payment methods should be demonstrated in the pharmacy's training program. Regardless of the form of payment, the pharmacy technician should always present the customer a payment receipt (the proof-of-purchase printout).

The various kinds of payment cards need to be verified with a card-swiping monitor for online transaction approval (pharmacy gift cards need in-house approvals of card amounts). Though sometimes you will do the swiping, the most common technology has the patient swipe the card and follow the prompts. If the amount submitted is declined, you will have to ask for an alternative card or form of payment. To decrease fraudulent use, most credit and debit cards are moving to **EMV chip** technology, or cards with an imbedded computer chip. Each time this card is used, the customer will enter a pin number and a one-time-only software code will be utilized to process the transaction. Any payment done with a credit card is added to the customer's overall credit card account, which is billed by the card company each month. The balance either must be paid off by the customer at the end of the month or it accrues interest as a finance charge.

Study Idea

A health savings account (HSA) is offered by some employers who provide insurance plans with high deductibles. The HSAs allow employees to put aside pre-tax money to use toward healthcare needs. The HSA cards look like credit cards when presented at the cash register. Smart registers are able to identify which purchases may be covered by the card.

Depending on pharmacy policy, patients may or may not need to sign for a credit card expense of less than $50. In most independent pharmacies, patients will sign for every credit card transaction. Credit and debit cards often allow customers the option to request cash back after the claim is processed. Cash-back options may be limited ($20 or less) or not available per store policy. Some chain pharmacies offer customers the **express pay option**, where the customer puts his or her credit card on file to be processed automatically at the time of each prescription filling.

Some independent pharmacies allow their most frequent customers to run a charge account and have the pharmacy bill them at the end of the month. This is a convenience for the customer but adds to operating expenses of the pharmacy, so it needs to be done with prudence, as decided by the owners.

Customers may elect to pay for their pharmacy purchases with personal checks, though this is becoming less common, and some businesses no longer accept checks. Procedures differ depending on the pharmacy. Larger pharmacies usually have a check reader connected to the cash register.

Finally, some customers will pay with cash, and you will need to be well versed in how to count the change back. Most cash registers will tell you the total amount due back, but you should also be able to count change from the purchase price.

Insurance Options

Study Idea

Know well the differences between the government plans—especially Medicare A, B, C, and D programs—by studying Table 10.1.

Most patients, though, have some sort of healthcare insurance to pay a portion or all their pharmaceutical costs. Healthcare coverage in the United States may be provided by commercial insurance paid by the individuals, be paid partially by employers (with shared premium costs), or be paid by one of the state or federal programs (see Table 10.1):

- **Medicare** (**A**, **B**, **C**, and **D**) for those over 64 or disabled, administered through the US Department of Health and Human Services and contracted private insurers
- **Medicaid** for low-income patients and their dependents, administered by individual states
- **Children's Health Insurance Program (CHIP)** and **Affordable Care Act Health Exchanges**, primarily administered by individual states
- **Tricare** for active military (including National Guard and Reserves), veterans, and military dependents, administered through the Defense Health Agency

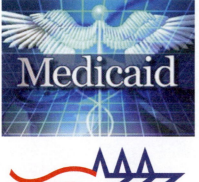

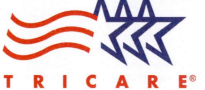

The employer-contracted programs can be administered by a private insurer or be contracted with a **health maintenance organization (HMO)**—which has its own providers and pharmacies. Another employer insurance option is a **preferred provider organization (PPO)**—which contracts with preferred providers for lower costs but still pays for claims for others only at higher costs. Both HMOs and PPOs use managed care to control costs, though all insurance organizations are working for these ends.

Commonly, patients have only one **primary health insurance plan**, which pays up to its coverage limits. Some patients also have a **secondary health insurance plan**, which pays what the primary insurance does not, if the service is covered under the secondary plan. The patient may still have out-of-pocket costs even with two insurance plans. Some patients who have excessive drug needs have to combine more than one healthcare insurance program with a specific prescription drug insurance policy.

TABLE 10.1 Insurance Providers and Benefits

Type of Provider	Description of Benefits	Special Considerations
Medicare		
• Medicare Part A	Covers 80% of hospital costs and limited coverage for skilled nursing and home health care; NO DRUG COVERAGE	Patients have a Medicare card, and program is run through the Centers for Medicare and Medicaid Services (CMS); enrollment period is mid-October through December.
• Medicare Part B	Covers 80% of costs for provider visits and some preventive medicine; COVERS SOME DURABLE MEDICAL EQUIPMENT (DME) if there are CMEs	Patients have same Part A Medicare card with additional line noting Part B coverage; need Certificate of Medical Necessity (CMN) form for DME claim processing; need the correct ICD-10 coding; need prescription for nebulizer; medication therapy management services also covered if through Medicare-approved pharmacy or health center.

• Medicare Part D	Drug insurance that enrollees of Medicare Parts A and B can add to their program(s); it pays 75% of drug costs up to annual limit; has "donut hole" of coverage between annual coverage cap and when the catastrophic coverage kicks in	Patients pick from a variety of insurance companies or PBMs that work with the government to offer Medicare Part D plans (such as Aetna, Humana, Blue Cross/Blue Shield)
• Medicare Part C	Comprehensive coverage—a combination plan that offers partial coverage of hospital, providers, and drugs; also known as Medicare Advantage	Patients pick from a variety of styles of plans through commercial carriers partially subsidized by the government.
Medigap Insurance Plans		
	Nongovernmental secondary insurance plans meant to supplement the gaps of costs not covered by Medicare	Patients pick from a variety of styles of plans through commercial carriers partially subsidized by the government.
Medicaid		
	Healthcare and drug subsidies for disabled, low-income, part-time, and unemployable citizens of all ages; some elderly disabled citizens are eligible for Medicare and Medicaid.	This is a program jointly run with states and often with commercial insurance providers; does not cover out-of-state costs.
Children's Health Insurance Program (CHIP)		
	Low-cost or free coverage for uninsured children from ages prenatal/birth to 19 (including pregnant women and their children in the womb) for parents who are over the poverty line but can't afford insurance.	This is a program jointly run with the states.
ACA Health Exchange Plans		
	Four plans available: platinum (90% coverage and highest monthly premium), gold (80%), silver (70%), and bronze (60% and highest deductible)	Enrollment period is November 1 through January 30th in next year; those who meet the income requirements are eligible; patients use the exchanges to pick among various subsidized programs from many carriers.

Insurance Claims and Payment Structures

Nearly all insurance companies and plans that handle prescriptions work with a **pharmacy benefits manager (PBM)** to establish the formulary and tiers, and administer and process its patients' prescription claims. Examples of PBMs include Merck-Medco, CVS Caremark, and Argus. The PBM is typically under contract with more than one insurance company and may have different rules for the different companies' insurance claims.

Each community pharmacy must negotiate a drug-provider contract with each PBM to work with it. Typically, pharmacies have annually renewable contracts with PBMs to provide prescription benefits at specified reimbursement rates to all the insurance enrollees managed by that PBM. Larger PBMs that can promise more business can negotiate lower rates of reimbursement. Technicians need to get used to the different rate schedules. In the community pharmacy, the very same drug may be billed at different rates to different patients depending on the PBM, insurance, and government program. The rates are generally based on **usual, customary, and**

Study Idea

The list of drugs the insurance company will pay for is called the preferred drug list or its formulary.

reasonable (UCR) charges for drugs plus a pharmacy dispensing fee. *The UCRs are based on the Average Warehouse Price (AWP) in the geographical region* for each drug. By law, the pharmacy cannot charge or negotiate a higher cost to the government programs than to a commercial user or PBM for the same prescription.

Deductibles

Most health insurance plans include some combination of individual and/or family annual deductible levels. The **deductible** is the designated amount of annual medical costs that must be paid by the patient *before* the full coverage by the insurance company kicks in. So in that sense, this amount is *deducted* from coverage benefits. For instance, if a plan designates a $6,000 deductible for an individual, the patient must pay for a large portion or all of the medical costs up to $6,000 before the insurance company starts paying the full or majority portion of each expense. In this high deductible plan, the patient may have numerous office visits and tests done and perhaps an emergency room visit before the insurance company will cover much or anything at all. The higher the deductible, the lower the monthly premium (or fee) for coverage, because the patient is assuming much of the risk.

Coinsurance Payments

For some policies, when patients receive a medical service or drug product, they must immediately pay a certain percentage of the retail cost of the drug, or **coinsurance** payment. For example, if a patient has an 80/20 coinsurance benefit, the patient pays 20% of the medication cost and the insurer pays 80%. The patient's portion of a $50 medication would be $10, but the patient would pay $30 for a medication that costs $150.

The Medicare Plan D program has a benefit donut hole. Each year, the patient pays 25% of prescription drug costs until the initial coverage limit is reached ($2,960 in 2015). After this, the patient must pay the full cost of prescriptions until reaching the cost ceiling ($7,062 in 2015) where the catastrophic insurance coverage kicks in—then the enrollee pays only 5%, the plan pays 15%, and Medicare pays 80%. Unfortunately, the donut hole is the time in which patients often stop taking their medications because they cannot afford them. Once the new year starts, the cycle begins again where the patient returns to paying 25%. To help patients through the donut hole of coverage, there are drug coupons and rebates available. This donut hole will be eliminated by 2019.

Copayments

A different shared approach to payment is the **copayment (copay)**. It is a flat out-of-pocket fee that the patient is required to pay for each drug product at time of delivery. For instance, a copay could be $20 per office visit and $10 per generic prescription. The remaining costs would either be covered by the insurance company or by the patient until the annual deductible level is reached, when the insurance will pay a higher percentage of the costs.

Prescription drug insurance companies also often have a tiered copay system, such as a **dual copay** with one flat fee for generic drugs versus another fee for brand name drugs. There can also be a three- or four-tiered copay program from least expensive to most, having different copays for generics, preferred brands, nonpreferred brands, and specialty drugs. (A drug not listed in the insurance formulary is most likely not covered at all.) For example, for the treatment of erectile dysfunction, a PBM may elect to cover the generic drug sildenafil at a $10 copay. However, Cialis (the

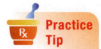
Practice Tip

You can direct patients to look for the most up-to-date information on their insurers' preferred drugs on the insurance websites.

preferred brand name drug) may have a $40 copay, and Levitra (the nonpreferred brand name drug), a $100 copay. Most insurance plans cover only a 30-day supply of a brand name medication in a community pharmacy. Sometimes a 90-day supply will be covered at a cost-saving copay if the PBM's mail-order pharmacy is used. Some PBMs have a maximum drug count for a 30-day supply; for example, triptans, prescribed for migraine headaches, are often limited to nine tablets per month.

Inputting Insurance Information

After reviewing a new prescription or refill order, the technician is responsible for updating any changes to the patient's demographic and insurance information. If a patient has more than one prescription insurance plan or coupons/manufacturer discounts, *the technician needs to enter all payment data before submitting the claim.* A new patient to the pharmacy should be asked for all payment sources prior to filling the prescription.

Verifying patient insurance information up front reduces unnecessary requests to insurers, which reduces the pharmacy's investment in terms of time and money, and decreases customer wait time. To begin the process, the technician asks for the customer's insurance card to input the information into the computer (or double-check it with the existing profile), including the following (see Figure 10.1):

FIGURE 10.1

Parts of an Insurance Identification Card

In this example, the mother is the primary insurance holder for her four children, the insurer is Central Healthcare, and the employer is UDrug.

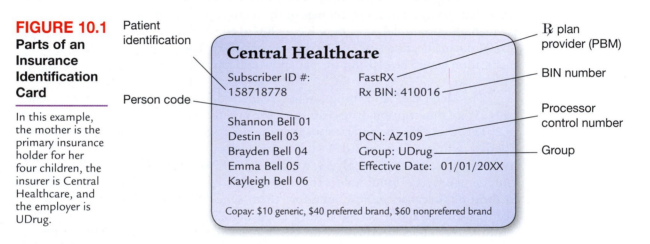

- name of the insured person and the primary insurance carrier along with other family members covered (sometimes)
- insurance carrier
- patient identification number (ID)—9 digits designating the insurance holder
- person code—2 or 3 digits indicating the relationship to insurance holder
- group number—designating the employer
- bank identification number (BIN)—6 digits designating the pharmacy benefits manager
- processor control number (PCN)—designating the kind of plan and processing flow
- the date coverage became effective
- the amount of the copay for generic and brand name prescriptions (and other tier payments)

Study Idea

Review the card information needed to process an insurance claim for a prescription.

The patients listed on the card all have the same first nine digits for their ID number. The primary insurance holder will have the person code after the ID of 01 (or 001), and the spouse will have the code of 02 (or 002). The numbers for dependent children would end with 03 (003), 04 (004), 05 (005), and so on, generally in their birth order. Always double-check that the right person code was entered. Most Medicare Part D and Medicaid cards, however, have a full patient-specific ID number, so there is no need for an additional person code.

Insurance card formats are not standardized, so getting all the necessary information may not be easy. For repeat or returning customers, you must ask if any information has changed, and if the card is still up-to-date, check the card's expiration date. If the cardholder's employment status has changed, the drug insurance on the profile will likely have changed. A patient may be dual eligible, having more than one insurer. If so, the information on both cards must be entered in the patient profile, *designating which insurer is the primary carrier and which is the secondary (and sometimes even tertiary).*

The BIN and PCN identify the correct pharmacy benefits manager (PBM) and the internal processing code for this patient's particular plan. (Some insurance cards do not list a PCN, making the technician's job a little more difficult.) Insurance and Medicaid-funded programs may switch PBMs within the calendar year without patient notice or issuance of a new insurance card, so *PBM information must be identified and updated with each patient visit.*

Study Idea

Coordination of benefits requires the technician to determine the sequence of billing for maximum reimbursement.

To electronically process a workers' compensation insurance claim, you must ask for additional information to enter into the patient profile. Besides the BIN, PCN, and group number, *you will need the Social Security number, date of injury, and name of compensating business.* Worker's compensation may not be billed to the same insurance as the employee's health insurance, and the technician will need to check with the employer for directions for billing the claim.

Coordination of Benefits

When the patients have more than one type of insurance, the technician has to make sure that both types of insurance are entered in the proper sequence in the patient profile to allow for the **coordination of benefits (COB)**, or proper order of claims processing. Once the primary insurance acknowledges acceptance and payment, the secondary insurance is automatically billed for further payment or to establish the patient's final copayment. Technicians need to remember that when a patient has two insurance policies and one is a state-funded Medicaid insurance program, *the Medicaid is always the secondary insurance* (or third). Legally, Medicaid cannot be billed until the primary insurance carrier has paid.

Coordinating benefits for workers' compensation can be even more complicated. The patient may have multiple claims to process at the same time—some drugs must be billed to workers' compensation, whereas other selected drugs must be sent to the patient's normal primary insurer's PBM, and if there is anything left, to the patient's original secondary insurance.

Online Claims Submission

When entering and submitting prescriptions into the pharmacy software for the drug utilization review (DUR), the software or technician transmits the prescription online to the PBM to complete the crucial online insurance **adjudication**. This process of adjudication electronically submits the prescription billing claims to the appropriate PBM for its judgment on whether or not it will provide reimbursement. The PBM online response then states the proportion of the pharmacy reimbursement as compared to the AWP and the patient's immediate portion. It usually takes less than 30 seconds to receive a reply. Usually, the message comes back from the PBM confirming payment of a claim, also known as **claim capturing**. The adjudication usually includes information on preferred formulary products that will lower the copayment or the adjusted copayment for certain choices. Pharmacy technicians and pharmacists *should look at the claim capture screen and make sure the pharmacy is not losing money on the transaction*. If this is the case, alert the pharmacist so another product or generic can be suggested or substituted based on the patient's policy.

Rejected Claims

Rejection messages can appear, often accompanied by a "reject code." Claims get rejected for many reasons, including problems with missing or mistyped information, wrong birthdate, wrong name, wrong dosages, or special medications requiring prior authorization (PA). Pharmacy and insurance software programs use the codes from the National Council for Prescription Drug Programs (NCPDP) linked with more specific codes and descriptive messages. For examples of the NCPCP codes that may appear on the screen with another software program, see Table 10.2. Each rejection message requires its own response action to resolve the problem. If such questions about coverage arise, the technician should use the appropriate (toll-free) insurance or PBM contact phone number.

Formulary Issues A common message for any brand or high-cost medication is *NDC Not Covered*. When this message or *Not an Option* appears on the screen in adjudication, it means that this particular drug with its National Drug Code is not covered by the PBM formulary. You can then present the following options to the patient: (1) he or she can pay the out-of-pocket costs if not too exorbitant, (2) you can keep the prescription on file for a later date, (3) the patient can call the prescriber and request a less costly alternative if available, or (4) the pharmacist can discuss the situation with the patient and then call the prescriber with recommendations for alternative options or prior authorization if that is needed.

Prior Authorization The alert *Requires Prior Authorization* may pop up. Then the pharmacy technician may need to notify the prescriber's office of the rejected claim to allow the prescriber to seek **prior authorization (PA)** from the insurance company or PBM for a nonformulary medication. For example, a prescriber might request prior authorization for the brand Lipitor because the patient had an allergic reaction to the generic atorvastatin. In this situation, the prescriber would contact the insurance plan either by phone, email, or in writing to request coverage of the more expensive brand name drug. The PBM has physician, nurse, and pharmacist consultants on staff who review each case to determine the merits and approve or deny payment.

Cases exist in which the medication selected by the physician is not covered by the insurance under any circumstances—not even with a prior approval. This lack of coverage often applies to new innovative drugs that are extremely expensive, drugs that promote weight loss or sleep, certain medications for anxiety or nervous disorders, certain cough syrups for adults, and drugs that have less costly alternatives or are available as OTC drugs. If the insurer denies coverage, the patient has the right to appeal by calling the appropriate (toll-free) insurance contact phone number. This is not done by the technician or pharmacist but by the patient (it takes time and much paperwork). However, the technician generally must break this news to the patient. In most cases, the patient pays cash or uses a discount card if eligible.

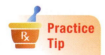

TABLE 10.2 Samples of Third-Party Payer Reject Error Codes from The National Council for Prescription Drug Programs (NCPDP)

NCPDP Error Code	NCPDP Error Code Description	PROMISe Code	Some of the PROMISe Electronic System Code Description Options for each NCPDP Code
1	M/I BIN	4178	Invalid bin number
5	M/I Pharmacy Number	201	Billing provider number is missing from claim
7	M/I Cardholder ID Number	203	Date of service prior to card issue date
		204	Recipient ID number is invalid or not found on CIS
16	M/I Prescription/Service Reference Number	212	Invalid Rx number submitted
		5021	Same provider, service location, dose & Rx # in history
17	M/I Fill Number	211	Refill number not valid
		5006	Maximum number of refills has been exceeded for Rx
19	M/I Days Supply	221	Days supply missing
		222	Days supply invalid
25	M/I Prescriber ID	206	Prescriber practitioner license number is not in valid format
		1025	Prescribing license not valid
75	Prior Authorization Required	3000	PA number invalid format
		4003	Drug indicated has been identified as less than effective
		4088	Prior authorization required for more than three tablets of OxyContin per day
		4266	Daily dosage exceeds limit for emergency claim
		7101	DUR plus Lipitor 80 mg

Often, only the information shown in red below is returned to pharmacies when billing electronically. M/I means "Missing/Invalid." PROMISe™ is a common claims processing and management information system that provides additional information and subcodes for each specific claim error type. The state of Pennsylvania uses NCPDP PROMISe and offers a guide to the crosswalk between the two systems. For complete listing, go to http://CertExam4e .ParadgimEducation.com/PROMISe.

Web

Prescribers' National Provider Identifier Issues The correct **National Provider Identifier (NPI) number** is required for the prescriptions from each physician, physician assistant, nurse practitioner, dentist, and pharmacist to be legitimate and processed. (Nurse practitioners or physician assistants may use the NPI number of their supervising physicians with their knowledge and approval.) These NPI numbers must always be carefully checked to ensure that they match up with the prescribers' names. In the case of controlled medications, the prescriber must also have a DEA (Drug Enforcement Administration) number on file in order for the claim to be processed and billed.

Out-of-Network Prescriber In rare cases, the claim can even be rejected because the prescriber is not contracted with the patient's insurance plan (as with Medicaid).

In this case, another prescriber or supervising physician in the network must be contacted by phone, and that prescriber must agree to put his or her name on the prescription (except for controlled substances) to process the claim. If the pharmacist or pharmacy technician can identify no alternative prescriber, the patient must pay cash for the prescriptions.

Drug Interactions and Combination Rejections There are also the DUR rejections where the PBM software compares the prescriptions with the patient's PBM medication profile and finds that the patient is receiving more than one similar medication, such as two antibiotics at the same time. Or it could be that the drug may interfere with another prescribed drug (a drug interaction) or produce an allergic reaction. In these cases, the technician must alert the pharmacist to carefully review the rejection. The pharmacist may choose to override the rejection with the computer software. If not, the PBM and/or prescriber must be notified.

Refill Too Soon Refills with most insurers can be processed within five to seven days of the end date of the current medication (based on days supply), but some plans are more restrictive. Then you may get the *Refill Too Soon* message. You can then tell the patient the exact date the insurance claim can be processed.

Incorrect Days Supply A rejection may also be due to an incorrect amount for **days supply**—the amount of medication required to last for the duration of the prescription. If you make a mistake in calculating or inputting the days supply, or if the PBM only permits a limited portion at a time, the claim will be rejected.

Calculating Days Supply

Calculating the days supply of a medication accurately is an important skill to prevent the rejection of claims. The following examples show how to calculate medication amounts and days supply for sample prescriptions.

Example 10.1

A prescription is received for:

> ℞ **Ciprofloxacin 500 mg.**
> **Take one tablet twice daily for 2 weeks**

What is the days supply?

2 tablets/day × 14 days = 28; This equals 28 tablets/14 days.
The days supply is 28 tablets for the two weeks.

Example 10.2

How many days will the following medication last?

> ℞ **Hydrocodone/APAP in a strength of 5 mg/325 mg #90.**
> **Take 1 tablet every 4 to 6 hours prn for pain.**

Step 1 Calculate the maximum number of tablets taken each day. If the patient takes 1 tablet every 4 hours for 24 hours, it means 24 ÷ 4 = 6. A maximum of 6 tablets could be taken in a day.

Step 2 Assuming the patient takes all 6 tablets per day, calculate the number of days the supply shall last.

$$90 \text{ tablets} \div 6 \text{ tablets/day} = 15 \text{ days}$$
$$\text{or} \quad 90 \text{ tablets} \times 1 \text{ day/6 tablets} = 15 \text{ days}$$

This means that a new prescription cannot be filled—or the claim processed—prior to 15 days from the date of initial dispensing.

Example 10.3

A patient is prescribed to take 40 units of Humulin N NPH insulin in the morning and 25 units before dinner. This insulin is U-100 and is available in a 10 mL vial (1,000 units per 10 mL, or 1,000 units per vial). The prescription is written to dispense 2 vials at a time. How many days will the prescribed medication last?

Step 1 Calculate the total daily dose of insulin.

40 units + 25 units = 65 units; 65 units are needed per day.

Step 2 Calculate the number of days that 2 vials will fulfill using dimensional analysis:

$$2 \text{ vials} \times \frac{1,000 \text{ units}}{\text{vial}} \times \frac{1 \text{ day}}{65 \text{ units}} = 30.769, \text{ or a 31 days supply.}$$

If you mistakenly input a 56-day supply in the prescription (28 days for each vial instead of 2 vials for 30 days) for insurance processing, the initial claim will be processed; however, the patient will not be able to get a needed refill after 30 days without the pharmacist calling the insurance provider to change and correct the original prescription claim.

Example 10.4

A prescription is received for:

> ℞ **Augmentin 250 mg/5 mL. Give 3/4 teaspoonful twice daily for 10 days.**

Augmentin is a brand suspension available as a generic suspension of amoxicillin and clavulanate potassium in quantities of 75 mL, 100 mL, and 150 mL. What is the days supply? What size bottle should be used? How much dispensed product will be unused?

Step 1 Calculate volume taken in each dose by converting 3/4 teaspoonful to milliliters (mL).

One tsp = 5 mL, and $^3/_4$ tsp = 0.75 tsp.

$$\frac{\text{1 tsp}}{\text{5 mL}} = \frac{\text{0.75 tsp}}{\textbf{\textit{y}} \text{ mL}}; \quad \textbf{\textit{y}} \textbf{ mL} = \textbf{5 mL} \times \textbf{0.75}; \quad y \text{ mL} = 3.75 \text{ mL}$$

Step 2 Calculate the amount of drug prescribed per day.

$$\frac{2 \text{ doses}}{\text{day}} \times \frac{3.75 \text{ mL}}{\text{dose}} = 7.5 \text{ mL/day}$$

Step 3 According to the prescription, the days supply is for 10 days. Calculate total volume needed for the days supply.

$$\frac{7.5 \text{ mL}}{\text{day}} \times 10 \text{ days} = 75 \text{ mL}$$

Step 4 Select the bottle size from the available stock, and determine how much product will remain after the patient takes the prescribed amount. Because Augmentin comes in 75 mL, 100 mL, and 150 mL bottles, the 75 mL bottle will be selected. Because the bottle amount equals the prescribed amount, none of the drug will be left over.

75 mL (dispensed amount) − 75 mL (prescribed amount) = 0 mL unused medication

Otic and Ophthalmic Calculation Challenges

Certain drug formulations, such as ear (otic) and ophthalmic solutions and suspensions, are particularly challenging to calculate when determining days supply. Many are available in both a solution and a suspension formulation. When calculating drops for a *solution*, the standard measure is equivalent to 20 drops per mL. For example, suppose that a prescription was written for Cortisporin otic solution, *4 drops into affected ear 3 times a day for 7 days*, or 12 drops daily for 7 days. That would equal 84 solution drops. The 5 mL package size (providing 100 drops) would be dispensed.

However, suspension drops, because they are thicker in density, have fewer drops per mL than solutions. In the past, the measure was 16 drops of suspension to 1 mL, but since IV drops go in rates of 10, 15, and 20 gtt (drops) per minute, there has been a movement toward standardization to round down the measurement to 15 drops of suspension per mL rather than round up to 16. The suspension drop rate now depends on individual pharmacy and insurance reimbursement policies, but most often it is 15 gtt/mL.

Study Idea

Practice calculating the number of drops in different solutions and suspension using 20 drops per mL of solution and 15 drops per mL of suspension.

Example 10.5

The pharmacy receives a prescription for:

> ℞ **Augmentin 125 mg/5 mL. 1 tsp tid for 7 days.**

The insurance will not cover this strength of 125 mg/5 mL but will cover Augmentin 250 mg/5 mL. Augmentin suspensions are available in 50 mL, 75 mL, and 100 mL bottles. If the substitution to the insured strength is made, which bottle size will be dispensed, what will the new sig be, and how much should remain after seven days?

Step 1 Since 1 tsp equals 5 mL, one dose of the prescribed Augmentin would equal the 125 mg. Calculate the volume of Augmentin 250 mg/5 mL needed to provide the prescribed 125 mg dose. Set up adimensional analysis equation multiplying the prescribed strength by the number of mL of insured concentration:

$$y \text{ mL} = 125 \text{ mg} \times \frac{5 \text{ mL}}{250 \text{ mg}} = 2.5 \text{ mL}$$

$$y \text{ mL} = 2.5 \text{ mL}$$

(measured with a dosing spoon instead of a teaspoon)

The sig in the computer prescription must be changed to read "Take 2.5 mL 3 times daily for 7 days."

Step 2 Calculate the volume needed per day for seven days.

$$2.5 \text{ mL} \times \frac{3}{\text{day}} \times 7 \text{ days} = 52.5 \text{ mL}$$

Step 3 Select the 75 mL bottle of Augmentin and subtract the days supply of 52.5 mL

$$75 \text{ mL} - 52.5 \text{ mL} = 22.5 \text{ mL}$$

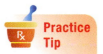

Practice Tip

A metric dosing spoon should be dispensed with oral solutions and suspensions.

That means 22.5 mL will remain. Some overage is allowed by insurance) so this bottle is appropriate. If you incorrectly chose the 50 mL size, there would not be enough and if you chose the 100 mL size, then 47.5 mL would be wasted, and the claim would likely not be processed. Or if it were approved, the claim could be reversed so the pharmacy would not be reimbursed for dispensing more medication than necessary.

Resolving Claim Issues

There are times when a claim is approved online, and the prescription is filled and picked up, but later the PBM refuses to pay the claim. The technician is often involved in resolving these "post-claim" functions: chargebacks and audits. With each reimbursement check, automatic deposit, or claim refusal, there comes an **explanation of benefits (EOB)** by the PBM to delineate what has been paid and what has not and why.

Study Idea

EOBs should each be reviewed for any listings of reversals of claims the pharmacy had thought were captured and for which the pharmacy was expecting money.

Chargebacks

If the PBM representative feels that it has overpaid or paid something in error, it may charge back or deduct this amount from what it owes the pharmacy in reimbursement. The notice comes in an EOB along with the pharmacy reimbursement check or automatic deposit receipt. Each EOB should be reviewed carefully for chargebacks. A chargeback is a post-claim rejection of a prescription claim by a PBM or insurance provider that must be investigated and, if possible, resolved by the pharmacy technician. A chargeback could occur for a number of reasons:

- The certificate of medical necessity for diabetic supplies was not completed properly (missing a diagnostic code or frequency direction, as for blood sugar testing strips), or a signed renewal from the doctor was not obtained for a Medicare Part B claim.

- Online processing was not functioning because of an Internet malfunction, and it was determined later that the patient was ineligible for drug insurance benefits.

- The primary insurer of a "dual eligible" patient was not billed or was billed second instead of first.

- A prescription was also filled at another pharmacy. (Then the patient may need to be billed, and a flag put on the patient file to prevent repetition of this.)

In each case, to challenge or resolve the chargeback, the technician must verify the details of the original prescription and supplemental documentation, patient profile, and adjudication process. You must retrieve documentation on whether or not the patient actually received the prescription (by written or computer receipt) to figure out the inconsistences and perhaps fix the errors. If the chargeback is not resolved in a timely manner, then the pharmacy loses that money.

Pharmacy Benefits Manager Audits

If there are a number of chargebacks or unresolved claims, the PBM might initiate an **audit**, or an assessment of the pharmacy's prescription records to challenge problems (as is done by the IRS in a tax audit). These challenges can be from prescriptions processed three to six months earlier or even two to three years ago. A community (or mail-order) pharmacy is also subject to periodic PBM medication audits. The audit is commonly conducted via the mail, but occasionally a PBM representative will personally investigate past claims on-site. Audits are intended to reduce fraud and waste.

Filing a false claim is considered **insurance fraud**. It is subject to civil and criminal penalties if it is confirmed, as well as employment termination. For example, a pharmacy technician cannot dispense a medication to a patient and then post or bill the insurance three days later when the prescription refill is allowed. Instead, you must direct the patient to return in three days to pick up the medication after the insurance approves it. If it is an emergency and the patient has (or will) run out of medication (because it was lost or spilled, or the patient will be on vacation) before the current prescription duration runs out, you may request an override from the PBM, or the patient can pay cash for a small supply of the medication.

Medication Assistance

As a technician, there are steps to take specifically when someone comes in with a prescription that he or she can't afford. Some technicians in large chain pharmacies even find themselves specializing in this area.

Sometimes drug companies offer discount coupons for their products to prescribers or providers. Pharmacy technicians, patients, or their family members can check at their store or online, or call the provider's office to see if they have any coupons available. In addition, many high-cost brand name drugs have "patient assistance" discount programs online to cover all or a portion of a drug's cost, often in combination with programs from the primary insurer.

There are also many prescription **discount cards** available in the mail or distributed as charity fund raisers. Many of these cards do not reimburse the pharmacy sufficiently to cover expenses, so they may not be accepted, depending on store policy. The conditions for the discount card or coupon (including expiration date, amount of drug allowed, and so on) must be carefully reviewed by the pharmacy technician. Some cards need to be activated by the patient prior to use.

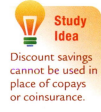

Some pharmacies occasionally advertise a list of "free" or low-cost ($4) prescriptions, usually for short-term antibiotic therapies. These medications are known within the trade as **loss leaders**—the community pharmacy chooses to lose or break even on these drugs offered at the lowered prices to entice consumers to visit the store and buy more groceries or merchandise. Technicians can watch for these loss leaders and inform their customers.

As a benefit to customers who pay for prescriptions on their own, some pharmacies offer a prescription savings club card for individuals and families (including pets). Many pharmacies offer senior citizen discounts for purchases not covered by insurance.

Technicians may also refer patients to free or low-cost charity clinics voluntarily staffed by doctors, nurses, dentists, and pharmacists, offering medical, dental, or even pharmacy services. If the community health center does have a pharmacy, the patient could qualify to get prescription drugs at government pricing through the federally funded 340B Drug Discount Program. Some clinics have drugs and services available for free or at low cost because of donor and grant support. The pharmacy technician can make the patient aware of the location and hours of operation of these clinics and encourage patients to see if they qualify for assistance.

It is estimated that one-third of patients are not taking their required medications to control their diseases. If patients stop refilling their prescriptions due to high costs, they may be not only jeopardizing their health but also increasing costs to the healthcare system. You may be able help some individuals who cannot afford to take care of their health by processing their insurance claims and finding them feasible ways to pay for the drugs they need.

STUDY SUMMARY

Billing and reimbursement are critical to the cash flow of the community pharmacy. Hospitals and other healthcare institutions have whole billing departments to deal with this, and the pharmacy technician does not get involved. However, in the community pharmacy, it is important for you to realize the importance of accurate cash register keying for the purpose of taxing products, reordering, and crediting correct departments. Since most patients have insurance to assist with the payment of their prescriptions, you must be able to identify key information on the insurance card, enter it into the patient's profile, and handle online adjudication messages.

The certification exam will expect you to know how to accurately calculate the days supply. Sometimes insurance companies will reverse the payment they provided for a prescription, and these chargebacks must be assessed for accuracy so they can be resubmitted as corrected claims in a timely manner, or the pharmacy will lose money. Insurance companies may audit the pharmacy if they have concerns about the accuracy of the claims billing. You will need to become versed in the requirements of the various insurance programs, especially those run by the government, and be ready to direct patients who do not have the ability to pay for their medications to assistance programs and options.

ADDITIONAL RESOURCES

For more in-depth explanations, check out *Pharmacy Practice for Technicians*, 6e from Paradigm Education Solutions. To master and extend the material presented in this chapter, take advantage of the resources available through the eBook resources links. These include digital supplements, study resources, and a practice exam generator with 1,000+ exam-style questions. End-of-chapter tests are accessible through the eBook for individuals using the self-study course and through Navigator+ for individuals enrolled in the instructor-guided course.

FINAL TEST AND EXAM GENERATOR

Once you've finished your last chapter test, take your final course test through the eBook (self-study students) or the Navigator+ Learning Management System. There is even more you can do to feel confident for your certification exam—test yourself with timed practice exams that simulate the same number of questions per domain as the PTCE with Paradigm's own exam generator (drawing from 1,000+ exam-like questions written by experts) accessed through the eBook link.

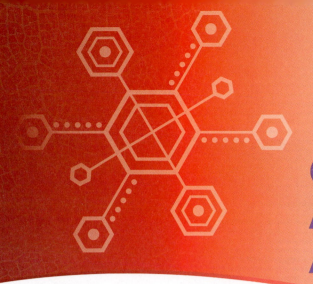

Appendix **A**

Common Pharmacy Abbreviations and Acronyms

The abbreviations with red lines through them are ones that are still in use but are discouraged by Institute for Safe Medication Practices (ISMP). The ISMP recommends the use of the correct words instead. Many of these discouraged abbreviations are also on The Joint Commission's Official "Do Not Use" List of Abbreviations.

Abbreviation	Meaning
A-B-C	
aaa	apply to affected area
ACA	Affordable Care Act (Patient Protection and Affordable Care Act)
~~ac; a.c.; AC~~	before meals
ACE	angiotensin-converting enzyme inhibitors
~~ad; a.d.; AD~~	right ear
ADD	attention-deficit disorder
ADH	antidiuretic hormone
ADHD	attention-deficit hyperactivity disorder
ADME	absorption, distribution, metabolism, and elimination
ADR	adverse drug reaction
AIDS	acquired immune deficiency syndrome
AM; a.m.	morning
ANDA	Abbreviated New Drug Application
APAP	acetaminophen; Tylenol
AphA	American Pharmacy Association
ARBs	angiotensin receptor blockers
~~as; a.s.; AS~~	left ear
ASA	aspirin
~~au; a.u.; AU~~	both ears; each ear
b.i.d.; BID	twice daily
BMI	Body Mass Index
BP	blood pressure
BUD	beyond-use date
°C	degrees centigrade; temperature in degrees centigrade
Ca⁺⁺	calcium

249

Abbreviation	Meaning
Cap; cap	capsule
CDC	Centers for Disease Control and Prevention
CF	cystic fibrosis
CHF	congestive heart failure
CNS	Central Nervous System
COPD	chronic obstructive pulmonary disease
CPR	cardio pulminary resuscitation
CSP	compounded sterile preparation
CV	cardiovascular
D-E-F	
D_5; D_5W; D5W	dextrose 5% in water
D_5 ¼; D5 1/4	dextrose 5% in ¼ normal saline; dextrose 5% in 0.225% sodium chloride
D_5 ⅓; D5 1/3	dextrose 5% in ⅓ normal saline; dextrose 5% in 0.33% sodium chloride
D_5 ½; D5 1/2	dextrose 5% in ½ normal saline; dextrose 5% in 0.45% sodium chloride
D_5LR; D5LR	dextrose 5% in lactated Ringer's solution
D_5NS; D5NS	dextrose 5% in normal saline; dextrose 5% in 0.9% sodium chloride
DAW	dispense as written
DC; d/c	discontinue
D/C	discharge
DCA	direct compounding area
Dig	digoxin
disp	dispense
EC	enteric-coated
Elix	elixir
eMAR	electronic medication administration record
EPO	epoetin alfa; erythropoietin
ER; XR; XL	extended-release
°F	degrees Fahrenheit; temperature in degrees Fahrenheit
$FeSO_4$	ferrous sulfate; iron
G-H-I	
g, G	gram
gr	grain
GI	gastrointestinal
GMP	good manufacturing practice
gtt; gtts	drop; drops
h; hr	hour
HC	hydrocortisone
HCTZ	hydrochlorothiazide
HIPAA	Health Insurance Portability and Accountability Act
HIV	human immunodeficiency virus
HMO	Health Maintenance Organization
HRT	hormone replacement therapy

Abbreviation	Meaning
h.s.; HS	bedtime (comes from Latin *hora somni* meaning "hour of sleep"); hs should also not be used
IBU	ibuprofen; Motrin
ICU	intensive care unit
IM	intramuscular
IND	Investigational New Drug Application
Inj; IJ	injection
IPA	isopropyl alcohol
ISDN	isosorbide dinitrate
ISMO	isosorbide mononitrate
ISMP	Institute for Safe Medication Practices
IV	intravenous
IVF	intravenous fluid
IVP	intravenous push
IVPB	intravenous piggyback
J-K-L	
K; K+	potassium
KCl	potassium chloride
kg	kilogram
L	liter
LAFW	laminar airflow workbench; hood
lb	pound
LD	loading dose
LVP	large-volume parenteral
JCAHO	Joint Commission on the Accreditation of Healthcare Organizations
M-N-O	
Mag; Mg; MAG	magnesium
MAR	medication administration record
mcg	microgram
MDI	metered-dose inhaler
MDV	multiple-dose vial
mEq	milliequivalent
mg	milligram
MgSO$_4$	magnesium sulfate; magnesium
mL	milliliter
mL/hr	milliliters per hour
mL/min	milliliters per minute

Abbreviation	Meaning
MMR	measles, mumps, and rubella vaccine
MRSA	methiciliin-resistant S. aureaus
MOM; M.O.M.	milk of magnesia
M.S.	morphine sulfate (save MS for multiple sclerosis)
MU†; mu	million units
MVI; MVI-12	multiple vitamin injection; multivitamins for parenteral administration
Na⁺	sodium
NABP	National Association of Boards of Pharmacy
NaCl	sodium chloride; salt
NDA	New Drug App
NDC	National Drug Code
NF; non-form	nonformulary
NKA	no known allergies
NKDA	no known drug allergies
NPO; npo	nothing by mouth
NR; d.n.r.	no refills; do not repeat
NS	normal saline; 0.9% sodium chloride
½ NS	one-half normal saline; 0.45% sodium chloride
¼ NS	one-quarter normal saline; 0.225% sodium chloride
NSAID	nonsteroidal anti-inflammatory drug
NTG	nitroglycerin
OC	oral contraceptive
od; o.d.; OD	right eye
ODT	orally disintegrating tablet
OPTH; OPHTH; Opth	ophthalmic
os; o.s.; OS	left eye
OTC	over the counter; no prescription required
ou; o.u.; OU	both eyes; each eye
oz	ounce
P-Q-R	
p.c.; PC	after meals
PCA	patient-controlled anesthesia
PCN	penicillin
pH	acid-base balance
PHI	protected health information
PM; p.m.	afternoon; evening
PN	paternal nutrition

Abbreviation	Meaning
PNS	peripheral nervous system
PO; po	orally; by mouth
PPE	personal protective equipment
PPI	proton pump inhibitor
PR	per rectum; rectally
PRN; p.r.n.	as needed; as occasion requires
PTSD	Post Traumatic Stress Disorder
PV	per vagina; vaginally
PVC	polyvinyl chloride
q	every
q.h.; qhour	every hour
q2h	every 2 hours
q4h	every 4 hours
q6h	every 6 hours
q8h	every 8 hours
q12h	every 12 hours
q24h	every 24 hours
q48h	every 48 hours
QA	quality assurance
QAM; qam	every morning
qDay; QD; Qd	every day
q.i.d.; QID	four times daily
QOD; Q other day; Q.O. Day	every other day
QPM; qpm	every evening
qs; qsad	quantity sufficient; a sufficient quantity to make
QTY; qty	quantity
qwk; qweek	every week
RA	rheumatoid arthritis
RDA	recommended daily allowance
Rx	prescription; pharmacy; medication; drug; recipe; take
S-T	
sig	write on label; signa; directions
SL; sub-L	sublingual
SMZ-TMP	sulfamethoxazole and trimethoprim; Bactrim
SNRI	serotonin nonrepinephrine reuptake inhibitor
SPF	sunburn protection factor

Abbreviation	Meaning
SR	sustained-release
~~SS; ss~~	one-half
SSRI	selective serotonin reuptake inhibitor (don't use for sliding scale insulins)
STAT; Stat	immediately; now
STD	sexually transmitted disease
~~Sub-Q; SC; SQ; sq,~~ subcut, SUBCUT	subcutaneous
SUPP; Supp	suppository
susp	suspension
SVP	small-volume parenteral
SW	sterile water
SWFI	sterile water for injection
Tab; tab	tablet
TB	tuberculosis
TBSP; tbsp	tablespoon; tablespoonful; 15 mL
TDS	transdermal delivery system
t.i.d.; TID	three times daily
~~t.i.w.; TIW~~	three times a week
TKO; TKVO; KO; KVO	to keep open; to keep vein open; keep open; keep vein open (a slow IV flow rate)
TNA	Total Nutrition Admixture
TPN	total parenteral nutrition
TSP; tsp	teaspoon; teaspoonful; 5 mL
U-V-W	
~~U or u~~	unit
~~u.d., UD, ut dictum~~	as directed
ung	ointment
USP	U.S. Pharmacopoeial Convention
USP-NF	*U.S. Pharmacopoeia-National Formulary*
UTI	urinary tract infection
UV	ultraviolet light
VAG; vag	vagina; vaginally
Vanco	vancomycin
VO; V.O.; V/O	verbal order
w/o	without
X-Y-Z	
Zn	zinc, but ~~$ZnSO_4$~~—should not be used for zinc sulfate
Z-Pak	azithromycin; Zithromax

Appendix B

Commonly Prescribed Controlled Substances

Commonly Prescribed Controlled Substances

Generic	Brand Examples	Used For
Schedule II		
amobarbital	Amytal, Tuinal	Sedative, analgesic
amphetamine/dextroamphetamine	Adderall	ADHD/narcolepsy
cocaine topical	C-Topical Solution	Nose bleed, vasoconstriction
codeine**		Analgesic
dexmethylphenidate	Focalin	ADHD
fentanyl	Duragesic, Sublimaze	Narcotic analgesic
fentanyl patch	Duragesic	Analgesic
glutethimide	Doriden, Dorimide	Hypnotic sedative
hydrocodone* (with cough/cold ingredients)	Vicotuss	Cough/cold relief
hydrocodone/APAP	Vicodin, Lortab, Norco	Analgesic
hydromorphone	Dilaudid, Exalgo, Palladone	Analgesic (for severe pain)
lisdexamfetamine	Vyvanse	ADHD
meperidine	Demerol	Narcotic analgesic
methadone	Dolophine	Analgesic
methadone	Methadose	Opioid maintenance
methamphetamine	Desoxyn	Weight reduction
methylphenidate CR	Concerta, Metadate, Ritalin LA	ADHD
methylphenidate	Ritalin	ADHD
morphine	MS Contin, Roxanol, Oramorph, RMS, MSIR	Analgesic

opium	Tincture of Opium	Antidiarrhea
oxycodone	OxyContin, ~~Percocet~~	Analgesic
oxycodone/APAP	Percocet, Tylox	Analgesic
Oxycodone/ASA	Percodan	Analgesic
oxymorphone	Opana	Analgesic
pentobarbital	Nembutal	Sedative, hypnotic, anti-anxiety, anticonvulsant
tapentadol	Nucynta	Analgesic

Schedule III

anabolic steroids (such as testosterone cypionate)	Depo-Testosterone	Various indications, depends on steroid
armodadinil	Nuvigil	Stimulant
ASA/butabital/caffeine	Fiorinal	Migraine relief
ASA/butabital/caffeine/Codeine	Fiorinal with codeine	Migraine relief
ASA/codeine	Empirin with Codeine	Analgesic
benzphetamine	Didrex, Recede	Appetite suppressant
buprenorphine	Subutex, Butrans	Opioid maintenance
buprenorphine/naloxone	Suboxone, Zubsolv	Opioid maintenance
butorphanol	Stadol	Analgesic
codeine/APAP	Tylenol No. 3	Analgesic
dronabinol	Marinol	Appetite stimulant
esterilfied estrogen/testosterone	Estratest	Hormone replacement
hydrocodone/chlorpheniramine	Tussionex	Cough suppressant, antihistamine
ketamine	Ketaset, Ketalar, Special K	Dissociative anesthetic
phendimetrazine	Plegine, Prelu-2, Bontril, Melfiat, Statobex	Appetite suppressant
testosterone	AndroGel, Testim	Low testosterone
thiopental	Pentothal	Anesthetic

Schedule IV

alprazolam	Xanax	Anti-anxiety, benzodiazepine
APAP/dichloralphenazone/isometheptane	Midrin, Epidrin	Migraine relief
carisoprodol	Soma	Muscle relaxer
chlordiazepoxide	Librium	Anti-anxiety, benzodiazepine
clidinium/chlordiazepoxide	Librax	GI antispasmotic
clonazepam	Klonopin	Anticonvulsant. Benzodiazepine

clorazepate	Tranxene	Sedative, anti-anxiety
diazepam	Valium, Diastat	Anti-anxiety, anticonvulsant, benzodiazepine
eszopiclone	Lunesta	Hypnotic
flurazepam	Dalmane	Hypnotic
lorazepam	Ativan	Anti-anxiety, benzodiazepine
meprobamate	Miltown, Equanil	Anti-anxiety
midazolam	Versed	Sedative
modafinil	Provigil	Stimulant
Oxazepam	Serax	Anti-anxiety, benzodiazepine
phenobarbital	Luminal	Anticonvulsant
phentermine	Adipex, Fastin	Appetite suppressant
propoxyphene	Darvon	Analgesic
propoxyphene/APAP	Darvocet	Analgesic
quazepam	Doral	Anti-anxiety, benzodiazepine
sibutramine	Meridia	Weight loss
suvorexant	Belsomra	Hypnotic
temazepam	Restoril	Hypnotic
tramadol	Ultram	Analgesic
triazolam	Halcion	Sedative, hypnotic
zaleplon	Sonata	Hypnotic
zolpidem	Ambien	Hypnotic

Schedule V

atropine/diphenoxylate	Lomotil	Antidiarrheal
codeine***	Robitussin AC, Phenergan with Codeine, and others	Cough suppressant, nasal congestion, upper respiratory tract concerns
ezogabine	Potiga	Anticonvulsant
lacosamide	Vimpat	Anticonvulsant
pregabalin	Lyrica	Neuropathic pain

Note: Information updated as of August 2016. New drugs come in often. Visit http://www.deadiversion.usdoj.gov/schedules/ for the updated list.

* Combination products containing hydrocodone are Schedule II as of 2014

** Products containing not more than 90 milligrams of codeine per dosage unit (ie tablet or capsule)are Schedule III

*** Cough preparations with one or more non-narcotic ingredients, containing not more than 200 milligrams of codeine per 100 milliliters or per 100 grams are Schedule V

INDEX

Locators for figures are indicated by *f,* tables by *t,* and photos by *p* following the page number.

A

abacavir, 37*t*

Abbreviated New Drug Application (ANDA), 182

abbreviations
  common pharmacy, 114–115, 115*t*
  Do Not Use abbreviations, 193*t,* 194
  dosages, 114–115, 115*t*
  drug delivery, 110*t*
  IV fluids and abbreviations, 129, 129*t*
  site of administration, 114–115, 115*t*
  time, 114–115, 115*t*
  time of administration, 114–115, 115*t*

ABC classification system, 223–224

Abilfy, 30*t,* 31

Absorica, iPLEDGE Program and, 187*t*

acarbose, 42*t*

accounting, inventory, 216–220
  estimating third party reimbursements, 216–219
  markup and profits, 217–219

Accreditation Council of Pharmacy Education (ACPE), 2

Accutane
  iPLEDGE Program and, 187*t*
  MedGuide for, 185*t*
  product package insert, 185

acetaminophen, 25*t,* 26, 27, 92

acetyl-para-aminophenol (APAP), 25*t,* 27

acquisition cost, 216

Actiq, 25*t*

Activase, 49*t*

Actos, 42*t,* 43

acyclovir, 37*t,* 40

Adalat CC, 113

Adalet, 34*t*

adalimumab, 50, 51*t*

Adderall, 31*t,* 32, 92, 94
  MedGuide for, 185*t*
  product package insert, 185

Addyi, 52
  as high-risk drug, 188

ADHD drugs, MedGuide for, 185*t*

adjudication, 196, 239–240

admitting order, 122

adrenaline, 33

Advair, 45, 45*t*

adverse drug reactions (ADRs)
  defined, 23, 190
  medication error prevention, 196
  reporting, 184

Adverse Event Reporting system (AERS), 184

Advil, 25*t,* 53*t*

aerosols, 109*t*

Affordable Care Act, 85*t,* 86

Affordable Care Health Exchanges, 235, 236*t*

Afrin, 53*t*

agglomeration, 140

air quality engineering equipment, 156–157, 156*f*

albuterol, 45, 45*t*

Aldactone, 48, 48*t*

alendronate, 43, 44*t*

Aleve, 25*t,* 53*t*

Align, 53*t*

Allegra, 46, 53*t*

allergy medication, 45–46, 45*t*

alligation, 146–148

allopurinol, 44, 44*t*

alpha-adrenergic blocker, 48

alpha blocker, 48*t*

alprazolam, 28*t*

Altace, 34*t*

alteplase, 49*t*

alternative medicine, 54

Amaryl, 42*t*

Ambien, 28, 28*t*

Ambisome, 37*t*

American Association of Pharmacy Technicians, 87

American Pharmacists Association (APhA), 87

American Pharmacy Association, 6

American Society of Health-System Pharmacists (ASHP), 2, 87
  Drug Information, 114

Amitiza, 47*t*

amitriptyline, 29*t,* 30

amlodipine, 33, 34*t*

Amnesteem, iPLEDGE Program and, 187*t*

amoxicillin, 37*t,* 38

amoxicillin-clavulanate, 37*t,* 38

Amoxil, 37*t,* 38

amphetamines, 32

amphetamine salts, 31*t,* 32

amphoteracin B, 37*t,* 40

ampicillin-sulbactam, 37*t,* 38, 39

ampule
  adding ingredients from, 170
  defined, 170

Anabolic Steroid Control Act, 85*t*

Anacin, 25*t*

analgesic medications, 25–27, 25*t*

anatomical classification of drugs, 23–50
  cardiovascular agents, 33–36
  central nervous system agents, 24–33
  endocrine and metabolic agents, 40–44
  gastrointestinal agents, 46–47
  hematologic agents, 48–50
  overview of, 23–24
  renal and genitourinary agents, 47–48
  respiratory agents, 45–46
  systemic anti-infective agents, 36–40

Ancef, 37*t,* 38

angiotensin-converting enzyme (ACE) inhibitors, 34, 34*t*

angiotensin receptor blockers (ARBs), 34, 34*t*

anteroom, 156, 157

antianxiety agents, 27–28, 28*t*

antibiotics, 37*t,* 38–39

anticholinergic, 45*t*

anticipatory compounding, 134

antidepressants, 28–30, 29*t*
  MedGuide for, 185*t*

antidiabetic agents, 41–43, 42*t*

antifungals, 37*t,* 40

antihistamines, 46

antihyperlipidemic drugs, 35, 35*t*

antihypertensive agents, 33–34, 34*t*

anti-infective agents
  common, 37*t*
  overview, 36

anti-inflammatory drugs, 25, 25*t,* 27, 44*t*

antiplatelet drug, 49*t*

antipsychotic drugs, 30–31, 30*t*

antivirals, 37*t,* 40

Apidra, 42*t*

apixaban, 49*t*

apothecary measurement system, 64–65

Aranesp, 50, 51*t*

Aricept, 32
aripiprazole, 30*t*, 31
Asacol, 47*t*
asepsis, 152
Aseptic Isolators, 175*t*
aseptic technique
    defined, 152
    for sterile compounding, 157, 157*t*
ASHP Drug Information, 114
Asmanex, 45*t*
asthma, 45, 45*t*
atazanavir, 37*t*
atenolol, 34*t*
Ativan, 28*t*, 32
atorvastatin, 35*t*
Atrovent, 45, 45*t*
attention-deficit hyperactivity disorder
    (ADHD), 94
audit, 246
Augmentin, 37*t*, 38
automated compounding devices (ACD),
    171, 212
automated dispensing system, 128*t*
    community pharmacy, 209–210
    institutional pharmacy, 212
automatic stop orders (ASO), 122
automation, for reducing medication
    errors, 194
Automation of Reports and
    Consolidated Orders System (ARCOS),
    100*t*
auxillary labels, 126
Avandia, product package insert, 185
average wholesale price (AWP), 216
avoirdupois measurement system, 64–65
AWARxE program, 178
axilliary labels, 59, 59*t*
Aygestin, 41*t*
azithromycin, 37*t*, 38–39
    storage, 228
Azulfidine, 47*t*

B

back orders, 225
Bactrim, 37*t*, 40
balance, 141–143
barcode, using, 122, 125–126, 125*f*, 126*f*
    reducing medication errors and, 195,
    195*f*, 195*t*
basal insulin, 42
base solutions, overfill of, 159–160
beakers, 143
Benadryl, 53*t*
benazepril, 34*t*
Benicar, 34*t*
benign prostatic hypertropy (BPH), 48
Bentyl, 47*t*
benzodiazepine (BZD) family, 28, 28*t*, 32
benzos, 28, 28*t*
Best Pharmaceuticals for Children Act
    (BPCA), 85*t*
beta-adrenergic blockers (beta blockers),
    33, 34*t*

beyond-use date (BUD)
    nonsterile compounding, 148, 149*t*
    sterile compounding, 171, 172*t*
biennial inventory count, 230
Bifidobacterium, 53*t*, 57
billing and reimbursement
    calculating third party reimburse-
    ments, 216–219
    charge-backs, 245–246
    coinsurance payments, 237
    coordination of benefits (COB), 239
    copays, 237–238
    days' supply calculations, 242–244
    deductibles, 237
    explanation of benefits (EOB), 245
    inputting insurance information,
    238–239
    insurance claims and payment
    structures, 236–238
    insurance providers and benefits,
    235, 235*t*–236*t*
    medication assistance, 246–247
    patient payment options, 234
    pharmacy benefits manager, 236, 246
    prior authorization, 240
    rejected claims, 240–242, 241*t*
    resolving claim issues, 245–246
    usual, customary, and reasonable
    (UCR) charges, 236–237
bioaccumulate, 28–29
bioequivalent, 111
biological drugs, 113
biological reference product, 113
Biological Safety Cabinets, 175*t*
biosimilar drugs, 113
biotechnology drugs, 50–51, 51*t*
birth control agents, 40–41, 41*t*
    MedGuide for, 127, 185*t*
bisacodyl, 53*t*
bisphosphonates, 43, 44*t*
black box warning, 127, 185
blending, 144
blood, hematologic agents, 48–50, 49*t*
bloodborne infection transmission,
    preventing, 200*t*
blood thinner, 49–50, 49*t*
body surface area (BSA), 74–75
body-weight ratios, 73–74
bolus insulin, 42
bone loss, 43
brand drug
    generic substitution for, 111–113
    requested by patient, 111
brand medically necessary, 111, 119
break ring, 170
brexpiprazole, 30*t*
bridging therapy, 50
bronchodilator, 45*t*
buccal dosage route, 108*t*
budesonide-formoterol, 45, 45*t*
buffer room, 156, 157
buprenorphine, 25*t*, 26, 90
    as high-risk drug, 188

buprenorphine-naloxone, 90
Byetta, 42*t*, 43
Bystolic, 34*t*

C

CADD-Prizm PCS II, 213
Calan, 34*t*
calcium, 56*t*
calcium channel blockers (CCBs), 33, 34*t*
calculations
    body surface area, 74–75
    body-weight ratios, 73–74
    child dosages, 74
    common measurement conversions,
    64–65
    compounding, 145–148
    concentration percentage ratios,
    145–146
    days' supply, 242–244
    dilution amounts, 77–79
    dimensional analysis, 69
    dosages, 70–77
    drug ratio strengths, 70–72
    liquid dosage amounts, 75–77
    metric system conversion, 65–66
    otic and ophthalmic challenges,
    244–245
    ratio-proportion equations, 67–70
    sterile compounding, 158–167
    tablet dosages, 72–73
    temperature conversions, 62–63
    test-taking tips for, 61–62
    third party reimbursement, 216–217
    time conversions, 63–64
    turnover ratio and rates, 220
capsule, 108*t*
    nonsterile compounding of, 139
carbamazepine, 32
cardiovascular agents, 33–36
    antihyperlipidemic drugs, 35, 35*t*
    antihypertensive agents, 33–34, 34*t*
    miscellaneous cardiovascular agents,
    36, 36*t*
    overview of, 33
Cardizem, 34*t*
carisoprodol, 31*t*, 32
cart unit fill*t*, 128
carvedilol, 36*t*
Catapres, 32
cefazolin, 37*t*, 38
cefdinir, storage, 228–229
ceftazidime, 37*t*, 38
ceftriaxone, 37*t*
Celebrex, 25*t*
celecoxib, 25*t*
Celexa, 29*t*
Celsius temperature, converting to
    Fahrenheit, 62–63
Center for Medicare Services (CMS), 87,
    182
centimeter, 66
Centralized Automated Dispensing
    Systems, 212

central nervous system agents, 24–33
    analgesic medications, 25–27, 25t
    antianxiety and hypnotic agents,
        27–28, 28t
    anti-inflammatory drugs, 25, 25t, 27
    antipsychotic and antidepressant
        agents, 28–30, 29t, 30t
    miscellaneous central nervous
        agents, 31–33, 31t
    overview, 24
cephalexin, 37t, 38
cephalosporins, 38
certification examinations. See also Exam
    for the Certification of Pharmacy
    Technicians (ExCPT); Pharmacy
    Technician Certification Exam (PTCE)
        described, 1
        eligibility for, 7–9
        reasons for taking, 2, 4
        test preparation strategies, 10–14
        title used after passing, 1
Certified Pharmacy Technician (CPhT),
    1
cetirizine, 53t
charge-backs, 245–246
chemotherapy agents, storage require-
    ment, 228
chemotherapy compounding mat, 175
chemotherapy dispensing pins, 175
Cheracol, 95
children
    child-resistant packaging, 84, 84t,
        189
    dosage calculations for, 74
    drug utilization review (DUR) and,
        198t
Children's Health Insurance Program
    (CHIP), 235, 236t
chlordiazepoxide, 28t
chlorpromazine, 30, 30t
chlorthalidone, 34t
cholecalciferol, 51t
cholesterol, 35
cholesterol-lowering drugs, 35, 35t
chondroitin, 56t
chronic obstructive pulmonary disease
    (COPD), 45, 45t
Cialis, 36, 48, 48t
Cipro, 37t, 39
ciprofloxacin, 37t, 39
    MedGuide for, 185t
citalopram, 29t
    MedGuide for, 185t
civil law, 101–102
claim capturing, 240
Claravis, iPLEDGE Program and, 187t
clarithromycin, storage, 228
Claritin, 46, 53t
Class III prescription balance, 141, 141p
cleanroom, 156–157
Cleocin, 37t
clindamycin, 37t, 39
clinical decision support system (CDSS),
    204

clonazepam, 28t, 32
clonidine, 32
clopidogrel, 49, 49t
closed formularies, 225
closed-system transfer devices, 175
clotrimazole, 53t
clozapine, as high-risk drug, 188
Clozaril, as high-risk drug, 188
codeine, 25t
Code of Conduct, for pharmacy techni-
    cians, 8
coinsurance payments, 237
Colace, 53t
colchicine, 44
Combat Methamphetamine Epidemic
    Act (CMEA), 85t, 86, 96
Combivent, 45
comminution, 143–144
common measurement, converting,
    64–65, 68–69
community pharmacy
    e-prescribing, 206–207
    point-of-sale cash registers, 210
    prescription processing, 207–209
    robotics and automated filling,
        209–210
    technology and, 206–211
compliance report, 224
compounded sterile preparations
    (CSPs), 152
    defined, 129
    label, 88t
compounding
    alligation, 146–148
    calculations, 145–148
    defined, 134
    documentation, 136, 138t, 139t
    good compounding practices,
        134–135, 134t
    hazardous compounding, 172–178
        engineering controls for,
            174–176
        medical surveillance, 174
        nuclear compounding, 176–177
        routes of exposure, 173, 173t
        waste handling and disposal,
            177–178
    nonsterile compounding, 133–150
        anticipatory compounding, 134
        beyond-use date (BUD), 148,
            149t
        calculations, 145–148
        comminution and blending
            techniques, 143–145
        documentation, 136, 138t, 139t,
            149
        dosage forms, 139–140
        equipment, 141–143, 141p
        label, 149, 149t
        location, 135
        steps in, 135–136, 137t
        types of, 134–135
    pharmacist checking, 149
    sterile compounding, 152–172

aseptic technique and protective
    garb, 157, 157t
beyond-use date (BUD), 171,
    172t
calculations, 158–167
cleanroom and air quality
    engineering equipment,
    156–157, 156f
compounding record, 154, 156
labels, 154, 154f, 155t
Master Formulation Record, 154,
    155t
medication orders for, 153–154
parenteral drug products,
    152–153
steps in, 167–172
USP chapter 797 guidelines, 152
waste disposal, 177–178
Compounding Aseptic Isolator (CAI),
    156, 156f
compounding record
    nonsterile compounding, 136, 138t,
        139t
    sterile compounding, 154, 156
compounding slab, 143
Comprehensive Drug Abuse Prevention
    and Control Act, 84t, 90
Comprehensive Methamphetamine
    Control Act, 85t
computer input devices, 206
computerized physician order entry
    (CPOE), 122, 211
concentration percentage ratios,
    145–146
Concerta, 31t, 32, 94
    MedGuide for, 185t
conjugated estrogen, 41t
Consumer Product Safety Commission
    (CPSC), 182
    Poison Prevention Packaging Act,
        189
Containment Primary Engineering
    Controls (C-PECs), 174, 175t
Containment Secondary Engineering
    Control (C-SEC), 174, 175t
continuation order, 122
continuous quality improvement (CQI),
    199
continuous quality improvement
    process, 149
contraindications, defined, 22
Controlled Substance Ordering System
    (CSOS), 92, 100t
controlled substances, 90–100
    classification and restrictions, 90–96,
        91t
    DEA number and, 118
    DEA role and, 90
    disposal of, 99–100
    e-presciptions, 93–94, 117
    forms used for, 100t
    inventory management, 229–230
    inventory requirements, 92, 92f, 93f,
        99–100

labels for, 127
narcotics as, 25
overview of, 91
prescription guidelines, 120
prescriptions for, 93–94
preventing forgeries and diversion, 98, 99t
refills, 94, 95, 121
restricted sale of certain OTC, 96, 97t, 98t
transferring prescriptions, 94–95
Controlled Substances Act (CSA), 90
conversions
common measurements, 64–65
dimensional analysis for, 68–69
metric system conversion, 65–66, 68–70
percent to strength ratio, 72
ratio-proportion equations for, 68–69
strength ratio to percent, 71
temperature, 62–63
time, 63–64
coordination of benefits (COB), 239
defined, 208–209
copayment (copay), 237–238
Cordarone, MedGuide for, 185t
Coreg, 36, 36t
coring, 170
corticosteroids, 27, 44, 44t
cortisol, 44
Cortizone-10, 53t
cough syrup with codeine, 95
Coumadin, 49, 49t, 119
MedGuide for, 185t
product package insert, 185
counterbalance, 141–143
Cozaar, 34t
creams, nonsterile compounding of, 140
Crestor, 35t
criminal law, 101
Culturelle, 53t
cyclobenzaprine, 29, 31t, 32
cylinders, 143
Cymbalta, 29t, 30

D

dabigatran, 49, 49t
daily order, 122
darbepoetin alfa, 50, 51t
darunavir, 37t
database management system (DBMS)
defined, 204
point-of-sale cash registers, 210
prescription process and, 207–209
safety and productivity reports, 211
DAW (dispense as written), 111, 119
DAW2, 111
days' supply
calculating, 242–244
incorrect, 242
DEA 41 form, 100t
DEA 106 form, 100t
DEA 222 form, 92, 92f, 100t

DEA 224 form, 100t
deactivation, 175
DEA number
controlled substances prescriptions and, 118
on prescription, 117, 118f
Decadron, 44
Decentralized Automated Dispensing Systems, 212
deductibles, 237
Deltasone, 44, 44t
Demadex, 34t
Demerol, 26
Depakote, 31t
Depo-Provera, 41t
dermal dosage form, 109t
Desyrel, 29t
dexamethasone, 44
dextroamphetamine, 32
dextroamphetamine-amphetamine, 92, 94
dextromethor-phan (DM), 54
DiaBeta, 42t, 43
diabetes
drugs for, 42–43, 42t
overview of, 41
Diastat, 28
diazepam, 28, 28t
dicyclomine, 47t
Dietary Supplement Health and Education Act (DSHEA), 55, 85t
dietary supplements, 55–56, 56t
FDA role and, 55
herbal and medicinal plants, 57
indications for common, 55, 56t
probiotics, 57
protein shakes and nutritional supplements, 57
vitamins and minerals, 55–56, 56t
Diflucan, 37t, 40
digital electronic analytical balance, 141
digoxin, 36, 36t
Dilacor, 34t
Dilaudid, 25t, 26
diltiazem, 34t
dilutions
calculating dilution amounts, 77–79
geometric, 144
weight-in-volume percents, 161
dimensional analysis calculation, 68–69, 74
Dipentum, 47t
diphenhydramine, 53t
diphenoxylate, 95
Direct Compounding Areas (DCAs), 156
discharge order, 122
discount cards, 247
dispense as written (DAW), 111, 119
disposal of medication
controlled substances, 99–100
of unused, 178
Dispose My Meds program, 178
dissolving, in nonsterile compounding, 144

diuretics, 33, 34t, 47–48, 48t
divalproex sodium, 31t, 32
docusate sodium, 53t
Dolophine, 25t, 26
donepezil, 32
Doryx, 37t, 39
dosage calculations, 70–77
body surface area, 74–75
body-weight ratios, 73–74
calculating dosage amounts, 75–77
for children, 74
dilution amounts, 77–79
drug ratio strengths, 70–72
tablet dosages, 72–73
dosage forms
commonly compounded, 139–140
overview of all, 108t–110t
dosages, abbreviations for, 114–115, 115t
doxepin, 29t
doxycycline, 37t, 39
drug abuse, of prescription drugs, 26
drug accountability record, 221
drug approval process, 183, 183t
drug classification, 90–96
drug delivery abbreviations, 110t
Drug Enforcement Administration (DEA)
controlled substance regulation, 90–96
established, 84t
as key oversight agency, 87
drug interactions
defined, 22
drug utilization review and, 204
Drug Listing Act, 85t
Drug Price Competition and Patent Term Restoration Act, 85t
Drug Quality and Security Act (DQSA), 85t, 87, 188–189
documentation, 227–228
drug ratio strengths, 70–72
drug reactions, tracking program, 183, 183t
drug recall, classification and procedures for, 89–90, 89t
drugs
anatomical classification of, 23–50
bioequivalent, 111
biological drugs, 113
biosimilar drugs, 113
biotechnology drugs, 50–51, 51t
generic substitutions for brand drugs, 111–113
interchangeable biological drug, 113
miscellaneous, 51–52, 51t
over-the-counter drugs, 52–54, 53t
routes of administration, 108t–110t
suffixes and prefixes, 58t
drug-seeking behavior, 99t
Drug Supply Chain Security Act, 188–189
drug supply chain security tracking, 188–189

drug utilization review (DUR)
  compounding process and checking, 136
  defined, 117
  medication error prevention, 196
  patient profile and, 117
  pharmacy software and, 204–205
  in prescription processing, 207–208, 208f
  requirement established, 86
  running, as step in filling prescription/medication order, 125
  special populations and, 198t
dry powder volume, calculating sterile compounding dilutions, 161–163
dual copay, 237–238
Ducolax, 53t
duloxetine, 29t, 30
dumb terminals, 206
Duragesic, 25t
Durham-Humphrey Amendments to FDCA, 84t
Dyazide, 47, 48t

E

early refill, 121
echinacea, 56t, 57
economic order quantity, 221
efavirenz, 37t
Effexor, 29t, 30
Elavil, 29t, 30
elderly patients, drug utilization review (DUR) and, 198t
electrolyte solutions, measuring, 163
electronic health records (EHRs), 211–212
electronic medical record (EMR), 207
electronic medication administration record (eMAR), 122, 212
Eliquis, 49t
eluxadoline, 47, 47t
emergency crash carts, 128
emergency refill, 121
EMV chip technology, 234
enalapril, 34t
Enbrel, 50, 51t
Endocet, 25t
endocrine and metabolic agents, 40–44
  antidiabetic agents, 41–43, 42t
  estrogens and birth control agents, 40–41, 41t
  miscellaneous, 43–44, 44t
  overview, 40
enoxaparin, 49t, 50
Environmental Protection Agency (EPA), 178
ephedrine
  over-the-counter limits, 85t, 86
  restricted sale of, 96, 97t, 98t
epinephrine, 33
epoetin alfa, 50, 51t
e-prescriptions
  advantages of, 117
  controlled substances, 93–94

process for, 207–209
  regulations for, 206–207
Epuris, iPLEDGE Program and, 187t
equivalent (Eq), 163
erectile dysfunction, 48, 48t
errors. See medication errors
ertapenem, 37t
escitalopram, 29t
  MedGuide for, 185t
Esidrix, 48t
esomeprazole, 46, 47t, 53t
Estrace, 41t
estradiol, 41t
Estring, 41t
estrogens, 40–41, 41t
eszopiclone, 28, 28t
etanercept, 50, 51t
ethics, 102
ethinyl estradiol-drospirenone, 41t
ethinyl estradiol-etonogestrel, 41t
ethinyl estradiol-norelgestromin, 41t
ethinyl estradiol-norethindrone, 41t
ethinyl estradiol-norgestimate, 41t
Exam for the Certification of Pharmacy Technicians (ExCPT), 1
  described, 7
  eligibility requirements and scheduling, 9
  grading, 15
  recertification, 15
  test preparation strategies, 10–14
  test-taking tips, 12–14
exenatide, 42t, 43
expired medication, 231
explanation of benefits (EOB), 245
express pay option, 234
extremes, 67
eyewash station, 136
ezetimibe, 35t

F

factor Xa inhibitor, 49t
Facts and Comparisons, 114
Fahrenheit temperature, converting to Celsius, 62–63
Failure Mode Effects Analysis (FMEA), 190
famotidine, 46, 47t, 53t
Fazacio, as high-risk drug, 188
FDA Modernization Act, 85t
Federal Drug Administration (FDA), dietary supplements and, 55
federal laws, timeline of, 84–87, 84t–85t
Federal Trade Commission (FTC), 87, 182
Femring, 41t
fenofibrate, 35, 35t
fentanyl, 25t
ferrous sulfate, 56t
fexofenadine, 46, 53t
fibrinolytic, 49t
filgrastim, 50, 51t
fill list, 125
filter needle, 170

filter straw, 170
finasteride, 48, 48t
5-alpha reductase inhibitor, 48t
Flagyl, 37t
Flexeril, 29, 31t, 32
flibanserin, as high-risk drug, 188
Flomax, 48, 48t
Flonase, 45t, 46, 53t
Flovent, 45t, 46
flow rate
  calculating
    flow rate based on volume delivered, 164–165
    flow rate in drops, 166–167
    time duration for infusion based on flow rate and 24-supply, 165–166
    time for new supply based on infusion rate, 167
    volume delivered with ordered flow rate, 164
  defined, 164
fluconazole, 37t, 40
fluoroquinolones, 39
fluoxetine, 29, 29t, 30
  MedGuide for, 185t
fluphenazine, 30t
fluticasone, 45t, 46, 53t
fluticasone-salmeterol, 45, 45t
folic acid, 51t, 52
Food, Drug, and Cosmetic Act (FDCA), 84t
  Durham-Humphrey Amendments, 84t
  Kefauver-Harris Amendment to, 84t
Food and Drug Administration (FDA)
  drug label requirements, 88t
  drug reaction tracking, 184
  drug recall classification and procedures, 89–90, 89t
  established, 84t
  Green Book, 114
  investigational drugs, 183
  as key oversight agency, 87
  MedGuide, 126, 127, 185, 186t
  MedWatch, 184
  new drug oversight, 182–183
  Orange Book, 113
  product label warnings, 185
  protective actions for released drugs, 184–188
  Purple Book, 113
  Risk Evaluation and Mitigation Strategies (REMS) medications, 186–188
Food Chemical Codex (FCC), 136
forgeries
  controlled substances and preventing, 98, 99t
  spotting, 121–122
Fortaz, 37t, 38
Fosamax, 43, 44t
furosemide, 34t, 47, 48t

G

gabapentin, 31t, 32
garlic, 56t, 57
gastrointestinal agents, 46–47
    common agents, 47t
    overview, 46–47
gels, nonsterile compounding of, 140
generic drug
    pharmaceutically equivalent, 111
    reference for substitutions, 113
    substituting for brand drug, 111–113
    therapeutically equivalent, 111
genitourinary agents, 47–48, 48t
gentamicin, 37t, 39
Geodon, 30t
geometric dilution, 144
Gianvi, 41t
ginger, 56t, 57
gingko, 56t, 57
glimepiride, 42t
glipizide, 42t, 43
Glucophage, 42t, 43
glucosamine, 56t
Glucotrol, 42t, 43
glyburide, 42t, 43
goldenseal, 57
good compounding practices (GCP),
    134–135, 134t
grain, 64–65
grams, 66
*Green Book: FDA Approved Animal Drug
    Products,* 114
gross profit, 218
guaifenesin, 53t
guanfacine, 32
gummies, nonsterile compounding of,
    140

H

H2 Blockers, 46, 47t
Haldol, 30t
haloperidol, 30t
hand washing
    for compounding, 136
    sterile compounding, 157, 157t
hardware, 206
hazardous compounding, 172–178
    automated, 213
    engineering controls for, 174–176
        containment primary engineer-
            ing controls, 174, 175t
        supplementary, 174–176
    hazardous drug criteria, 172
    labeling, 175
    medical surveillance, 174
    nuclear compounding, 176–177
    routes of exposure, 173, 173t
    spill kit, 175–176, 176t
    waste handling and disposal,
        177–178
hazardous drug, criteria for, 172
Hazardous Drug Label, 88t
hazardous waste, 177, 177t
HDL (high-density lipoprotein), 35

Health and Human Services,
    Department of (HHS), 87
healthcare-associated infections (HAIs),
    152
Health Care Financing Administration
    (HCFA), 87
Health Exchange Plans, 235, 236t
health insurance. *See also* insurance
    reimbursement
        options for, 235, 235t–236t
Health Insurance Portability and
    Accountability Act (HIPAA)
    confidentiality, 86
    overview of, 86
    patient profile and privacy, 116t, 117
    provisions, 85t
health maintenance organization
    (HMO), 235
heating, in nonsterile compounding, 144
Helicobacter pylori infections, 46
hematologic agents, 48–50, 49t
heparin, 49t
heparinarin, 50
herbals, 57
high-efficiency particulate airflow
    (HEPA), 156
HMG-CoA reductase inhibitors, 35
holistic health medications, 54–57
homeopathic medications, 54–55
homeopathy, 54–55
hood, 156, 156f
horizontal laminar airflow workbench
    (H-LAFW), 156, 156f
hormonal agents, 40–41, 41t
hormone-replacement therapy, 40, 41t
household measurement system, 64–65
Humalog, 42
Humira, 50, 51t
Humulin, 42, 42t, 54
Humulin N, 42t
hydrochlorothiazide, 34t, 47, 48t
hydrocodone, 25t, 26, 92
hydrocortisone, 53t
Hydrodiuril, 34t
HydroDIURIL, 48t
hydromorphone, 25t, 26
Hygroton, 34t
hypercalcemia, 44t
hyperthyroidism, 44, 44t
hypnotic agents, 27–28, 28t
hypoglycemia, 43
hypothyroidism, 44, 44t

I

ibuprofen, 25t, 53t
ICD-10, 209
Imdur, 36, 36t
imipramine, 29t
Imitrex, 31t, 32
Imodium, 53t
implant dosage form, 110t
Inderal, 34t
infections, healthcare-associated infec-
    tions (HAIs), 152

Inflectra, 50
Inflextr, 51t
infliximab, 50, 51t
informatics, 204
informed consent form, 183
infusions
    calculating time duration for, 167
    time for new supply based on rate of,
        167
inhalation dosage form, 109t–110t
inhaled solutions, 110t
inhalers, type of, and dispensing tips,
    109t–110t
inline filter, 170
inscription, on prescription, 117, 118f,
    119
insert dosage form, 110t
Institute for Safe Medication Practices
    (ISMP), 182
    programs for minimizing medica-
        tion errors, 192–193
institutional pharmacies
    automated dispensing system, 128t
    dispensing robots and automated
        dispensing, 212
    electronic health records and admin-
        istrative tracking, 211–212
    medication order
        checking for completion,
            123–125
        receiving, 122
        types of, 122
    robotic systems, 123
    technology and, 211–213
Institutional Review Board (IRB), 123,
    183
insulin
    action and classification of, 42–43,
        42t
    storage of, 229
insulin aspart, 42t
insulin determir, 42t
insulin glargine, 42, 42t
insulin glulisine, 42t
insulin lispro, 42t
insurance fraud, 246
insurance identification card, 238–239,
    238f
insurance reimbursement
    calculating third party reimburse-
        ments, 216–219
    charge-backs, 245–246
    coinsurance payments, 237
    coordination of benefits (COB), 239
    copays, 237–238
    days' supply calculations, 242–244
    deductibles, 237
    explanation of benefits (EOB), 245
    inputting insurance information,
        238–239
    insurance claims and payment
        structures, 236–238
    insurance providers and benefits,
        235, 235t–236t

medication assistance, 246–247
online claims submission, 239–242
pharmacy benefits manager, 236, 246
prior authorization, 240
resolving claim issues, 245–246
usual, customary, and reasonable
(UCR) charges, 236–237
integrative medicine, 54
interchangeable biological drug, 113
International Federation of Pharmacy
Technicians, 87
interoperability, 204–206, 205f
intradermal (ID) route, 110t, 153
intramuscular (IM) route, 110t, 153
intrauterine device, 110t
intravenous compatibility data, 204
intravenous dosage form, 110t, 153
calculating flow rates and volumes,
164–167
IV fluids and abbreviations, 129, 129t
patient-controlled analgesia (PCA)
device, 213
preparing premade IV solutions, 171
vial-and-bag system, 171
Intuniv, 32
Invanz, 37t
inventory management
ABC classification system for,
223–224
acquisition costs vs. pharmacy
reimbursement, 216
controlled substances, 92, 99–100,
229–230
drug returns and credits, 230–231
estimating profit, 217–219
estimating third party reimbursements, 216–219
handling purchasing orders,
226–227
importance of, 215–216
inventory value and turnover,
219–220
of investigational drugs, 221
out-of-stock medications, 229
partially-filled medications, 229
periodic automatic replenishment
levels, 221–222
perpetual inventory, 219–220
posting orders, 227
purchasing relationships and
contracts, 224–225
receiving orders, 227
shelf maintenance and rotating
stock, 224
storage, 228–229
inventory value, 219–220
investigational drugs, 183
inventory management of, 221
Investigational New Drug Application
(INDA), 84t, 183
iPLEDGE Program, 187, 187t
ipratropium, 45, 45t
ipratropium-albuterol, 45t
Ismo, 36, 36t

Isoptin, 34t
Isordil, 36, 36t
isosorbide, 36, 36t
isotretinoin
as high-risk drug, 187
iPLEDGE Program, 187, 187t
Isotroin, iPLEDGE Program and, 187t
IV Bolus Injections, 153
IV medication orders, 129, 129t
IV piggyback (IVPB), 153

J
Janumet, 43
Januvia, 42t, 43
Joint Commission, 87, 182
Do Not Use abbreviations, 193t, 194
just-in-time (JIT) ordering, 221

K
Kapvay, 32
K-Dur, 51t, 52
Kefauver-Harris Amendment to FDCA,
84t
Keflex, 37t, 38
Kenalog, 51t
kilogram, 66
Klonopin, 28t, 32
Klorcon, 51t, 52

L
labels
auxillary labels, 59, 59t, 126
black box warnings, 127, 185
for controlled substance, 127
drug stock, 125, 125f
FDA requirements for, 88t
hazardous agents, 175
medication label components, 170f
nonsterile compounding, 149, 149t
patient, 125
product package insert, 185
sterile compounding, 154, 154f, 155t
tall man lettering, 193
warning for pregnant/lactating
women, 185, 185t
lactating women
drug utilization review (DUR) and,
198t
label warnings for, 185, 185t
Lactobacillus, 53t, 56t, 57
Lactobacillus acidophilus, 57
Lamictal, 31t
lamotrigine, 31t, 32
Lanoxin, 36, 36t
lansoprazole, 46, 47t, 53t
Lantus, 42, 42t
large volume parenterals solutions
(LVPs), 129, 153
overfill and, 160
Lasix, 34t, 47, 48t
Latuda, 30t
laws and regulation. See also specific laws
controlled substance regulations,
90–100

criminal and civil court cases,
101–102
drug label requirements, 88t
drug recall procedures, 89–90, 89t
e-prescriptions, 206–207
ethics, 102
oversight agencies and organizations, 87
restricted sale of certain OTC, 96,
97t, 98t
standard of care, 102
state laws, 100–101
timeline of federal laws, 84–87,
84t–85t
LDL (low-density lipoprotein), 35
lead time, 223
least weighable quantity (LWQ),
142–143
levalbuterol, 45, 45t
Levaquin, 37t, 39
Levemir, 42t
levigation, 144
Levitra, 36, 48t
levofloxacin, 37t, 39
levonorgestrel, 41t
levothyroxine, 44, 44t
Levoxyl, 44t
Lexapro, 29t
Lialda, 47t
Librium, 28t
licensure, of pharmacy technicians, 3
lidocaine, 25t, 27
Lidoderm, 25t, 27
linaclotide, 46, 47t
Linzess, 47t
lipids, 35
Lipitor, 35t
liquids, calculating dosage amounts,
75–77
liraglutide, 42t, 43
lisdexamfetamine, 31t, 32
lisinopril, 34t
liter, 66
local area network (LAN), 206
Loestrin 24 Fe, 41t
lolipops, nonsterile compounding of,
140
Lomotil, 95
loop diuretic, 48t
loperamide, 53t
Lopressor, 34t
loratadine, 46, 53t
lorazepam, 28t, 32
Lorcet, 92
Lortab, 25t, 26, 92
Losarten, 34t
loss leaders, 247
Lotensin, 34t
lotions, nonsterile compounding of, 140
Lotrimin, 53t
lovastatin, 35t
Lovaza, 35, 35t
Lovenox, 49t, 50
lubiprostone, 46, 47t

Lunesta, 28, 28*t*
lurasidone, 30*t*
lutein, 56*t*
Lyrica, 31*t*, 32, 95

M

Maalox, 32
mainframe, 206
malpractice, 102
manufacturing, reducing medication
    errors, 194
marijuana, 91
markup, 217–219
Master Formulation Record
    nonsterile compounding, 136, 138*t*
    sterile compounding, 154, 155*t*
Material Safety Data Sheet (MSDS), 136
Maxzide, 47, 48*t*
means, 67
measurement
    abbreviations for, 114–115, 115*t*
    common, 64–65
    measuring equipment for
        compounding, 141–143
    metric, 65–66, 67*f*, 68–69
    percentage of error, 141–142
MedGuides, 126, 127
    for high risk medication, 185, 186*t*
mediation therapy management (MTM),
    207
Medicaid, 235, 236*t*
medical coding, 209
Medicare Modernization Act, 85*t*, 86
Medicare Part A, 235, 235*t*
Medicare Part B, 235, 235*t*
Medicare Part C, 235, 236*t*
Medicare Part D, 86, 235, 236*t*, 237
medication(s)
    disposing of unused, 178
    high risk and MedGuides, 185, 186*t*
    Risk Evaluation and Mitigation
        Strategies (REMS) medications,
        186–188
Medication Error Reporting Program
    (MERP), 192–193
medication errors
    adverse drug reaction and, 190
    categories and causes, 191*t*–192*t*
    defined, 190
    Do Not Use abbreviations, 193*t*, 194
    Failure Mode Effects Analysis
        (FMEA), 190
    incidence of, 189
    NDC numbers and bar codes, 195,
        195*f*, 195*t*
    patient rights and, 189, 190*f*
    pharmacist interventions, 196
    quality control and assurance
        programs, 199–201
    resources to fight, 192–194
    safety process at every step, 197–198
    technology to reduce, 194
medication history, 117
medication labels, 57

medication orders
    automatic stop orders, 122
    checking for completion, 123–124
    compared to prescriptions, 122–123
    computerized prescriber order entry
        (CPOE), 122
    electronic medication administra-
        tion record (eMAR), 122
    filling, 125–130
        drug utilization review, 125
        NDC confirmation, 125–126
        pharmacist final check, 130
        steps in, 112*f*, 128*t*
    final check by pharmacist, 130
    overview, 122, 127
    parenteral medication order,
        129–130, 129*t*
    receiving, 122
    repackaging drugs for unit doses,
        128–129
    for sterile compounded products,
        153–154
    types of, 122
medication safety. *See also* medication
    errors
    agencies efforts for, 182
    drug reaction tracking, 184
    drug supply chain security tracking,
        188–189
    investigational drugs, 183
    MedGuides for high risk medication,
        185, 186*t*
    new drug oversight, 182–183
    product label warnings, 185
    protective actions for released drugs,
        184–188
    Risk Evaluation and Mitigation
        Strategies (REMS) medications,
        186–188
medicinal plants, 57
Medrol dosepak, 44, 44*t*
medroxyprogesteron, 41*t*
MedWatch, 184
melatonin, 56*t*
Mellaril, 30
meloxicam, 25*t*
memantine, 31*t*, 32
meperidine, 26
meropenem, 37*t*, 39
Merrem, 37*t*, 39
mesalamine, 47*t*
metabolic agents, 40–44
meter, 66
metered dose inhalers, dispensing
    description and tips, 109*t*
metformin, 42*t*, 43
methadone, 25*t*, 26
    registration to dispense, 90
methamphetamine, Combat
    Methamphetamine Epidemic Act, 85*t*,
    86
methicillin-resistant Staphylococcus
    aureus (MRSA), 39, 152
methimazole, 44, 44*t*

methotrexate (MTX), 52
methylphenidate, 31*t*, 32, 92
    MedGuide for, 185*t*
methylprednisolone, 44, 44*t*
metoclopramide, 31*t*, 33
metoprolol, 34*t*
metoprolol succinate, 33
metric system
    conversions, 65–66, 68–69
    overview, 65–66
    units of, in steps, 67*f*
metronidazole, 37*t*, 39
Mevacor, 35*t*
miconazole, 53*t*
Micronase, 42*t*, 43
micronized powders, 110*t*
Micronor, 41*t*
military time, 63–64
milking technique, 170
milliequivalents (mEq), 163
milliliter, 65–66
minerals, 55–56, 56*t*
minicomputer, 206
Miralax, 53*t*
mirtazapine, 29*t*
miscellaneous drugs, 51–52, 51*t*
mixing instruments, 143
Mobic, 25*t*
Model State Pharmacy Act and Model
    Rules initiative, 8
modems, 206
mometasone, 45*t*, 46
Monistat, 53*t*
montelukast, 45*t*, 46
morphine, 25*t*, 26
mortar and pestle, 143
Motrin, 25*t*, 53*t*
MS Contin, 25*t*
Mucinex, 53*t*
multiple-dose vials (MDVs), 169
Mylanta, 32
Myorisan, iPLEDGE Program and, 187*t*

N

nafcillin, 37*t*, 39
naloxone, 25*t*, 26
Namenda, 31*t*, 32
Naprosyn, 25*t*
naproxen, 25*t*, 53*t*
narcotics, 25–26, 25*t*
Nardil, 29*t*
Nasacort, 53*t*
nasal dosage form, 109*t*
Nasonex, 46
National Association of Boards of
    Pharmacy (NABP), 6, 8, 87
National Association of Chain Drug
    Stores, 7
National Childhood Vaccine Injury Act,
    184
National Community Pharmacists
    Association, 7
    AWARxE program, 178
    Dispose My Meds program, 178

National Coordinating Council for Medication Error Reporting and Prevention (NCC MERP), 182
National Council for Prescription Drug Programs (NCPDP), 207
   rejected claims error codes, 240, 241t
National Drug Code (NDC) number, 85t
   barcode, 125, 125f
   FDA requirements, 88t
   parts of, 126, 126f
   reducing medication errors and, 195, 195f, 195t
National Formulary (NF), 136
National Healthcareers Association (NHA), 7
   code of conduct, 8
National Institute for Occupational Safety and Health (NIOSH), 173
National Percursor Log Exchange (NPLEx), 96
National Pharmacy Technician Association, 87
National Provider Identifier (NPI), 118
national provider identifier (NPI) number, insurance reimbursement and, 241
Navane, 30t
nebivolol, 34t
nebulizers, 110t
needles, parts of, 168–169, 169f
negative pressure, 174
negative profit, 219
negligence, 102
Neosporin, 53t
net profit, 218
Neulasta, 51t
Neupogen, 50, 51t
Neurontin, 31t, 32
new drug dispensing kiosks, 210
Nexium, 46, 47t, 53t
Next Choice, 41
niacin, 35t
Niaspan, 35, 35t
nicotinic acid, 35
nifedipine, 34t, 113
nitrates, 36
nitroglycerin, 36, 36t
   storage requirements, 228
Nitrolingual, 36t
Nitrostat, 36t
nonaerosolized inhalers, 110t
non-narcotic analgesic, 25t, 27
non-nucleoside reverse transcriptase inhibitors (NNRTIs), 40
Nonsterile Compounded Products Label, 88t
nonsterile compounding, 133–150
   anticipatory compounding, 134
   beyond-use date (BUD), 148, 149t
   calculations, 145–148
      alligation, 146–148
      concentration percentage ratios, 145–146
      comminution, 143–144

compounding record, 136, 138t, 139t
defined, 134
documentation, 136, 138t, 139t, 149
dosage forms, 139–140
equipment for, 141–143, 141p
good compounding practices, 134–135, 134t
ingredient preparation and blending techniques, 143–145
label, 149, 149t
location, 135
Master Formulation Record, 136, 138t
pharmacist checking, 149
steps in, 135–136, 137t
types of, 135
nonsteroidal anti-inflammatory drugs (NSAIDs), 25t, 27
   MedGuide for, 186t
nontaxable items, 234
Norco, 25t, 26
norethindrone, 41t
Normal Saline (NS), 153
Nor-QD, 41t
nortriptyline, 29t
Norvasc, 33, 34t
Norvir, 37t
Novalin N, 42t
Novolin, 42, 42t, 54
Novolog, 42
nuclear compounding, 176–177
nuclear pharmacy technician (NPT), 176
nucleoside/nucleotide revers transcriptase inhibitors (NRTIs), 40
nutritional supplements, 57
NuvaRing, 41, 41t
   storage requirement, 228

O

OBRA-90, 86
Occupational Safety and Health Administration (OSHA), 87
oil-in-water (o/w) emulsion, 140
ointments, nonsterile compounding of, 140
olanzapine, 30t, 31
   as high-risk drug, 188
olmesartan, 34t
olsalazine, 47t
omega-3 fatty acid, 35, 35t
omega-3 fatty acids, 56t
omeprazole, 46, 47t, 53t
Omnibus Budget Reconciliation Act (OBRA), 85t, 86
ondansetron, 31t, 33
online adjudication, 208–209
open formularies, 225
ophthalmic dosage form, 109t
   calculation challenges, 244–245
opiates, 25–26, 25t
opiods, 25t, 26
oral dosage form, 108t
oral liquid dosage form, 108t

Orange Book: Approved Drug Products with Therapeutic Equivalence Evaluations, 113
Oretic, 48t
Orphan Drug Act, 85t
Ortho Evra, 41, 41t
oseltamivir, 37t, 40
osteoporosis, 43, 44t
otic dosage form, 109t
   calculation challenges, 244–245
out-of-stock (OOS) items, 226, 229
overfill of base solutions, 159–160
overhead, 218
over-the-counter drugs
   FDA requirements for, 88t
   herbal medicine and, 57
   overview of common, 52–54, 53t
   pseudoephedrine regulations, 86
   restricted sale of certain, 96, 97t, 98t
oxcarbazepine, 32
oxycodone, 25t, 26, 92
oxycodone-acetaminophen, 91
OxyContin, 25t, 26, 52, 92
oxymetazoline, 53t

P

packaging, child-resistant packaging, 84, 84t, 189
Pamelor, 29t
Panadol, 25t
pantoprazole, 46, 47t
parenteral dosage form, 110t
   types of, 152–153
parenteral medication order, 129–130, 129t
parenteral route of administration, 152
Parnate, 29t
paroxetine, 29, 29t
   MedGuide for, 185t
partial refill, 121
Patient-Controlled Analgesia (PCA) devices, 213
patient education
   essential medication information for, 198t
   labels, 57
   medication information for prescription, 126–127
   by pharmacist, 127, 196
patient information
   patient profile, 116, 116t
   on prescription, 117, 118f
patient label, 125
Patient Package Insert, 88t
patient profile, 207
   checking, 117
   components of, 116, 116t
   defined, 116
   drug utilization review (DUR) and, 117
   medication history, 117
   patient privacy and HIPAA regulations, 116t, 117
Patient Protection and Affordable Care Act (ACA), 85t, 86

patient rights, 189, 190*f*
Patient Safety and Quality Improvement
  Act (PSQI), 85*t*, 199
Patient Safety Organizations (PSOs), 85*t*,
  199
patient satisfaction, measuring, 201
Paxil, 29, 29*t*
  product package insert, 185
Pediatric Research Equity Act (PREA),
  85*t*
pegfilgrastim, 51*t*
penicillin, 37*t*, 38
  storage, 228
Pentasa, 47*t*
Pen VK, 37*t*, 38
Pepcid, 46, 47*t*, 53*t*
percent, strength ratio conversions,
  71–72
Percocet, 25*t*, 91
Periodic Automatic Replenishment
  (PAR) level, 221–222
perpetual inventory, 219–220
  Schedule II drugs, 230
personal protective equipment (PPE),
  152, 153*t*
  garbing and handwashing, 157, 157*t*
pharmaceutical alternative drug products, 112
pharmaceutically elegant product, 140
pharmaceutically equivalent, 111
pharmaceutics, 22
pharmacist
  checking compounding process, 149,
    172, 172*p*
  final check of prescription by, in
    filling process, 127, 130
  patient education by, 127, 196
  role in reducing medication errors,
    196
pharmacodynamics, 22
pharmacognosy, 22
pharmacokinetics, 22
pharmacology
  anatomical classification, 23–50
  auxiliary labels, 59, 59*t*
  biotechnology drugs, 50–51, 51*t*
  defined, 22
  drug suffixes and prefixes, 58*t*
  holistic health medications and
    dietary supplements, 55–57
  miscellaneous drugs, 51–52, 51*t*
  over-the-counter drugs, 52–54, 53*t*
  overview of, 22–23
pharmacy benefits manager (PBM), 236,
  246
pharmacy software interoperability,
  204–206, 205*f*
Pharmacy Technician Certification
  Board (PTCB), 1
  code of conduct, 8
Pharmacy Technician Certification
  Exam (PTCE), 1
  described, 6–7
  eligibility requirements, 7–8

grading, 14–15
recertification, 15
scheduling, 8–9
test preparation strategies, 10–14
test-taking tips, 12–14
Pharmacy Technician Initiative, 2
pharmacy technicians
  benefits to certification, 2, 4
  Code of Conduct for, 8
  filing and dispensing roles, 111–114
  licensure, 3
  reducing medication errors, 194–198
  registration of, 3
phenelzine, 29*t*
Phenergan, 31*t*, 33
phenylpropanolamine, over-the-counter
  limits, 85*t*, 86
phenytoin, 32
phosphodiesterase inhibitor, 48*t*
Physician's Desk Reference (PDR), 185
pioglitazone, 42*t*, 43
pipettes, 143
Plan B, 41, 41*t*
Plavix, 49, 49*t*
point-of-sale cash registers, 210
Poison Prevention Packaging Act, 84,
  84*t*, 189
policosanol, 56*t*
Policy and Procedures (P&P) Manual,
  123
polyethylene glycol, 53*t*
polypharmacy, 204
posting inventory orders, 227–228
postinjection delirium/sedation
  syndrome (PDSS), 188
potassium chloride, 51*t*, 52
potassium-sparing diuretic, 48*t*
powders, 108*t*
powder volume (pv), 161
Pradaxa, 49, 49*t*
Pravachol, 35*t*
pravastatin, 35*t*
Praxbind, 49
Precose, 42*t*
prednisone, 44, 44*t*
preferred provider organization (PPO),
  235
prefixes, drug, 58*t*
pregabalin, 31*t*, 32, 95
pregnant women
  drug utilization review (DUR) and,
    198*t*
  high-risk medication cautions, 187
  label warnings for, 185, 185*t*
  teratogenicity, 187
Premarin, 41*t*
prescriber
  legal, 120
  on prescription, 117, 118*f*
prescription drug abuse, 26
Prescription Drug Marketing Act, 85*t*
prescriptions
  abbreviations, common, 114–115,
    115*t*

accuracy check, 118–120
biologically comparable drugs,
  113–114
compared to medication order,
  122–123
container, 127
controlled substance, 93–94, 118, 120
DAW (dispense as written), 111, 119
e-prescribing, 117
filling, 125–130
  automated filling, 209–210
  DBMS system and processing,
    207–209, 208*f*
  drug utilization review, 125,
    207–208, 208*f*
  final check by pharmacist, 127,
    130
  NDC confirmation, 125–126
  overview of steps, 112*f*
  patient education material,
    126–127
  safety processes for, 197–198
  steps in, 126–127, 197–198
final check by pharmacist, 130
forgeries, 121–122
generic substitutions for brand
  drugs, 111–113
labeling, 57, 88*t*
legality of, 120–121
parts of, 117, 117*t*, 118*f*
patient profile updating, 116–117
pharmaceutical alternative drug
  products, 112
preventing forgeries and diversion,
  98, 99*t*
refills, 121
storage information, 127
submitting, 117
transfer in/out, 121
Prevacid, 46, 47*t*, 53*t*
Prezista, 37*t*
Prilosec, 46, 47*t*, 53*t*
primary engineering controls (PECs), 156
primary health insurance plan, 235
primary indications, 22
primary wholesaler purchasing contract,
  225
prime vendor purchasing contract, 225
Prinivil, 34*t*
prior authorization, 240
  issues of, 196
privacy, patient profile and HIPAA
  regulations, 116*t*, 117
ProAir, 45, 45*t*
Probcysbi, 52
probiotics, 57
Procardia, 34*t*, 113
processor, 206
Procrit, 50, 51*t*
productivity reports, 211
product package insert (PPI), 185
profit, 216
  estimating, 218–219
profit and loss statement, 216

progesterone, 40
progestin, 40
Prolixin, 30*t*
promethazine, 31*t*, 33
proportions
    converting to metric, 68–69
    defined, 67
    with means and extremes, 67
    steps for solving, 68
propranolol, 34*t*
Proscar, 48, 48*t*
prostate disorder, 48*t*
protease inhibitors, 40
protein shakes, 57
Protonix, 46, 47*t*
proton pump inhibitors (PPIs), 46, 47*t*
Proventil, 45, 45*t*
Provera, 41*t*
Prozac, 29, 29*t*
pseudoephedrine
    over-the-counter limits, 85*t*, 86
    restricted sale of, 96, 97*t*, 98*t*
psychoactive drugs, 27–28, 28*t*
pulverization by intervention, 143–144
punch method, 139
purchasing. *See* inventory management
Pure Food and Drug Act, 84*t*
Purple Book: Lists of Licensed Biological Products with Reference Product Exclusivity and Biosimilarity or Interchangeability Evaluations, 113
Push Injections (IVP), 153

Q

quality control and assurance
    continuous quality improvement process, 199
    staff quality and safety, 199–200
quetiapine, 30*t*, 31

R

radiopharmaceuticals, 176
ramipril, 34*t*
ranitidine, 46, 47*t*, 53*t*
ratio equations
    concentrations with weight-in-volume percentage strength, 71–72
    converting strength ratio to percent, 71
    converting to metric, 68–69
    defined, 67
    drug strengths, 70–72
    with means and extremes, 67
    steps for solving with, 68
ratio strength, 70
    compounding and, 145
    concentrations with weight-in-volume percentage strength, 71–72
    converted to percent, 71
    converting percentage to, 72
real-time claims adjudication, 208–209
recalled medication
    classification and procedures for, 89–90, 89*t*

pharmacy returning, 231
receiving inventory orders, 227
recertification, 15
recommended daily allowance (RDA), 55
rectal dosage form, 109*t*
red yeast rice, 56*t*
refills
    controlled substances, 94, 95, 121
    early, 121
    emergency fill, 121
    overview, 121
    partial, 121
    refill too soon message, 242
    transfer in/out, 121
registration, of pharmacy technicians, 3
Reglan, 31*t*, 33
regulation. *See* laws and regulation
reimbursement, insurance. *See* insurance reimbursement
Remeron, 29*t*
Remicade, 50, 51*t*
Remisima, 50, 51*t*
renal and genitourinary agents, 47–48, 48*t*
reorder point, 223
Repackaged Medication Label, 88*t*
repackaging control log, 129, 129*f*
repacking drugs, for unit doses, 128–129
Repatha, 52
Requip, 31*t*, 33
respiratory agents, 45–46
    common agents, 45*t*
    overview, 45–46
Restoril, 28*t*
reteplase, 49*t*
Retevase, 49*t*
reverse distributors, 231
Rexulti, 30*t*
Reyataz, 37*t*
Risk Evaluation and Mitigation Strategies (REMS) medications, 186–188
Risk Management Authorization (RMA) number, 187
Risperdal, 30*t*, 31
risperidone, 30*t*, 31
Ritalin, 31*t*, 32, 92, 94
    MedGuide for, 185*t*
ritonavir, 37*t*
rivaroxaban, 49, 49*t*
Robitussin A-C, 95
robotic systems, 123
    in hospitals, 212
Rocephin, 37*t*, 38
ropinirole, 31*t*, 33
rosuvastatin, 35*t*
rotating stock, 224
routes of drug administration, 108*t*–110*t*
Rowasa, 47*t*
Roxicodone, 25*t*, 26

S

safety. *See* medication safety
Safety Data Sheet (SDS), 136, 173

safety reports, 211
safety stock, 223
St. John's wort, 56*t*, 57
saw palmetto, 56*t*
Schedule I (C-I) drugs, 91–94, 91*t*
Schedule II (C-II) drugs
    biennial inventory count, 230
    disposal of, 230
    inventory requirements, 92, 92*f*, 93*f*, 99–100
    ordering and purchasing, 92
    overview, 91*t*
    perpetual inventory record, 230
    prescriptions for, 93–94
    purchasing, 229–230
    receiving and documentation, 230
    refills, 94
Schedule III (C-III) drugs
    inventory management, 100, 229
    overview, 91*t*, 94–95
    refills, 95
    transferring prescriptions, 94–95
Schedule IV (C-IV) drugs
    inventory, 100
    inventory management, 229
    overview, 91*t*, 94–95
    refills, 95
    transferring prescriptions, 94–95
Schedule V (C-V) drugs
    inventory management, 229
    overview, 91*t*, 95–96
    restrictions on sale of, 95–96
Schimmelm, William, 1
SCRIPT standards, 207
Sealed Sterile Compounding Isolators, 175*t*
Seasonale, 41
Seasonique, 41
secondary engineering controls, 156
secondary health insurance plan, 235
selective serotonin reuptake inhibitors (SSRIs), 29*t*, 30
    MedGuide for, 186*t*
Senakot, 53*t*
senna, 53*t*
sensitivity range, 141–142
Septra, 37*t*, 40
Seroquel, 30*t*, 31
serotonin, 29–30
sertraline, 29, 29*t*
    MedGuide for, 185*t*
shadow, 168
shortage cost, 223
side effects, defined, 22
sifting, 144
signa, on prescription, 117, 118*f*, 120
sildenafil, 48, 48*t*
    MedGuide for, 185*t*
simvastatin, 35*t*
simvastatin-ezetimibe, 35*t*
Sinequam, 29*t*
single-dose vials (SDVs), 169
Singulair, 45*t*, 46
sitagliptin, 42*t*, 43

site of administration, abbreviations, 114–115, 115*t*

small volume parenteral solutions (SVPs), 153

smart terminals, 206

software, pharmacy, 204–206, 205*f*

solute, 140

solutions
    nonsterile compounding of, 140
    overfill of base solutions, 159–160

solvent, 140

Soma, 31*t*, 32

Sotret, iPLEDGE Program and, 187*t*

spatula, 143

spatulation, 144

spill kit, 175–176, 176*t*

Spiriva, 45, 45*t*

spironolactone, 48, 48*t*

Spritam, 52

standard of care, overview of, 102

standing order, 122

state laws and regulations
    licensure requirements, 3
    overview, 100–101
    registration requirements, 3

statins, 35

stat order, 122, 128*t*

Stelazine, 30*t*

STEPS (System for Thalidomide Education and Prescribing Safety), 187

sterile, defined, 152

sterile compounding, 152–172
    aseptic technique and protective garb, 157, 157*t*
    automation for, 212–213
    beyond use date, 171, 172*t*
    calculations, 158–167
        combining two different concentrations, 158–159
        dilutions, 161–163
        dry powder volume and dilutions, 161–163
        electrolytes solutions, 163
        IV administration flow rates, 164–167
        overfill of base solutions, 159–160
        overview, 158
        weight-in-volume percents, 161
    cleanroom and air quality engineering equipment, 156–157, 156*f*
    compounding record, 154, 156
    labels, 154, 154*f*, 155*t*
    Master Formulation Record, 154, 155*t*
    medication orders for, 153–154
    parenteral drug products, 152–153
    products used in, 155*t*
    skills proficiencies, 153*t*
    steps in, 167–172
        adding ingredients from ampule, 170
        adding ingredients from vial, 169–170

automated compounding device (ACD), 171
        manipulating needles and syringes, 168–171
        overview, 167–168, 168*t*
        pharmacist checking, 172, 172*p*
        preparing premade IV solutions, 171
    USP chapter 797 guidelines, 152
    waste disposal, 178

steroids, 27

storage
    by patients, 228–229
    in pharmacies, 228–229

Strattera, MedGuide for, 185*t*

study skills, 10–11

subcutaneous dosage form, 110*t*

subcutaneous (SUBCUT) route, 153

sublingual dosage route, 108*t*

Suboxone, 25*t*, 26, 90
    as high-risk drug, 188

subscription, on prescription, 117, 118*f*

Subutex, 25*t*, 90
    as high-risk drug, 188

suffixes, drug, 58*t*

sulfa drugs, 40

sulfamethoxazole, 37*t*, 40

sulfasalazine, 47*t*

sulfonylureas, 43

sumatriptan, 31*t*, 32

supplementary engineering controls, 175–176

suppositories, nonsterile compounding of, 140

suspensions, nonsterile compounding of, 140

Sustiva, 37*t*

SVP chemotherapy medication, 160

Symbicort, 45, 45*t*

Synjardy, 52

Synthroid, 44, 44*t*

syringes, parts of, 168–169, 169*f*

systemic anti-infective agents, 36–40
    antibiotics, 37*t*, 38–39
    antifungals, 37*t*, 40
    antivirals, 37*t*, 40
    common agents, 37*t*
    overview, 36
    sulfa drugs, 40

T

tablets
    dispensing description and tips, 108*t*
    dosages calculations, 72–73
    nonsterile compounding of, 139

tadalafil, 48, 48*t*

Take Action, 41

tall man lettering, 193

Tamiflu, 37*t*, 40

tamsulosin, 48, 48*t*

Tapazole, 44, 44*t*

Tazicef, 37*t*, 38

tea tree oil, 56*t*

tech-check-tech (TCT), 130, 199

technology
    automated dispensing system, 128*t*
    barcode, 122, 125–126, 125*f*, 126*f*, 195, 195*f*, 195*t*
    community pharmacy practice and, 206–211
    computerized prescriber order entry (CPOE), 122
    drug utilization review (DUR), 116
    electronic medication administration record (eMAR), 122
    e-presciptions, 117, 206–209
    institutional pharmacy practice, 211–213
    online adjudication, 208–209
    online claims submission, 239–242
    pharmacy software interoperability, 204–206, 205*f*
    reducing medication errors, 194
    robots, 123, 209–210, 212

telepharmacy, 210

temazepam, 28*t*

temperature, conversion formulas, 62–63

tenecteplase, 49*t*

Tenex, 32

tenofovir, 37*t*

Tenormin, 34*t*

teratogenicity, 187

test-taking tips, 12–14

thalidomide, as high-risk drug, 187

therapeutically equivalent, 111

therapeutic drug duplications, 204

therapeutics, defined, 22

thiazide diuretic, 48*t*

thioridazine, 30

thiothixene, 30*t*

Thorazine, 30, 30*t*

thrombin inhibitor, 49*t*

thyroid hormones, 43–44, 44*t*

time
    abbreviations for, 114–115, 115*t*
    conversions, 63–64

tiotropium, 45, 45*t*

tizanidine, 31*t*, 32

TNKASE, 49*t*

Tofranil, 29*t*

Topamax, 31*t*

topical dosage form, 109*t*

topiramate, 31*t*, 32

Toprol, 34*t*

torsamide, 34*t*

torts, 101–102

totes, 227

toxicology, 22

tramadol, 25*t*, 27, 29

transdermal adhesives, 109*t*

transdermal gel or lotion, 109*t*

transfer in, 121

transfer out, 121

transmucosal dosage form, 109*t*

Transmucosal Immediate-Release Fentanyl, as high-risk drug, 187–188

Transmucosal Immediate-Release Fentanyl (TIRF), MedGuide for, 185*t*
trazodone, 29*t*, 30
triamcinolone, 51*t*, 53*t*
triamterene-hydrochlorothiazide, 48*t*
Tricare, 235
TriCor, 35, 35*t*
tricyclic antidepressant (TCA), 29*t*, 30
trifluperazine, 30*t*
triglycerides, 35
trimethoprim, 37*t*, 40
TriNessa, 41*t*
Trintellix, 29*t*
triple antibiotic, 53*t*
Tri-Sprintec, 41*t*
trituration, 143
troches, nonsterile compounding of, 140
tumbling, 144
tumeric, 56*t*
Tuojeo, 42*t*
turbulence, 168
turnover, inventory, 219–220
Tylenol, 25*t*, 27

U

Ultracet, 25*t*
Ultram, 25*t*, 27, 29
Unasyn, 37*t*, 38, 39
unique patient identifier, 211
unit calculation, 68–69
unit dose, repacking drugs for, 128–129
Unit Dose Label, 88*t*
United States Pharmacopeia and National Formulary (USP-NF), storage and handling requirements, 228
Universal Precautions, 200*t*
USP Chapter <795>, 134–135
USP Chapter <797>, 135, 152, 156, 157, 171
USP Chapter <800>, 173–174
USP Chapter <823>, 176–177
US Pharmacopeial Convention (USP), 87
    cleanroom, 156, 157
    compounding guidelines, 134–135, 152
    good compounding practices, 134–135, 134*t*
    hazardous compounding, 173–174
    medication safety efforts, 182
    National Formulary (NF), 136, 193
    nuclear compounding guidelines, 176–177
    personal protective equipment (PPE), 152, 153*t*

safety recommendations, 193
usual, customary, and reasonable (UCR) charges, 236–237

V

Vaccine Adverse Event Reporting System (VAERS), 184
vaccines
    government program to monitor adverse reactions, 184
    storage requirements, 228
Vagifem, 41*t*
vaginal dosage form, 109*t*
vaginal ring, 110*t*
valacyclovir, 37*t*, 40
Valium, 28, 28*t*
Valtrex, 37*t*, 40
Vancocin, 37*t*, 39
vancomycin, 37*t*, 39
vardenafil, 48*t*
vasodilator, 36
Vasotec, 34*t*
Veetids, 37*t*, 38
venlafaxine, 29*t*, 30
    MedGuide for, 185*t*
vented needle, 170
Ventolin, 45, 45*t*
verapamil, 34*t*
Versacloz, as high-risk drug, 188
vertical airflow, 174
Viagra, 36, 48, 48*t*
vial
    adding ingredients from, 169–170
    defined, 169
    single-dose and multiple-dose, 169
vial-and-bag system, 171
Viberzi, 47*t*
Vibramycin, 37*t*
Vicodin, 25*t*, 26, 92
Victoza, 42*t*, 43
Viread, 37*t*
vitamins, 55–56, 56*t*
    C, 56*t*
    D, 52, 55, 56*t*
    E, 56
volatiles, 110*t*
vorioxetine, 29*t*
Vytorin, 35*t*
Vyvanse, 31*t*, 32

W

warfarin, 49, 49*t*
waste
    hazardous waste disposal, 177, 177*t*

sterile and general compounding, 178
water, for compounding, 136
water-in-oil (w/o) emulsion, 140
weighing instruments, 141–143
    least weighable quantity (LWQ), 142–143
    percentage of error, 141–142
weight-in-volume percentage strength, 71–72
    calculating sterile compounding dilutions, 161
    compounding and, 145
    types of, 141, 141*p*
weight-in-weight, 145
withdrawal symptoms, 28–29

X

Xanax, 28*t*
xanthine oxidase inhibitor, 44, 44*t*
Xarelto, 49, 49*t*
    MedGuide for, 185*t*
Xopenex, 45, 45*t*
Xulane, 41*t*
Xylocaine, 27

Z

Zanaflex, 31*t*, 32
Zantac, 46, 47*t*, 53*t*
Zenatane, iPLEDGE Program and, 187*t*
Zestril, 34*t*
Zetia, 35*t*
Ziagen, 37*t*
zinc, 56*t*
ziprasidone, 30*t*
Zithromax, 38
Zocor, 35*t*
Zofran, 31*t*, 33
Zoloft, 29, 29*t*
zolpidem, 28, 28*t*
    MedGuide for, 185*t*
zone of turbulence, 168
Zostavax, storage requirements, 228
Zovirax, 37*t*, 40
Z-Pak, 37*t*, 38
Zubsolv, 52
Zyloprim, 44*t*
Zyprexa, 30*t*, 31
Zyprexa Relprevv, as high-risk drug, 188
Zyrtec, 53*t*

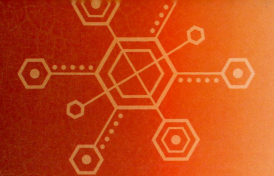

PHOTO CREDITS